Phyto-Oxylipins

Oxylipins are an important class of signaling molecules in plants, which play an important role in plant defense and innate immunity. Oxylipins have critical roles in plant growth and plant responses to physical damage caused by herbivores, insects, and pathogenic microbes. Over the last decade, our understanding of oxylipin production, metabolism, and function, particularly jasmonates has advanced considerably. Jasmonates have provided further mechanistic insights into enzyme function and signaling cascades. Other oxylipins, such as hydroxy fatty acids, have recently been shown to exhibit individual signaling features and crosstalk with other phytohormones.

There is scant literature on plant oxylipins and their relevance to our understanding and therefore, understanding oxylipin production, metabolism, and function is pivotal. As a result, researchers, students, professors, and other book readers will have a thorough understanding of plant oxylipin biosynthesis, structure, and function, assisting in the improvement of plant science.

Plant oxylipins: metabolism, physiological roles, and profiling techniques address the mechanism, metabolism, and roles of oxylipins in plant resistance to various biotic and abiotic stimuli in detail. This book covers fundamental ideas in oxylipin production, metabolism, structural biochemistry, and signaling pathways. It also discusses cutting-edge methodologies for oxylipin metabolic profiling, with an emphasis on computing applications. This book is an excellent resource for plant scientists, plant biochemists, biotechnologists, botanists, phytochemists, toxicologists, chemical ecologists, taxonomists, and other scholars in those subjects. The book is written by a global team of professionals.

Features

- Presents concrete and extensive information about a basic and applied aspect of plant oxylipins as well as expanded coverage of signaling mechanisms.
- Highlights the fundamental concepts of the biosynthesis, metabolism, structural biochemistry, and signaling pathway of oxylipins.
- Details the state-of-the-art methods and techniques in metabolic profiling of oxylipins in plants.
- Presents insights on computational applications in the evaluation and study of oxylipins in plants.

Current Developments in Agricultural Biotechnology and Food Security

Series Editor: Charles Oluwaseun Adetunji

This series intends to provide comprehensive coverage of sustainable modern technologies, aimed at improvement of food production via agriculture and food biotechnological techniques. Proposed suite of books focusses on topics in agricultural microbiology, biotechnology, food science, crop production, post-harvest management, aimed at both basic and advance food and agricultural biotechnology. The series seeks to discuss and provide foundational content from bench to bedside in food microbiology, agricultural and food biotechnology. The Series' goal is to enhance knowledge, and present update on hot topics in the field of the Agricultural Biotechnology specifically, the series aims to translate results and recent findings of studies into enhanced food production. This is primarily intended for researchers, students in Food and Agricultural Biotechnology at the graduate level and above, including those working in academic, corporate, or non-profit settings.

Agricultural Biotechnology
Food Security Hot Spots
Edited by Charles Oluwaseun Adetunji, Deepak Gopalrao Panpatte and Yogeshvari Kishorsinh Jhala

Phyto-Oxylipins
Metabolism, Physiological Roles, and Profiling Techniques
Edited by Sheikh Mansoor, Chukwuebuka Egbuna and Charles Oluwaseun Adetunji

For more information about this series, please visit: www.routledge.com/Current-Developments-in-Agricultural-Biotechnology-and-Food-Security/book-series/CRCABFS

Phyto-Oxylipins

Metabolism, Physiological Roles, and Profiling Techniques

Edited by
Sheikh Mansoor, Chukwuebuka Egbuna and
Charles Oluwaseun Adetunji

CRC Press
Taylor & Francis Group
Boca Raton London New York

CRC Press is an imprint of the
Taylor & Francis Group, an **informa** business

First edition published 2023
by CRC Press
6000 Broken Sound Parkway NW, Suite 300, Boca Raton, FL 33487–2742

and by CRC Press
4 Park Square, Milton Park, Abingdon, Oxon, OX14 4RN

CRC Press is an imprint of Taylor & Francis Group, LLC

ISBN: 9781032327556 (hbk)
ISBN: 9781032327587 (pbk)
ISBN: 9781003316558 (ebk)

DOI: 10.1201/9781003316558

Typeset in Times New Roman
by Newgen Publishing UK

Contents

Contributors

Aatifa Rasool
Division of Fruit Sciences, SK- University of Agricultural Sciences and Technology of Shalimar Srinagar Kashmir, J&K India.

Abdul Hamid
Department of Horticulture, University of Poonch Rawalakot, 12350, Azad Jammu and Kashmir, Pakistan, and Vice Chancellor, Women University of Azad Jammu and Kashmir Bagh, Pakistan.

Abdul Mujib G. Yusuf
King Saud University, College of Food and Agriculture, Plant Protection Department.

Abdul Qadir Khan
Department of Botany, University of Poonch Rawalakot, 12350, Azad Jammu and Kashmir, Pakistan.

Ali Muhammad
Department of Zoology, University of Poonch Rawalakot, 12350, Azad Jammu and Kashmir, Pakistan.

Ambreen Hamadani
Sher-e-Kashmir University of Agricultural Sciences and Technology of Kashmir, Srinagar, J&K, India.

Ansar Mehmood
Department of Botany, University of Poonch Rawalakot, 12350, Azad Jammu and Kashmir, Pakistan.

Babatunde Oluwafemi Adetuyi
Department of Natural Sciences, Faculty of Pure and Applied Sciences, Precious Cornerstone University, Ibadan.

Banke Ogundipe
Department of Biochemistry, Covenant University, Ota, Ogun State.

Barbara Krochmal-Marczak
Department of Food Production and Safety, Krosno State College, 00–635 Warsaw, Poland.

Barbara Sawicka
Department of Plant Production Technology and Commodity Science, University of Life Sciences in Lublin, 20–950 Lublin, Poland.

Baseerat Afroza
Division of Vegetable Science; Faculty of Horticulture, Sher e Kashmir University of Agricultural Sciences and Technology of Kashmir, Shalimar-190025, Jammu and Kashmir, India.

Bazilla Mushtaq
Division of Fruit Science; Faculty of Horticulture, Sher e Kashmir University of Agricultural Sciences and Technology of Kashmir, Shalimar-190025, Jammu and Kashmir, India.

Bismat un Nisa
Division of Entomology, Faculty of Horticulture, SKUAST-Kashmir.

Charles O. Adetunji
Applied Microbiology, Biotechnology and Nanotechnology Laboratory, Department of Microbiology, Edo State University Uzairue, Edo State, Nigeria.

Dominika Skiba
Department of Plant Production Technology and Commodity Science, University of Life Sciences in Lublin, 20–950 Lublin, Poland.

Fahim Nawaz
Department of Agronomy, MNS, University of Agriculture, Multan, Pakistan.

Farhood Yeganehpoor
Department of Plant Eco-Physiology, University of Tabriz, 51368 Tabriz, Iraq.

Firdose A. Malik
College of Temperate Sericulture, Mirgund, Sher-e-Kashmir University of Agricultural Sciences and Technology of Kashmir (SKUAST-K), Srinagar, India.

Gazala Gulzar
Division of Plant Pathology; Faculty of Horticulture, Sher e Kashmir University of Agricultural Sciences and Technology of Kashmir, Shalimar, Jammu and Kashmir, India.

Hamayun Shabir
Division of Horticulture, Sher-e-Kashmir University of Agricultural Sciences and Technology of Kashmir (SKUAST-K), Shalimar, Srinagar, India.

Ifshan Malik
Division of Basic Sciences and Humanities, Sher e Kashmir University of Agricultural Sciences and Technology, Kashmir.

Ikra Manzoor
Division of Fruit Science, Faculty of Horticulture, SKUAST-Kashmir.

Iqra Farooq
CSIR- Indian Institute of Integrative Medicine, Jammu, J&K, 180001, India.

Kamoru A. Adedokun
King Saud University Medical City, DUH, Oral Pathology Department.

Kehinde Abraham Odelade
Department of Natural Sciences, Faculty of Pure and Applied Sciences, Precious Cornerstone University, Ibadan.

Khair Ul Nisa
Department of Environmental Science, University of Kashmir, Srinagar, India, 190006.

Khawaja Shafique Ahmad
Department of Botany, University of Poonch Rawalakot, 12350, Azad Jammu and Kashmir, Pakistan.

Labiba Riyaz Shah
Division of Vegetable Science; Faculty of Horticulture, Sher e Kashmir University of Agricultural Sciences and Technology of Kashmir, Shalimar-190025, Jammu and Kashmir, India.

Mehrun Nisa
Department of Botany, University of Kashmir, Srinagar, India.

Mohd Ashraf Bhat
Division of Plant Biotechnology, Sher-e-Kashmir University of Agricultural Sciences and Technology of Kashmir (SKUAST-K), Shalimar, Srinagar, India.

Momin Showkat Bhat
Division of Floriculture and Landscape Architecture, Sher e Kashmir University of Agricultural Sciences and Technology, Kashmir.

Mudasir A Mir
Division of Plant Biotechnology, Sher-e-Kashmir University of Agricultural Sciences and Technology of Kashmir (SKUAST-K), Shalimar, Srinagar, India.

Nadia Gul
School of Biosciences and Biotechnology, Baba Ghulam Shah Badshah University, Rajouri, India.

Najeebul Tarfeen
Centre of Research for Development, University of Kashmir, Srinagar, India, 190006.

Nawreen Mir
Division of Plant Pathology; Faculty of Horticulture, Sher e Kashmir University of Agricultural Sciences and Technology of Kashmir, Shalimar, Jammu and Kashmir, India.

Nazir A. Ganai
Sher-e-Kashmir University of Agricultural Sciences and Technology of Kashmir, Srinagar, J&K, India.

Nazir Suliman
Department of Pharmacy, University of Poonch Rawalakot, 12350, Azad Jammu and Kashmir, Pakistan.

Navneet Kaur
Division of Biochemistry, FBSc, Sher-e-Kashmir University of Agricultural Sciences & Technology of Jammu, India.

Neha Sharma
Division of Vegetable Science, IARI, Pusa, New Delhi, Pin-110012.

O.C.U. Adumanya
Department of Biochemistry, the University of Agriculture and Environmental Sciences, Umuagwo, Imo State, Nigeria.

Olubanke Olujoke Ogunlana
Department of Biochemistry, Covenant University, Ota, Ogun State.

Olugbemi T. Olaniyan
Laboratory for Reproductive Biology and Developmental Programming, Department of Physiology, Rhema University Aba, Abia State, Nigeria.

Oluwakemi Semiloore Omowumi
Department of Natural Sciences, Faculty of Pure and Applied Sciences, Precious Cornerstone University, Ibadan.

Oluwatosin Adefunke Adetuyi
Department of Biochemistry, Osun State University, Osogbo, Osun State.

Oluwabusayo Odunola Oluyide
School of Basic medical sciences, Department of Biomedical Engineering College of Health Sciences and Technology, PMB 316 Epe road, Ijero Ekiti.

Omotayo Opemipo Oyedara
Department of Microbiology, Osun state University, Nigeria.

Owais Ali Wani
Division of Soil Science, SKUAST Kashmir.

Peter Onyebuagu
Department of Physiology, Federal University of Technology, Owerri, Nigeria.

Pravin Kumar A.
CSIR- Indian Institute of Integrative Medicine, Jammu, J&K, 180001, India.

Piotr Barbaś,
Department of Potato Agronomy, Institute of Plant Breeding and Acclimatization—National Research Institute, 05–870 Błonie, Poland.

Piotr Pszczółkowski
Experimental Station for Cultivar Assessment of Central Crop Research Centre, Uhnin, 20–950 Lublin, Poland.

Qadrul Nisa
Division of Plant Pathology, SKUAST-K, Shalimar, India, 190025.

Rizwan Rashid
Division of Vegetable Science; Faculty of Horticulture, Sher e Kashmir University of Agricultural Sciences and Technology of Kashmir, Shalimar-190025, Jammu and Kashmir, India.

Sabba Khan
Division of Vegetable Science; Faculty of Horticulture, Sher e Kashmir University of Agricultural Sciences and Technology of Kashmir, Shalimar-190025, Jammu and Kashmir, India.

Sadaf Rafiq
Division of Floriculture and Landscape Architecture, SKUAST-Kashmir, Srinagar, J&K 190025, India.

Sajad un Nabi
ICAR - Central Institute of Temperate Horticulture, Rangreth Srinagar Kashmir.

Shahjahan Rashid
Division of Plant Pathology; Faculty of Horticulture, Sher e Kashmir University of Agricultural Sciences and Technology of Kashmir, Shalimar-190025, Jammu and Kashmir, India.

Sheikh Mansoor
Division of Biochemistry, Faculty of Basic Sciences, Sher-e-Kashmir University of Agricultural Sciences & Technology of Jammu, India.

Shilpa Raina
Division of Biochemistry, Faculty of Basic Sciences, Sher-e-Kashmir University of Agricultural Sciences & Technology of Jammu, India.

Sweeta Manhas
Division of Biochemistry, Faculty of Basic Sciences, Sher-e-Kashmir University of Agricultural Sciences & Technology of Jammu, India.

Tabinda Wani
Division of Floriculture and Landscape Architecture, Sher e Kashmir University of Agricultural Sciences and Technology, Kashmir.

Tamana Khan
Division of Vegetable Science; Faculty of Horticulture, Sher e Kashmir University of Agricultural Sciences and Technology of Kashmir, Shalimar-190025, Jammu and Kashmir, India.

Temidayo Oluyomi Elufisan
Centro de Ciencia Genomica, Universidad Nacional Autonoma de Mexico.

Usma Jan
Division of Vegetable Science, Faculty of Horticulture, SKUAST-Kashmir.

Yathish VC
Division of Vegetable Crops, ICAR-IIHR, Bengaluru-560089.

Zaffar Bashir
Department of Microbiology, University of Kashmir, Srinagar, India.

Preface

According to the number of studies now being published on the topic, there has been a substantial increase in interest in the study of Plant Oxylipins in recent years. Since oxylipin signaling networks were discovered 50 years ago, significant progress has been made in our comprehension of them. There has been a resurgence in oxylipin research as a result of recent developments in mass spectrometry. With the use of this technique, it is now possible to test hundreds of distinct oxylipins during intricate signaling processes in plants.

The book starts with the classification of oxylipins, their signaling pathways, and the enzymes involved. The importance of oxylipins in plant physiology and under biotic and abiotic stress has been emphasized. The book has explained the role of oxylipins in resistance and after a pathogen attack, physiological processes, which play a part in maturation, reproduction, and ultimately senescence. Thus, authors have made every effort to touch on and link the function of oxylipins with every element of the plant. Additionally, the book will teach readers various methods for plant oxylipin profiling. Finally, the book's originality is enhanced by the various databases and instruments required for plant oxylipins profiling. Written by a global team of experts, *Phyto-Oxylipins: Metabolism, Physiological Roles, and Profiling Techniques* is an ideal resource for plant scientists, plant biochemists, biotechnologists, botanists, phytochemists, toxicologists, chemical ecologists, taxonomists, and other researchers in those fields. It will also be very valuable to professors, students, and researchers in the domain of plant sciences and pathology.

Phyto-Oxylipins: Metabolism, Physiological Roles, and Profiling Techniques presents complete coverage of the mechanism, metabolism, and roles of oxylipins in plant resistance to different biotic and abiotic stresses. Oxylipins play important roles in plant development and responses to physical damage caused by herbivores, insects, and attacks by pathogenic microorganisms. As described above, almost everyone working in the area of plant sciences will find this book useful. In addition, this book will also be useful to medicinal chemists and drug developers. The book will be used by students, researchers, and scientists as it covers the most basic and interesting topics related to oxylipins, their biosynthesis, metabolism, role in different signaling pathways, defense, role in resistance, etc. The most likely users of the book are the post-pharmaceutical institutions (R&D), biotechnology companies, academic institutions: graduate students and senior academic researchers, etc.

Editor Biographies

Sheikh Mansoor is currently a postdoctoral researcher. Previously he was working as project associate-I at the CSIR- Indian Institute of Integrative Medicine Jammu (IIIM). He has obtained his BSc from SP College of Science (University of Kashmir), an MSc from HNBGU Uttarakhand, and a PhD degree from Sher-e-Kashmir University of Agricultural Sciences and Technology of Jammu. Dr. Mansoor has made important contributions to his field and has been working hard to shape himself as an impressive and contributive scientist of the highest intellectual caliber. He has an impressive lab experience in biochemistry, molecular biology, and genetics to his credit. He has collaboratively worked and published more than thirty research and review papers in highly reputed journals like *Frontiers*, *PLOS One*, *Scientific Reports*, *Journal of Fungi*, *Molecules* (MDPI), etc. He has published two books, ten book chapters and he has filed one patent application, which was published on April 1, 2022. Dr. Mansoor has delivered many guest lectures on sequence alignment, submission tools, and phylogenetic analysis. He has submitted more than 150 sequences to the NCBI GenBank. He has attended several national and international conferences, and workshops like European Molecular Biology Organisation (EMBO), and also received hands-on training on Advance Techniques in Modern Biology at Jamia Hamdard University New Delhi. Dr. Mansoor is a review editor for *Frontiers in Ethnopharmacology* and is also the reviewer of several reputed journals like *3 biotech*, *Cell Reports*, *Frontiers*, *PLOS ONE*, MDPI journals, etc.

Chukwuebuka Egbuna is a chartered chemist and academic researcher. He is a member of the Institute of Chartered Chemists of Nigeria (ICCON), the Nigerian Society of Biochemistry and Molecular Biology (NSBMB), and the Royal Society of Chemistry (RSC) (United Kingdom). Egbuna is the founder and editor of the Elsevier book series on Drug Discovery Update. The series includes books, monographs and edited collections from all areas of drug discovery including emerging therapeutic claims for the treatment of diseases. He has been engaged in a number of roles at New Divine Favor Pharmaceutical Industry Limited, Akuzor Nkpor, Anambra State, Nigeria, and Chukwuemeka Odumegwu Ojukwu University (COOU) in Nigeria. Egbuna has published research articles in many international journals of repute and is ranked among the top 500 Nigerian scientists, in SciVal/SCOPUS. He has edited over twenty books with Elsevier, Springer, Wiley, and Taylor & Francis. His most recent book is a 3-volume book on Coronavirus Drug Discovery. Egbuna is also the founder and the publishing director of IPS Intelligentsia Publishing Services. He is a reviewer and editorial board member of various journals. His primary research interests cut across biochemistry, phytochemistry, pharmacology, nutrition and toxicology, food and medicinal chemistry, and analytical biochemistry.

Charles Oluwaseun Adetunji is presently a faculty member at the Microbiology Department, Faculty of Sciences, Edo State University Uzairue (EDSU), Edo State,

Nigeria, where he utilized the application of biological techniques and microbial bioprocesses for the actualization of sustainable development goals and agrarian revolution, through quality teaching, research, and community development. He was formally the Acting Director of Intellectual Property and Technology Transfer, the Head of Department of Microbiology, Sub Dean for Faculty of Science and currently the Chairman Grant Committee and the Ag Dean for Faculty of Science, at EDSU. He is a visiting professor and the Executive Director for the Center of Biotechnology, Precious Cornerstone University, Ibadan. He is presently an external examiner to many academic institutions around the globe. He has won several scientific awards and grants from renowned academic bodies. He has published many scientific journal articles and conference proceedings in refereed national and international journals with over 390 manuscripts. Since 2019 he has been ranked among the top 500 prolific authors in Nigeria, by SciVal/SCOPUS. His research interests include microbiology, biotechnology, post-harvest management, food science, bioinformatics, and nanotechnology. He is presently a series editor with Taylor & Francis, USA, editing several textbooks on agricultural biotechnology, nanotechnology, pharmafoods, and environmental sciences. He is an editorial board member of many international journals and serves as a reviewer to many double-blind peer review journals like Elsevier, Springer, Taylor & Francis, Wiley, *PLOS One*, *Nature*, *Journal of the American Chemistry Society*, Bentham Science Publishers, etc.

Acknowledgements

This book is dedicated to all those people who change the lives of others by living as an example and empowering others.

First and foremost, praises and thanks to God, the Almighty for showering His blessings. We would like to thank all those who have contributed to the project. It would have been difficult without the help and encouragement of all who were professionally or unprofessionally involved with us. We would like to thank our mentors for being an inspiration to us and to other students. I, Dr. Sheikh Mansoor, am highly indebted to Dr. Vikas Sharma, Dr. Khalid Z Masoodi, Dr. Javid Iqbal Mir, Dr. Parvaiz Ahmad, and Dr. Mudasir A Mir for their valuable suggestions, continuous support, and encouragement. I would also like to thank Dr. Chukwuebuka Egbuna and Dr. Charles Oluwaseun Adetunji (co-authors) for initiating this project by developing a roadmap for designing this proposal and for their valuable input in the compilation of this book.

Last but not least, my special and sincere thanks to my loving parents (Mrs and Mr Mohammad Shafi Sheikh), siblings (Sheikh Sajad, Sheikh Kulsum, Rifat Ara, and Sheikh Ab Hanan), and fiancée (Aqeelah Ammatullah) for their consistent guidance and support throughout my career. Thank you for showing me how to stand my ground and have the kind of career that I can be proud of. I will forever be grateful for your support and kindness.

1 Plant Oxylipins

Types and Classifications

Sheikh Mansoor[1], Sweeta Manhas[1], Aatifa Rasool[2], Navneet Kaur[1], and Mudasir A. Mir[3]
[1]Division of Biochemistry, FBSc, SK-University of Agricultural Sciences & Technology of Jammu, India
[2] Division of Fruit Sciences, SK-University of Agricultural Sciences & Technology of Kashmir (SKUAST-K), Shalimar, Srinagar, India
[3]Division of Plant Biotechnology, Sher-e-Kashmir University of Agricultural Sciences and Technology of Kashmir (SKUAST-K), Shalimar, Srinagar, India

CONTENTS

1.1 INTRODUCTION

Oxylipins consist of a number of products that are physiologically active and whose structural diversity is formed by the coordinated action of lipases, lipoxygenases, and cytochromes P450 specialized in the metabolism of fatty acids of hydroperoxide [1, 2]. Oxylipin research has largely been conducted to examine the formation of plant-reported jasmonic acid molecules and their involvement in the control of developmental and defensive processes. Recent genetic research has shown that metabolic constituents of jasmonate operate as signals for themselves and that jasmonate production and perception is crucial for systemic protective reactions caused by wound [3, 4]. In all aerobic species, the oxylipins signal molecules are synthesized enzymatically or spontaneously from unsaturated fatty acids. Oxylipins govern metabolism, growth, and reactions to microorganisms' external stimuli. The oxylipin biosynthesis pathway in plants consists of several parallel branches designated after their branch's initial enzyme: allene oxide, lyases of hydroperoxides, divinyl ether synthase, peroxygenase, alcohol synthases of epoxy, etc. As a result of oxygenation by free radicals and reactive oxygen species, oxylipins can be produced non-enzymatically

DOI: 10.1201/9781003316558-1

[5, 6, 7]. Phytoprostane is called spontaneously produced oxylipin. Various studies have described the involvement of oxylipins in biotic stress reactions [8, 9]. The role of oxylipins in plant adaptation to the circumstances of abiotic stress has been less researched; the data gathering and analysis accessible in this field are also obviously absent. In this review we have discussed biosynthesis of oxylipins, functions in the adaptation of plants to abiotic stress circumstances, for example wounds, temperature, drought, and salinity impacts. The roles of oxylipins are outlined in the signal transduction, gene expression regulation, and interaction with other signal translation pathways. Analysis of more specific responses regulated by oxylipins solely under particular situations of stress is followed by oxylipin-driven mechanisms that assist plants to adapt to a wide range of stress events.

1.2 PLANT OXYLIPIN TYPES

Phyto-oxylipins (PO) are a diverse class of lipid metabolites derived from unsaturated fatty acids oxidation. Plant oxylipins include hydroxy-, oxo-, or keto fatty acids, fatty acid hydroperoxides, volatile aldehydes, divinyl ethers or the plant hormone jasmonic acid (JA), and 12-oxo-phytodienoic acid (OPDA) [10]. The PO family is highly versatile structurally, with several geometric isomers. Regioisomers having similar oxylipin structure may have varied biological effects. Changes in the epoxy or hydroxyl groups drastically change the corresponding oxylipin biological activity. Pathways of PO synthesis result in the production of metabolites which are structurally diverse and have key biological activities. One such phyto-oxylipin is jasmonic acid (JA), which acts as a vital signaling molecule in growth and development of plants, such as pollen, flower development, and seed maturation, along with its role in plant stress responses. Derivatives of JA are well-characterized lipooxygenase-derived metabolites that accumulate rapidly in damaged plants. A methyl derivative of JA is released as a volatile compound signaling mutual danger response between plants both inter as well as intra species communication [11]. Both a-DOX and 9-LOX pathways-derived oxylipins possess strong antibacterial properties. A major product from LA (linoleic acid), 9-LOX is potentially active against tomato bacterial pathogen P. syringae [12]. Four downstream pathways majorly exist leading to the biosynthesis of POs: (i) the AOS pathway (allene oxide synthase) which results in the biosynthesis of jasmonic acid, ketol, 12-oxo-phytoenoic acid, KODA (9-hydroxy-10-oxo-12(Z), 15(Z)-octadecadienoic acid) and OPDA; (ii) the hydroperoxide lyase pathway for the synthesis of C12 derivatives and green leaf volatiles; (iii) the peroxygenase pathway and epoxy alcohol synthase for the production of hydroxy and epoxy fatty acids; and (iv) the divinyl ether biosynthesis pathway.

An α-ketol oxylipin (KODA), is produced from α-linolenic acid through the action of AOS and 9-LOX following a non-enzymatic reaction. KODA promotes reshooting after dormancy, rooting, and flowering, in plants. It also enhances the resistance mechanism in some herbaceous plants against pathogens [13]. A class of POs formed spontaneously called phytoprostanes is also known. In a study on tobacco plants, pretreatmeant of plants with phytoprostanes resulted in reduced cell death response induced by copper sulfate [14]. Another well-studied class of oxylipins are GLVs (green leaf volatiles) comprising of alcohols, esters, and C6 aldehydes. This class of oxylipins is formed via HPL (hydroperoxide lyase) branch of lipooxygenase pathway. The compounds are known to play major roles in plant-herbivore and plant-plant interactions. The examples of this class include (3E)-hexenal and (2E)-hexenal possessing antibacterial properties whereas (2E)-hexenal and (2E)-nonenal inhibit hyphal growth thus exhibiting antifungal properties. Besides GLVs, traumatic acid involved in wound healing is formed by the HPL pathway DES (divenyl ether synthase), and EAS (epoxyalcohol synthase) are another branch of LOX pathway which are less studied. The participation of divinyl ethers in pathogen protection against oomycetes, bacteria, and fungi has been described [15].

1.3 OXYLIPINS BIOSYNTHESIS

Oxylipins are oxygenated polyunsaturated fatty acid metabolites found in abundance in bacteria, fungi, algae, mosses, and flowering plants. The term oxylipin is generally used for plant tissue fatty acid derivatives whereas animal fatty acid metabolites are referred to as eicosanoids. They are signaling molecules that regulate developmental processes such as pollen formation, mediate wound healing responses and also play a role in defensive reactions due to their antimicrobial properties [16, 17]. The release of fatty acids from lipid bilayer membrane initiates oxylipin biosynthesis followed by an oxidation reaction carried out by different enzymes at distinct positions of the fatty acid backbone. The biosynthetic origin of oxylipins has divulged an array of different enzymes and a radical pathway. This diverse molecular group can be generated through autoxidation (non-enzymatic) or enzymatic oxidation [18].

1.3.1 Non-Enzymatic Routes of Lipid Oxidation

Non-enzymatic or enzymatic formation of compounds is based on the higher abundance of enantiomers or racemic mixtures (S or R configurations of hydroperoxides) catalyzed by lipoxygenases or chemical oxidation that results in the formation of different positional isomers of fatty acids (hydroxy). Out of all fatty acids, linoleic and linolenic acid, being most abundant, can easily undergo oxidation due to free radicals resulting into the formation of peroxy fatty acid racemic mixtures or esterified fatty acid hydroperoxides [19]. Peroxy radicals and hydroperoxides of polyunsaturated fatty acids having more than double bonds thus formed, can further be oxidized to generate bicyclic hydroperoxides having a shorter half life similar to PPG1 (phytoprostane). Phytoprostanes having structural similarity to that of animal isoprostanes, can be created by other sequences of spontaneous reactions taking place. Esterified phytoprostanes are found in higher levels in the membranes of some species of plants than free phytoprostanes; there is an increase in overall levels of phytoprostranes after an oxidative stress exposure in plants [20]. During oxidative stress, many of the oxidized lipids are generated that act as ligands for lipidation of proteins that profoundly effects the patterns of gene expression thus representing mediators of oxidant injury [21]. Alkenals, ketodienes, ketotrienes, epoxy alcohols, di and tri-hydroxy fatty acids are well defined products formed by peroxy radicals. In plants, keto fatty acids and phytoprostanes are the major oxylipins that are involved in protein lipidation.

Non-enzymatic oxylipins formation in plants also takes place when there is pathogen attack which results in an increase in esterified hydroxy fatty acids with a significant increase in F1 phytoP in esterified lipids which is more abundant (30 times) than the free oxylipins. This suggests that they are largely formed in the membranes from which it can be released. In studies using A1-PhytoP from Arabidopsis it has been revealed that PhytoP is the signaling compound modulating Arabidopsis proteome with over 35% of the affected proteins being found in the chloroplast. In a recent study it has been found that B1-PhytoP products which are derivatives of alpha linolenic (18:3 Δ 9,12,15) can affect oligodendrocyte progenitors and neuroblasts (immature brain cells) and can confer neuroprotection when there is oxidant injury thus promoting myelation [22].

1.3.2 Enzymatic Routes of Lipid Oxidation

Linoleic and linolenic acid are majorly involved in the enzymatic routes of oxylipins formation. Biosynthetic pathway of oxylipins generally starts when oxygen is added to the acyl chain of PUFAs (linoleic and linolenic acid) through lipooxygenases action or through the action of dioxygenases. Lipoxygenase-non haeme proteins generally catalyze stereo and region specific deoxygenation reactions of polyunsaturated fatty acids, having 4Z and 1Z pentadiene motifs based on their activity; they are classified as 9 or 13 lipoxygenases (LOXs) (Figure 1.1) thus generating 9-hydroperoxy and 13-hydroperoxy derivatives [11, 13]. A substitution of histidine 608 by valine can result in the conversion of 13-LOX into 9-LOX. A stereospecific deoxygenation at the C9 position can be facilitated by demasking guanidino group (positively charged) which is close to the active site thus, forcing an inverse orientation (head to tail) of fatty acid substrate, which results in stereospecific dioxygenation. Lipoxygenases are capable of utilizing both unesterified as well as esterified acyl chains in phospholipids or triacylglycerols. Six lipoxygenases in Arabidopsis and at least 14 lipoxygenases have been identified in potato from the multigene families of lipoxygenes which suggests their role in physiological and developmental aspects for the generation of hydroperoxy pools serving specific functions [23]. Specific isomers of LOX seem to control metabolites directional flow determining the initiation of downstream signaling pathways [24].

Studies with overexpression of LOXH1 of potato leaf revealed its localization to the chloroplast and a high specific activity to PG (phosphatidyglycerol) which is a phospholipid specific to chloroplast and a possible target for inducing plastid signaling pathway. Antisense induced co-suppression of LOXH1 showed no effect on wound induced or basal levels of jasmonates which are 13-hydroperoxylinolenic acid derivatives but there was a marked reduction in the aliphatic C6 aldehydes production. The perception of jasmonic acid oxygenated precursors in the chloroplast galactolipids (DGDG and MGDG) put forward that lipoxygenase may act on these substrates as well, which has been confirmed by in vitro studies using soybean LOX recently. Study of *Arabidopsis* mutant lines deficient of 13-LOX revealed that LOX6 amongst the four 13-lipoxygenases accounts for root accumulation of jasmonate

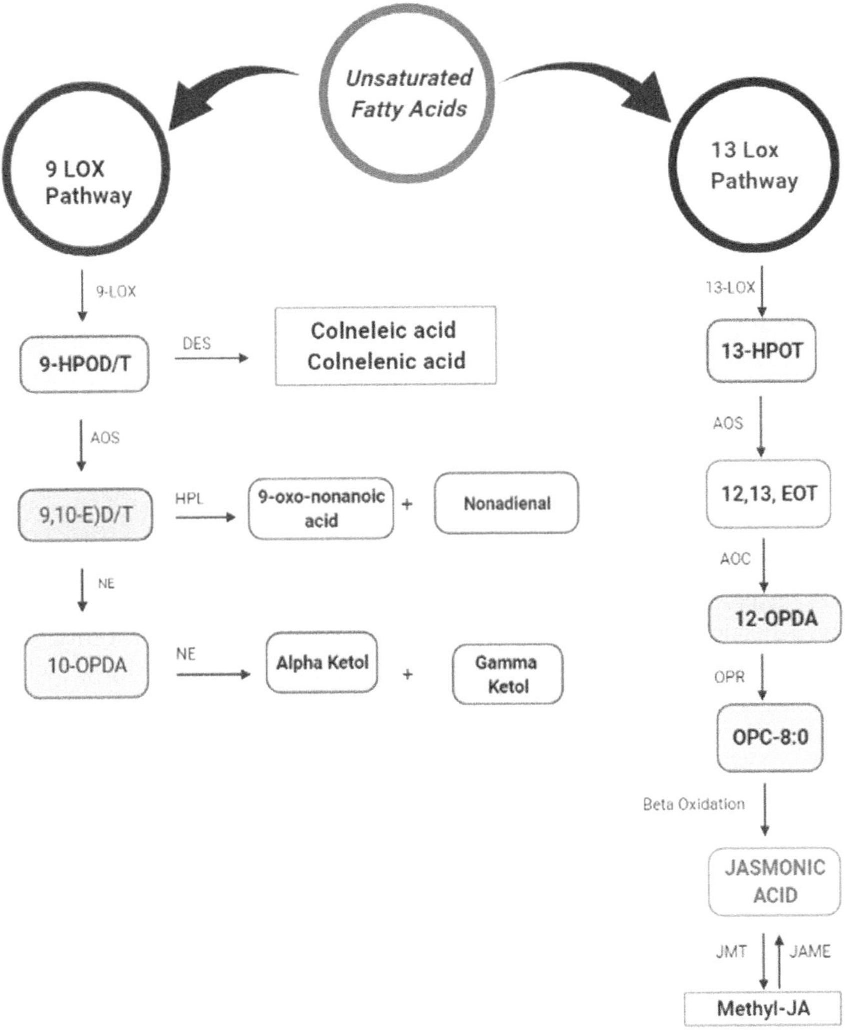

FIGURE 1.1 Diagrammatic representation of 9-LOX and 13-LOX pathways, where HPOD: 9 or 13-hydroperoxide linolenic acid; 13(S) or 9(S)-hydroperoxylinolenic acid; OPDA: 12-oxo-phytodienoic acid; LOX: Lipoxygenase; AOS: Allene oxide synthase; AOC: Allene oxide cyclase; OPR: Oxo-phytodienoic acid reductase; JMT: Jasmonic acid carboxyl methyltransferase; JAME: Methyl jasmonate esterase; HPL: Hydroperoxide lyase; DES: Divinyl ether synthase. NE: Non-enzymatic.

under stress. LOX6 was also necessary for 12-oxo-phutodienoic acid in rots and leaves. High sensitivity to drought stress was observed in LOX6 loss of function mutants which indicates that oxylipins derived from LOX6 plays crucial for biotic and abiotic stress mediated responses [25].

The jasmonates family of oxylipins includes jasmonic acid (JA) which is enzymatically produced when α-linoleic acid and hexadecatrienoic acid are transformed into JA and its derivatives. Jasmonates are known for their role in plant defensive and developmental roles. Derivatives of JA and few of its precursors can modulate gene regulation, thus leading to defensive and developmental changes that are necessary. Jasmonates help in promoting defensive action against insects in plants. 11-HPHT and 13-HPOT hydroperoxides also acts as substrates for hydroperoxide lyase (HPL), which cleaves the bond between C12-C13, producing (9Z)-traumatin (3Z)-hexenal and from (3Z)-hexenal and 13-HPOT. Also, (7Z)-dinortraumatinis produced from 11-HPHT [26]. It has recently been shown that hemiacetals are the initial products of HPL. Hemiacetals are unstable compounds that rapidly transform into oxoacids and aldehydes [27]. Oxidized derivatives (divinyl ethers) are produced by the consecutive action of divinyl ether synthase and LOX on fatty acids, primarily on LA and LEA. Amongst these compounds, colnelenic and colneleic acids are synthesized from 9-hydroperoxides of LA and LEA, respectively. 13-hydroperoxides of LA and LEA produce etherolenic and etheroleic acids in turn [17].

1.4 TRANSCRIPTIONAL REGULATION

The term transcriptional regulation is used for a change at gene expression level with an alteration in transcription rate, which mainly relies on the consolidated effects that mainly include transcriptional factors and their properties. Plant oxylipins include mainly jasmonic acid and many of its derivatives, together known as jasmonates (JAs). These oxylipins are oxygenated fatty acids formed either enzymatically or non-enzymatically through lipoxygenase and alpha-dioxygenases, respectively. These are biologically active signaling molecules that function in plant immunity and development [17, 28]. JA has been extensively investigated in several dicot plants, such as *A. thaliana, S. lycopersicum*, and *N. tabacum*, but only to a very limited level in monocot plants, such as *H. vulgare* and *O. sativa*. Extensive studies in particularly Arabidopsis demonstrated F-box protein i.e., CORONATINE insensitive 1(COI1), which comprises a functional ubiquitin ligase complex [29, 30] with a class of JAZ (jasmonate ZIM-domain) proteins that act as transcriptional repressors [31, 32], a set of transcription factors that modulate/regulate many of the JA responses [28]. The foremost transcriptional factor, MYC-2, contains a basic helix-loop helix (BHLH) module and is known to regulate the two branches of JA-responsive genes [33]. JA-Ile (jasmonyl-isoleucine) is the bioactive form of JA, the level of which is very low in cell cytoplasm. Due to the low level of JA-Ile, transcription factors are unable to activate the promoters of JA-responsive genes. In many of the cases, TFs get repressed by a series of ZIM (zinc-finger inflorescence meristem) domain proteins i.e., JAZ which act as transcriptional repressors. Thereafter, to inhibit the effect of JAZ repressors, both topless protein (TPL) and adaptor protein novel interactor of JAZ (NINJA) get combined to create an effective repression complex by converting an open complex to a closed one *via* histone deacetylase 6 (HDA6) and HDA19 [34, 5] many transcription factors like NAC, ERF, and WRKY play their key roles in JA signaling thereby leads to activation of calcium channel, MAPK cascade, interaction with SA and ABA in case of stress conditions [35]. MYC2, a BHLH transcription factor binds to G-box and its associated hexamers, can interact with members of JAZ repressors. The DNA-binding domain of the other two TFs, i.e., MYC3 and MYC4, are similar whereas MYC5 also related to MYC2 promotes stamen development and seed production [36]. Apart from MYC, several other JA-associated proteins—BHLH3/JAM3, BHLH13/JAM2, BHLH14 and BHLH17/JAM1—facilitate anthocyanin accumulation, chlorophyll loss, leaf senescence [37, 36].

1.5 CONCLUSION

The diversity, occurrence, biosynthesis, and activity of jasmonates have all been greatly expanded. Furthermore, unique signaling features for various oxylipins, such as the hydroxy fatty acids, have recently been discovered for biotic and abiotic stress responses, as well as in development. The equilibrium of active and inactive molecules following synthesis and metabolic conversion maintains these signaling properties. Increased spatial and temporal resolution, as well as transcriptomic, proteomic, and metabolomic approaches, will help researchers better understand the roles of oxylipins in plant stress responses and development. The identification of novel oxylipin-forming genes will add to our understanding of the various oxylipins. Regulatory issues and system biology methodologies will be especially important.

REFERENCES

1. Fujita Y, Fujita M, Shinozaki K, Yamaguchi-Shinozaki K. ABA-mediated transcriptional regulation in response to osmotic stress in plants. Journal of plant research. 2011 Jul;124(4):509–25.
2. Hanif S, Saleem MF, Sarwar M, Irshad M, Shakoor A, Wahid MA, Khan HZ. Biochemically triggered heat and drought stress tolerance in rice by proline application. Journal of Plant Growth Regulation. 2021 Feb;40(1):305–12.
3. Feys BJ, Benedetti CE, Penfold CN, Turner JG. Arabidopsis mutants selected for resistance to the phytotoxin coronatine are male sterile, insensitive to methyl jasmonate, and resistant to a bacterial pathogen. The Plant Cell. 1994 May;6(5):751–9.
4. Reinbothe C, Springer A, Samol I, Reinbothe S. Plant oxylipins: role of jasmonic acid during programmed cell death, defence and leaf senescence. The FEBS Journal. 2009 Sep;276(17):4666–81.
5. Wasternack C, Strnad M. Jasmonates are signals in the biosynthesis of secondary metabolites—Pathways, transcription factors and applied aspects—A brief review. New Biotechnology. 2019 Jan 25;48:1–1.
6. Zhang G, Zhao F, Chen L, Pan Y, Sun L, Bao N, Zhang T, Cui CX, Qiu Z, Zhang Y, Yang L. Jasmonate-mediated wound signalling promotes plant regeneration. Nature Plants. 2019 May;5(5):491–7.
7. Erb M, Kliebenstein DJ. Plant secondary metabolites as defenses, regulators, and primary metabolites: the blurred functional trichotomy. Plant Physiology. 2020 Sep 1;184(1):39–52.
8. Farmer EE, Ryan CA. Octadecanoid-redived signals in plants. Trends in Cell Biology. 1992 Aug 1;2(8):236–41.
9. Partridge M, Murphy DJ. Roles of a membrane-bound caleosin and putative peroxygenase in biotic and abiotic stress responses in Arabidopsis. Plant Physiology and Biochemistry. 2009 Sep 1;47(9):796–806.

10. Ihara Y, Wakamatsu T, Yokoyama M, Maezawa D, Ohta H, Shimojima M. Developing a platform for production of the oxylipin KODA in plants. Journal of Experimental Botany. 2022 May 13;73(9):3044–52.
11. Deboever E, Deleu M, Mongrand S, Lins L, Fauconnier ML. Plant–pathogen interactions: underestimated roles of phyto-oxylipins. Trends in Plant Science. 2020 Jan 1;25(1):22–34.
12. Vicente J, Cascón T, Vicedo B, García-Agustín P, Hamberg M, Castresana C. Role of 9-lipoxygenase and α-dioxygenase oxylipin pathways as modulators of local and systemic defense. Molecular Plant. 2012 Jul 1;5(4):914–28.
13. Wang KD, Borrego EJ, Kenerley CM, Kolomiets MV. Oxylipins other than jasmonic acid are xylem-resident signals regulating systemic resistance induced by Trichoderma virens in maize. The Plant Cell. 2020 Jan;32(1):166–85.
14. Jablonkai I. Molecular defense mechanisms in plants to tolerate toxic action of heavy metal environmental pollution. In: Kimatu, JN, editor. *Plant Defense Mechanisms* [Internet]. London: IntechOpen; 2022 [cited 2022 Oct 17]. Available from: https://www.intechopen.com/chapters/80091 doi: 10.5772/intechopen.102330
15. Gorina S, Ogorodnikova A, Mukhtarova L, Toporkova Y. Gene Expression Analysis of Potato (Solanum tuberosum L.) Lipoxygenase Cascade and Oxylipin Signature under Abiotic Stress. Plants. 2022 Mar 2;11(5):683.
16. Griffiths G. Biosynthesis and analysis of plant oxylipins. Free Radical Research. 2015 May 4;49(5):565–82.
17. Genva M, Obounou Akong F, Andersson MX, Deleu M, Lins L, Fauconnier ML. New insights into the biosynthesis of esterified oxylipins and their involvement in plant defense and developmental mechanisms. Phytochemistry Reviews. 2019 Feb;18(1):343–58.
18. Jikumaru Y, Seo M, Matsuura H, Kamiya Y. Profiling of jasmonic acid-related metabolites and hormones in wounded leaves. In *Jasmonate Signaling* 2013 (pp. 113–122). Humana Press, Totowa, NJ.
19. Babenko LM, Shcherbatiuk MM, Skaterna TD, Kosakivska IV. Lipoxygenases and their metabolites in formation of plant stress tolerance. The Ukrainian Biochemical Journal. 2017;89(1):5–21.
20. Böttcher C, Weiler EW. Cyclo-oxylipin-galactolipids in plants: occurrence and dynamics. Planta. 2007 Aug;226(3):629–37.
21. Andersson MX, Larsson KE, Tjellström H, Liljenberg C, Sandelius AS. Phosphate-limited oat: the plasma membrane and the tonoplast as major targets for phospholipid-to-glycolipid replacement and stimulation of phospholipases in the plasma membrane. Journal of Biological Chemistry. 2005 Jul 29; 280(30):27578–86.
22. Creelman RA, Mulpuri R. The oxylipin pathway in Arabidopsis. The Arabidopsis Book/American Society of Plant Biologists. 2002;1.
23. Vu HS, Tamura P, Galeva NA, Chaturvedi R, Roth MR, Williams TD, Wang X, Shah J, Welti R. Direct infusion mass spectrometry of oxylipin-containing Arabidopsis membrane lipids reveals varied patterns in different stress responses. Plant Physiology. 2012 Jan;158(1):324–39.
24. Grebner W, Stingl NE, Oenel A, Mueller MJ, Berger S. Lipoxygenase6-dependent oxylipin synthesis in roots is required for abiotic and biotic stress resistance of Arabidopsis. Plant Physiology. 2013 Apr;161(4):2159–70.
25. Davoine C, Abreu IN, Khajeh K, Blomberg J, Kidd BN, Kazan K, Schenk PM, Gerber L, Nilsson O, Moritz T, Björklund S. Functional metabolomics as a tool to analyze Mediator function and structure in plants. PloS one. 2017 Jun 22;12(6):e0179640.

26. Koo AJ. Metabolism of the plant hormone jasmonate: a sentinel for tissue damage and master regulator of stress response. Phytochemistry Reviews. 2018 Feb;17(1):51–80.
27. Mukhtarova LS, Brühlmann F, Hamberg M, Khairutdinov BI, Grechkin AN. Plant hydroperoxide-cleaving enzymes (CYP74 family) function as hemiacetal synthases: structural proof of hemiacetals by NMR spectroscopy. Biochimica et Biophysica Acta (BBA)-Molecular and Cell Biology of Lipids. 2018 Oct 1;1863(10):1316–22.
28. Zhai Q, Li C. The plant Mediator complex and its role in jasmonate signaling. Journal of Experimental Botany. 2019 Jun 15;70(13):3415–24.
29. Devoto A, Nieto-Rostro M, Xie D, Ellis C, Harmston R, Patrick E, Davis J, Sherratt L, Coleman M, Turner JG. COI1 links jasmonate signalling and fertility to the SCF ubiquitin–ligase complex in Arabidopsis. The Plant Journal. 2002 Nov;32(4):457–66.
30. Xu L, Liu F, Lechner E, Genschik P, Crosby WL, Ma H, Peng W, Huang D, Xie D. The SCFCOI1 ubiquitin-ligase complexes are required for jasmonate response in Arabidopsis. The Plant Cell. 2002 Aug;14(8):1919–35.
31. Thines B, Katsir L, Melotto M, Niu Y, Mandaokar A, Liu G, Nomura K, He SY, Howe GA, Browse J. JAZ repressor proteins are targets of the SCFCOI1 complex during jasmonate signalling. Nature. 2007 Aug;448(7154):661–5.
32. Yan Y, Stolz S, Chételat A, Reymond P, Pagni M, Dubugnon L, Farmer EE. A down-stream mediator in the growth repression limb of the jasmonate pathway. The Plant Cell. 2007 Aug;19(8):2470–83.
33. Kazan K, Manners JM. MYC2: the master in action. Molecular Plant. 2013 May 1;6(3):686–703.
34. Chini A, Gimenez-Ibanez S, Goossens A, Solano R. Redundancy and specificity in jasmonate signalling. Current Opinion in Plant Biology. 2016 Oct 1;33:147–56.
35. Li Y, Qin L, Zhao J, Muhammad T, Cao H, Li H, Zhang Y, Liang Y. SlMAPK3 enhances tolerance to tomato yellow leaf curl virus (TYLCV) by regulating salicylic acid and jasmonic acid signaling in tomato (Solanum lycopersicum). PLoS One. 2017 Feb 21;12(2):e0172466.
36. Qi T, Huang H, Song S, Xie D. Regulation of jasmonate-mediated stamen development and seed production by a bHLH-MYB complex in Arabidopsis. The Plant Cell. 2015 Jun;27(6):1620–33.
37. Nakata M, Mitsuda N, Herde M, Koo AJ, Moreno JE, Suzuki K, Howe GA, Ohme-Takagi M. A bHLH-type transcription factor, ABA-inducible BHLH-type transcription factor/JA-associated MYC2-LIKE1, acts as a repressor to negatively regulate jasmonate signaling in Arabidopsis. The Plant Cell. 2013 May;25(5):1641–56.

2 Oxylipin Mediated Signaling

Iqra Farooq[1], Pravin Kumar A.[1], and Sadaf Rafiq[2]
[1]CSIR- Indian Institute of Integrative Medicine, Jammu, J&K, India
[2]Division of Floriculture and Landscape Architecture, SKUAST- Kashmir, Srinagar, J&K, India

CONTENTS

2.1 INTRODUCTION

Phyto-oxylipns act as vital signaling molecules in carrying out the key biological activities for plant growth and development, and responses against abiotic and biotic stresses. The signaling and signature of oxylipins depend on the plant species, kind of stressor, and the affected organ and life cycle of the insect and pathogen [1–6] as shown in the studies conducted on potato infected by *Phytophthora infestans* having high levels of 9(S)- and 13(S)-polyunsaturated fatty acid (FA) (PUFA) hydroperoxides (HPOs) (Fauconnier et al., 2008), tobacco leaves having an infection of *Pseudomonas syringae* have higher α-dioxygenase (a-DOX) levels and 9-lipoxygenase (LOX) products [7].

DOI: 10.1201/9781003316558-2

2.2 SYNTHESIS

Oxylipins are the compounds that are derived from lipids due to polyunsaturated fatty acid (PUFA) oxidation, like hexadecatrienoic acid, linoleic acid and octadecatrienoic acid [8–9], and oxidized by lipoxygenases (LOX) resulting in the hydroperoxides formation [10–11]. A study on the synthesis of an oxylipid, jasmonic acid, showed that octadecanoid pathway in *Arabidopsis thaliana* starts from the oxidation of octacatrienoic acid by 13-LOX forming 13-hydroperoxylinolic acid. This process takes place in the plastids. Later, allene oxide cyclase (AOC) and allene oxide synthase (AOS) react on 13-hydroperoxylinolic acid to form cis-(+)-12-oxo-phytodienoicacid (cis-OPDA) which then localizes to peroxisome through cytosol mediated by ABC (ATP binding cassette) transporter protein, COMATOSE. After cis-OPDA reaches peroxisome, it is then reduced to get activated to CoA ester [12–13] followed by three β-oxidation processes to form JA [14–16].

Another pathway initiating from hydroperoxides of plastids with the action of divinyl ester synthases (DES) producing divinyl ether oxylipins has proved to play a role in plant stress and defense responses [17]. Other alternate pathways are hydroperoxide lyases (HPL), epoxy alcohol synthase (EAS), or peroxygenases (PXG). The products formed are oxylipin-JA and phytohormones with characteristic reactive epoxide, a,b-unsaturated carbonyl, or aldehyde functionalities.

2.2.1 Signaling and Defense Mechanisms in Plants

Plants have evolved a defense mechanism for protection against stress and diseases and phyto-oxylipins have proven to play a key role in these defense mechanism systems. The responses against biotic and abiotic stresses include the synthesis of particular oxylipjns having various biological functions. They act as agents for wound healing and act as signal molecules for antibacterial and antifungal activities [18]. The distinctive oxylipins are jasmonic acid (JA) and the precursor 12-oxo-phytodienoicacid (OPDA) formed enzymatically which get accumulated in reaction to various stresses [19]. Additionally, the oxylipins are also formed non-enzymatically in response to the activity of reactive oxygen species (ROS) as a reaction to the various kinds of stresses and it has been established that the oxylipins formed non-enzymatically play an important role as signaling molecules in plant stress responses [20].

The roles of JA and OPDA have been evaluated and recent studies have depicted that both the biomolecules act as the significant signaling molecules for expression of certain genes that contribute to stress responses. The signaling mechanism of jasmonic acid is known to be the transcriptional control of jasmonic acid-responsive genes. In Arabidopsis, JA is believed to be associated with amino acids by the enzyme encoded by the gene *JAR1* to form conjugates like jasmonoyl-L-isoleucine (JA-Ile) that play a significant role in transcriptional control through jasmonate ZIM domain repressor proteins [21]. The signaling of jasmonic acid results in the interaction of the F-box ubiquitin ligase CORONATINE-IN SENSITIVE1 (COI1) and JAZ transcriptional repressors, and thus degrading downstream JA-induced gene repressors, most of which depend on MYC2/JIN1, the key transcription factor [22]. JA-Ile gets metabolized to 12OH-JA-Ile by a cytochrome P450 [23] having a lesser effect than JA-Ile for the promotion of COI1-JAZ binding thus advocating the part played by this enzyme in the inhibition of JA-Ile activity and attenuation of the jasmonate response [12].

However, it has been established that OPDA induces COI1-independent genes [24]. Another subclass of oxylipins, phytoprostanes, have also been shown to carry out the response activities [25]. OPDA, as well as phytoprostanes, belong to the group of oxylipins viz., reactive electrophile species (RES) for the fact that they possess active α, β-unsaturated carbonyl structure that has a role to play in bio-physiological activities carried out by RES. RES has the ability to reshape the proteins by associating them to free thiol groups. Many studies have suggested that RES have the property of inducing a common set of genes responsible for defense mechanisms in the plants [26–28].

2.3 KEY ENZYMES

2.3.1 Acyl-Lipid Hydrolases

Attempts to change the biosynthesis of oxylipins by the over expression of one of the enzymes participating in the biosynthesis process have been published [29]. It is clear that oxylipin production is triggered by external stimuli and is primarily influenced by one of the substrates, LA, roughanic acid, or α-LeA [30]. In this respect, it is worth noting that Arabidopsis' phospholipases DAD1 and DGL, present in plastids, appear to play a role in oxylipin signaling, as evidenced by research on *dad1* and *dgl* mutants [31–32]. Another family of acyl-lipid hydrolases, the patatins, appears to be involved in feeding substrates to the oxylipin biosynthesis pathway [33]. Despite these examples, enzymes involved in delivering free PUFAs to the LOX pathway are still poorly understood, and additional research is required.

2.3.2 Lipoxygenases

LOXs catalyze the PUFA dioxygenation with a (1Z,4Z)-pentadiene system, such as LA, a-LeA, or roughanic acid, in a regio- and stereo-specific manner. Plant LOXs are characterized according to the position of LA oxygenation, occurring at carbon atom 9 (9-LOX) or carbon atom 13 (13-LOX) of the hydrocarbon in the case of an 18-carbon fatty acid [34]. The creation of two sets of molecules, the (13S)-hydroperoxy and (9S)-hydroperoxy derivatives of PUFAs, is due to the differing specificities [35]. Cyanobacteria have recently been found to produce a (9R)-hydroperoxide-forming LOX [36]. Genes encoding the LOXs are found as multigene families in every plant species studied, with six groups in Arabidopsis and almost 14 in potatoes. It is likely that distinct subcellular localizations of LOX-isoforms produce diverse pools of hydroperoxy PUFAs, which serve as substrates for alternate conversion pathways having different physiologic effects [35].

2.3.3 CYP74-Enzymes

Several critical enzymes in the metabolism of oxylipin belong to the CYP74-enzymes, an unusual family of cytochrome P450 monooxygenases. AOS, HPL, and DES belong to CYP74 enzymes that do not require molecular oxygen or NAD(P)H-dependent cytochrome P450-reductase as cofactors, unlike other P450 enzymes [17, 37–38]. CYP74-enzymes employ acyl hydroperoxides to act as substrate and as well as an oxygen donor to generate carbon-oxygen bonds.

2.3.3.1 AOS

AOS is a crucial enzyme in the octadecanoid pathway that leads to JA production, with formation of unstable allylic fatty acid epoxides by conversion of fatty acid hydroperoxides [39]. Membrane-associated AOSs are found in all AOSs isolated from plants. While Arabidopsis, *Linum usitatissimum*, *Parthenium argentatum*, and *Medicago truncatula* each have a single AOS gene, tomato has two AOSs [40–43] and potato is shown to have three AOSs [44]. The structures of AOS from Parthenium and Arabidopsis were also revealed, defining more about the mechanism of the reaction for these enzymes [31, 45].

2.3.3.2 HPL

HPL catalyzes the splitting of hydroperoxides in fatty acids and (3Z)-alkenals, resulting in aggregates of C6 volatiles known as green leaf volatiles (GLVs), including hexanol, hexanal, (3Z)-hexenal, (2E)-hexenol and (2E)-hexenal. The formation of the kind of GLVs depends on the available substrate. As a result, the pools of fatty acid hydroperoxides accessible for alternate jasmonate synthesis decrease. C6 volatiles produced from HPL have previously been hypothesized to play a function in signaling during plant defense mechanisms [46]. A study on the defense mechanism against sucking insect pests by the action of these oxylipins has been conducted, for example, for GLVs generated by 13-HPL in transgenic potato plants by antisense-mediated depletion of this specific 13-HPL [47]. Aphid performance was also improved when hazardous HPL-derived volatiles was reduced [48]. Arabidopsis, corn, barley, guava), bell pepper, melon, potato, and tomato have all produced single cDNA-clones for HPLs [49–51]. AOS and HPL have been found in chloroplasts of leaves in several studies [52]. The fact that many CYP74-cDNAs encode plastidial transit peptides suggests a plastidial site [44]. 13-HPL was detected in the outer membrane of tomato mesophyll chloroplasts, while 13-AOS was found in the inner membrane [53]. 13-HPL is integrally produced in potato leaves and at the time of floral development, producing (3Z)-hexenal and (3Z)-hexenol preferentially [47].

2.3.3.3 DES

Fatty acid hydroperoxides are converted to divinyl ether fatty acids by the enzyme DES. Tobacco (*Nicotiana tabacum*) [54] and potato [55] have all produced DES cDNA. While the enzymes from tomatoes, tobacco, and potatoes are highly specific for 9-hydroperoxide substrates, a garlic enzyme (*Allium sativum*) prefers 13-hydroperoxide substrates (13-DES) [56]. A study revealed colneleic acid and colnelenic acid that are conjugated fatty acids to increase in potato and tobacco during infection [54, 57] offered the first hints for a function in defense mechanism againt plant infections such as *Phytophthora*. Although there are transgenic lines that overexpress DES, they have not been thoroughly studied. The evolution of oxylipin synthesis is linked to the evolution of CYP74-enzymes that have evolved from previous enzymes to have a diverse set of specialized functions thereby exhibiting catalytic versatility. The discovery of enzymes having multiple functions suggests that the structural backbone of CYP74-enzymes can support a variety of fatty acid hydroperoxide substrate transformations [58]. It has also been established using x-ray crystallography data that only a few amino acid alterations are required to convert an AOS enzyme into an HPL or vice versa, revealing close structural relationships [31].

The role of HPL and AOS in the generation of GLVs and jasmonates respectively, shows that the development of these signaling components occurs as a result of just minor genetic differences. It has been claimed that enzymes essential for oxylipin production existed in the last common ancestor of plants and animals, but now have been lost in metazoan lineages with just a few exceptions, using bioinformatics methods and biochemical data.

2.3.4 Dioxygenases

α-DOX catalyzes the PUFA conversion to their equivalent 2-hydroperoxy fatty acids, providing source for fatty acid hydroperoxides other than LOXs [59]. Two isoforms of α-DOX have been identified in Arabidopsis. In Arabidopsis, studies on the cellular signals that activate α-DOX1 indicated that salicylic acid, intracellular superoxide, and nitric oxide, three signaling molecules that mediate cell death, all promote gene expression [7, 60]. In leaves subjected to artificial senescence by leaf detachment, the accumulation of α-DOX2 transcripts was increased [61]. Within the plastid and later in the peroxisome, the octadecanoid pathway employs a number of enzymes that convert AOS-products into physiologically active oxylipins. Allene oxides (allylic epoxides) supplied by AOS can convert chemically to cyclopentenones [62] or, in the case of the allene oxide derived from 13-hydroperoxy α-LeA, via conversion by enzymatic action by allene oxide cyclase (AOC, EC 5.3.99.7), generate chiral OPDA [63].

2.4 REGULATION OF THE OXYLIPIN PATHWAY

Plants possess the pools of phyto-oxylipin of varied sizes, which impose an oxylipin signature on any organelle, tissue, plant, or species. The type of stress, like pathogen attack, insect attack, or wound formation, influences the composition of oxygenated fatty acid derivatives based on the response to the damage. In barley leaves for instance, salicylic acid, causes nearly exclusively the synthesis of hydroxy fatty acid derivatives. Methyl jasmonate, on the other hand, causes aldehyde buildup in these plants [64].

All the plant species do not possess the various oxylipin biosynthetic enzymes, contrary to popular belief. The *CYP74D* (divinyl ether synthase) gene, for example, is lacking from the genome of Arabidopsis, and its acitivity has only been discovered in the Solanaceae family. However, besides the requirement of these enzymes, the spatial and temporal expression of the various oxylipin biosynthetic enzymes appears to be crucial. Several plant species have been documented to produce LOXs in response to wounding, mechanical stress, or pathogen infection. Some of the LOXs for which inductions have been linked to the de novo synthesis of jasmonic acid against wounding and insect bites create the required precursor (13S-hydroperoxylinolenic acid). As a result, transgenic plants of potato with lower levels of specific LOX-isoforms have been found to be more susceptible to insect attacks [65].

The compartmentalization of the many biosynthetic enzymes is another important factor in the regulation of phytooxylipin pathways. In the envelope of spinach plastids with LOX activity, for example, at least two CYP74s (AOS and hydroperoxide lyase) are found [18]. Furthermore, it was also shown that AOS was localized to the inner envelope of tomato plastids, although the hydroperoxide lyase is found in the outer membrane of the same envelope [53], raising doubts concerning the origin and manner of release of the fatty acids that are substrates of such enzymes. Many lipases, including phospholipases A and D, galactolipases, and acyl hydrolases, can release polyunsaturated fatty acids from membranes.

2.5 CONCLUSION

It has been established that phyto-oxylipins have a major role to execute in the biotic and abiotic stress response mechanism. They act as signaling agents for the functions like wound healing, and antifungal and antibacterial activities. Jasmonic acid, a distinctive oxylipin and its precursor OPDA has been proven as to induce certain gene expressions responsible for the stress management mechanism that are formed both by enzymatic and non-enzymatic pathways. Various Key enzymes responsible for the regulation of the oxylipin pathway viz., acyl-lipid hydrolases, LOX, DOX, and CYP74-enzymes have been explored. Oxylipin biosynthesis is extremely dynamic and takes place both constitutively and as a result of different stressors. Since oxylipin signals are involved in so many different signaling pathways, they are essential parts of the network of plant signals. While the production, sensing, and physiological functions of molecules like OPDA or JA, for example, are well understood, the significance of other oxylipins for plant function is only now starting to become clear. The most recent developments in oxylipin analysis technology open the door for non-targeted metabolomic techniques, which might offer additional insights into the roles that lesser known oxylipin species play in plant function and development.

REFERENCES

1. Wasternack, C., & I. Feussner. (2018), The oxylipin pathways: biochemistry and function. Annual Review of Plant Biology, 69 363–386.
2. Wasternack, C., & Song, S. (2017). Jasmonates: biosynthesis, metabolism, and signaling by proteins activating and repressing transcription. Journal of Experimental Botany, 68(6), 1303–1321.
3. Delaplace, P., Rojas-Beltran, J., Frettinger, P., Du Jardin, P., & Fauconnier, M. L. (2008). Oxylipin profile and antioxidant status of potato tubers during extended storage at room temperature. Plant Physiology and Biochemistry, 46(12), 1077–1084.

4. Gosset, V., Harmel, N., Göbel, C., Francis, F., Haubruge, E., Wathelet, J. P., ... & Fauconnier, M. L. (2009). Attacks by a piercing-sucking insect (Myzus persicae Sultzer) or a chewing insect (Leptinotarsa decemlineata Say) on potato plants (Solanum tuberosum L.) induce differential changes in volatile compound release and oxylipin synthesis. Journal of Experimental Botany, 60(4), 1231–1240.
5. León Morcillo, R. J., Ocampo, J. A., & García Garrido, J. M. (2012). Plant 9-lox oxylipin metabolism in response to arbuscular mycorrhiza. Plant Signaling & Behavior, 7(12), 1584–1588.
6. Tsitsigiannis, D. I., & Keller, N. P. (2007). Oxylipins as developmental and host–fungal communication signals. Trends in Microbiology, 15(3), 109–118.
7. Hamberg, M., Sanz, A., Rodriguez, M. J., Calvo, A. P., & Castresana, C. (2003). Activation of the fatty acid α-dioxygenase pathway during bacterial infection of tobacco leaves: formation of oxylipins protecting against cell death. Journal of Biological Chemistry, 278(51), 51796–51805.
8. Mosblech, A., Feussner, I., & Heilmann, I. (2009). Oxylipins: structurally diverse metabolites from fatty acid oxidation. Plant Physiology and Biochemistry, 47(6), 511–517.
9. Wasternack, C., & Kombrink, E. (2010). Jasmonates: structural requirements for lipid-derived signals active in plant stress responses and development. ACS Chemical Biology, 5(1), 63–77.
10. Vick, B. A., & Zimmerman, D. C. (1983). The biosynthesis of jasmonic acid: a physiological role for plant lipoxygenase. Biochemical and Biophysical Research Communications, 111(2), 470–477.
11. Bell, E., Creelman, R. A., & Mullet, J. E. (1995). A chloroplast lipoxygenase is required for wound-induced jasmonic acid accumulation in Arabidopsis. Proceedings of the National Academy of Sciences, 92(19), 8675–8679.
12. Koo, A. J., Cooke, T. F., & Howe, G. A. (2011). Cytochrome P450 CYP94B3 mediates catabolism and inactivation of the plant hormone jasmonoyl-L-isoleucine. Proceedings of the National Academy of Sciences, 108(22), 9298–9303.
13. Kienow, L., Schneider, K., Bartsch, M., Stuible, H. P., Weng, H., Miersch, O., ... & Kombrink, E. (2008). Jasmonates meet fatty acids: functional analysis of a new acyl-coenzyme A synthetase family from Arabidopsis thaliana. Journal of Experimental Botany, 59(2), 403–419.
14. Theodoulou, F. L., Job, K., Slocombe, S. P., Footitt, S., Holdsworth, M., Baker, A., ... & Graham, I. A. (2005). Jasmonic acid levels are reduced in COMATOSE ATP-binding cassette transporter mutants. Implications for transport of jasmonate precursors into peroxisomes. Plant Physiology, 137(3), 835–840.
15. Stintzi, A., Weber, H., Reymond, P., Browse, J., & Farmer, E. E. (2001). Plant defense in the absence of jasmonic acid: the role of cyclopentenones. Proceedings of the National Academy of Sciences, 98(22), 12837–12842.
16. Schilmiller, A. L., Koo, A. J., & Howe, G. A. (2007). Functional diversification of acyl-coenzyme A oxidases in jasmonic acid biosynthesis and action. Plant Physiology, 143(2), 812–824.
17. Itoh, A., & Howe, G. A. (2001). Molecular cloning of a divinyl ether synthase: identification as a CYP74 cytochrome P-450. Journal of Biological Chemistry, 276(5), 3620–3627.
18. Blée, E., & Joyard, J. (1996). Envelope membranes from spinach chloroplasts are a site of metabolism of fatty acid hydroperoxides. Plant Physiology, 110(2), 445–454.
19. Block, A., Schmelz, E., Jones, J. B., & Klee, H. J. (2005). Coronatine and salicylic acid: the battle between Arabidopsis and Pseudomonas for phytohormone control. Molecular Plant Pathology, 6(1), 79–83.

20. Sattler, S. E., Mene-Saffrane, L., Farmer, E. E., Krischke, M., Mueller, M. J., & DellaPenna, D. (2006). Nonenzymatic lipid peroxidation reprograms gene expression and activates defense markers in Arabidopsis tocopherol-deficient mutants. The Plant Cell, 18(12), 3706–3720.
21. Thines, B., Katsir, L., Melotto, M., Niu, Y., Mandaokar, A., Liu, G., ... & Browse, J. (2007). JAZ repressor proteins are targets of the SCFCOI1 complex during jasmonate signalling. Nature, 448(7154).
22. Chini, A., Fonseca, S.G.D.C., Fernandez, G., Adie, B., Chico, J.M., Lorenzo, O., García-Casado, G., López-Vidriero, I., Lozano, F.M., Ponce, M.R. and Micol, J.L., 2007. The JAZ family of repressors is the missing link in jasmonate signalling. Nature, 448(7154), 666–671.
23. Heitz, T., Widemann, E., Lugan, R., Miesch, L., Ullmann, P., Désaubry, L., ... & Pinot, F. (2012). Cytochromes P450 CYP94C1 and CYP94B3 catalyze two successive oxidation steps of plant hormone jasmonoyl-isoleucine for catabolic turnover. Journal of Biological Chemistry, 287(9), 6296–6306.
24. Taki, N., Sasaki-Sekimoto, Y., Obayashi, T., Kikuta, A., Kobayashi, K., Ainai, T., ... & Ohta, H. (2005). 12-oxo-phytodienoic acid triggers expression of a distinct set of genes and plays a role in wound-induced gene expression in Arabidopsis. Plant Physiology, 139(3), 1268–1283.
25. Thoma, I., Krischke, M., Loeffler, C., & Mueller, M. J. (2004). The isoprostanoid pathway in plants. Chemistry and Physics of Lipids, 128(1–2), 135–148.
26. Alméras, E., Stolz, S., Vollenweider, S., Reymond, P., Mène-Saffrané, L., & Farmer, E. E. (2003). Reactive electrophile species activate defense gene expression in Arabidopsis. The Plant Journal, 34(2), 205–216.
27. Weber, H., Chételat, A., Reymond, P., & Farmer, E. E. (2004). Selective and powerful stress gene expression in Arabidopsis in response to malondialdehyde. The Plant Journal, 37(6), 877–888.
28. Farmer, E. E., & Davoine, C. (2007). Reactive electrophile species. Current Opinion in Plant Biology, 10(4), 380–386.
29. Miersch, O., Weichert, H., Stenzel, I., Hause, B., Maucher, H., Feussner, I., & Wasternack, C. (2004). Constitutive overexpression of allene oxide cyclase in tomato (Lycopersicon esculentum cv. Lukullus) elevates levels of some jasmonates and octadecanoids in flower organs but not in leaves. Phytochemistry, 65(7), 847–856.
30. Wasternack, C. (2007). Jasmonates: an update on biosynthesis, signal transduction and action in plant stress response, growth and development. Annals of botany, 100(4), 681–697.
31. Lee, D. S., Nioche, P., Hamberg, M., & Raman, C. S. (2008). Structural insights into the evolutionary paths of oxylipin biosynthetic enzymes. Nature, 455(7211), 363–368.
32. Matsui, K., Fukutomi, S., Ishii, M., & Kajiwara, T. (2004). A tomato lipase homologous to DAD1 (LeLID1) is induced in post-germinative growing stage and encodes a triacylglycerol lipase. FEBS letters, 569(1–3), 195–200.
33. Dhondt, S., Geoffroy, P., Stelmach, B. A., Legrand, M., & Heitz, T. (2000). Soluble phospholipase A2 activity is induced before oxylipin accumulation in tobacco mosaic virus-infected tobacco leaves and is contributed by patatin-like enzymes. The Plant Journal, 23(4), 431–440.
34. Schneider, C., Pratt, D. A., Porter, N. A., & Brash, A. R. (2007). Control of oxygenation in lipoxygenase and cyclooxygenase catalysis. Chemistry & Biology, 14(5), 473–488.
35. Liavonchanka, A., & Feussner, I. (2006). Lipoxygenases: occurrence, functions and catalysis. Journal of Plant Physiology, 163(3), 348–357.

36. Zheng, Y., Boeglin, W. E., Schneider, C., & Brash, A. R. (2008). A 49-kDa mini-lipoxygenase from Anabaena sp. PCC 7120 retains catalytically complete functionality. Journal of Biological Chemistry, 283(8), 5138–5147.
37. Mita, G., Quarta, A., Fasano, P., De Paolis, A., Di Sansebastiano, G. P., Perrotta, C., ... & Santino, A. (2005). Molecular cloning and characterization of an almond 9-hydroperoxide lyase, a new CYP74 targeted to lipid bodies. Journal of Experimental Botany, 56(419), 2321–2333.
38. Utsunomiya, Y., Nakayama, T., Oohira, H., Hirota, R., Mori, T., Kawai, F., & Ueda, T. (2000). Purification and inactivation by substrate of an allene oxide synthase (CYP74) from corn (Zea mays L.) seeds. Phytochemistry, 53(3), 319–323.
39. Tijet, N., & Brash, A. R. (2002). Allene oxide synthases and allene oxides. Prostaglandins & Other Lipid Mediators, 68, 423–431.
40. Laudert, D., Pfannschmidt, U., Lottspeich, F., Holländer-Czytko, H., & Weiler, E. W. (1996). Cloning, molecular and functional characterization of Arabidopsis thaliana allene oxide synthase (CYP 74), the first enzyme of the octadecanoid pathway to jasmonates. Plant Molecular Biology, 31(2), 323–335.
41. Harms, K., Atzorn, R., Brash, A., Kuhn, H., Wasternack, C., Willmitzer, L., & Pena-Cortes, H. (1995). Expression of a flax allene oxide synthase cDNA leads to increased endogenous jasmonic acid (JA) levels in transgenic potato plants but not to a corresponding activation of JA-responding genes. The Plant Cell, 7(10), 1645–1654.
42. Pan, Z., Durst, F., Werck-Reichhart, D., Gardner, H. W., Camara, B., Cornish, K., & Backhaus, R. A. (1995). The major protein of guayule rubber particles is a cytochrome P450: characterization based on cDNA cloning and spectroscopic analysis of the solubilized enzyme and its reaction products. Journal of Biological Chemistry, 270(15), 8487–8494.
43. Hughes, R. K., Belfield, E. J., & Casey, R. (2006). CYP74C3 and CYP74A1, plant cytochrome P450 enzymes whose activity is regulated by detergent micelle association, and proposed new rules for the classification of CYP74 enzymes. Biochemical Society Transactions 34(6), 1223–1227.
44. Stumpe, M., Göbel, C., Demchenko, K., Hoffmann, M., Klösgen, R. B., Pawlowski, K., & Feussner, I. (2006). Identification of an allene oxide synthase (CYP74C) that leads to formation of α-ketols from 9-hydroperoxides of linoleic and linolenic acid in below-ground organs of potato. The Plant Journal, 47(6), 883–896.
45. Li, L., Chang, Z., Pan, Z., Fu, Z. Q., & Wang, X. (2008). Modes of heme binding and substrate access for cytochrome P450 CYP74A revealed by crystal structures of allene oxide synthase. Proceedings of the National Academy of Sciences, 105(37), 13883–13888.
46. Shiojiri, K., Kishimoto, K., Ozawa, R., Kugimiya, S., Urashimo, S., Arimura, G., ... & Takabayashi, J. (2006). Changing green leaf volatile biosynthesis in plants: an approach for improving plant resistance against both herbivores and pathogens. Proceedings of the National Academy of Sciences, 103(45), 16672–16676.
47. Vancanneyt, G., Sanz, C., Farmaki, T., Paneque, M., Ortego, F., Castañera, P., & Sánchez-Serrano, J. J. (2001). Hydroperoxide lyase depletion in transgenic potato plants leads to an increase in aphid performance. Proceedings of the National Academy of Sciences, 98(14), 8139–8144.
48. Eigenbrode, S. D., Ding, H., Shiel, P., & Berger, P. H. (2002). Volatiles from potato plants infected with potato leafroll virus attract and arrest the virus vector, Myzus persicae (Homoptera: Aphididae). Proceedings of the Royal Society of London. Series B: Biological Sciences, 269(1490), 455–460.

49. Bate, N. J., Sivasankar, S., Moxon, C., Riley, J. M., Thompson, J. E., & Rothstein, S. J. (1998). Molecular characterization of an Arabidopsis gene encoding hydroperoxide lyase, a cytochrome P-450 that is wound inducible. Plant Physiology, 117(4), 1393–1400.
50. Tijet, N., Wäspi, U., Gaskin, D. J., Hunziker, P., Muller, B. L., Vulfson, E. N., ... & Whitehead, I. M. (2000). Purification, molecular cloning, and expression of the gene encoding fatty acid 13-hydroperoxide lyase from guava fruit (Psidium guajava). Lipids, 35(7), 709–720.
51. Fukushige, H., & Hildebrand, D. F. (2005). Watermelon (Citrullus lanatus) hydroperoxide lyase greatly increases C6 aldehyde formation in transgenic leaves. Journal of Agricultural and Food Chemistry, 53(6), 2046–2051.
52. Kuroda, H., Oshima, T., Kaneda, H., & Takashio, M. (2005). Identification and functional analyses of two cDNAs that encode fatty acid 9-/13-hydroperoxide lyase (CYP74C) in rice. Bioscience, Biotechnology, and Biochemistry, 69(8), 1545–1554.
53. Farmaki, T., Sanmartín, M., Jiménez, P., Paneque, M., Sanz, C., Vancanneyt, G., ... & Sánchez-Serrano, J. J. (2007). Differential distribution of the lipoxygenase pathway enzymes within potato chloroplasts. Journal of Experimental Botany, 58(3), 555–568.
54. Froehlich, J. E., Itoh, A., & Howe, G. A. (2001). Tomato allene oxide synthase and fatty acid hydroperoxide lyase, two cytochrome P450s involved in oxylipin metabolism, are targeted to different membranes of chloroplast envelope. Plant Physiology, 125(1), 306–317.
55. Fammartino, A., Cardinale, F., Göbel, C., Mene-Saffrané, L., Fournier, J., Feussner, I., & Esquerré-Tugayé, M. T. (2007). Characterization of a divinyl ether biosynthetic pathway specifically associated with pathogenesis in tobacco. Plant Physiology, 143(1), 378–388.
56. Stumpe, M., Kandzia, R., Göbel, C., Rosahl, S., & Feussner, I. (2001). A pathogen-inducible divinyl ether synthase (CYP74D) from elicitor-treated potato suspension cells. FEBS letters, 507(3), 371–376.
57. Stumpe, M., Carsjens, J. G., Göbel, C., & Feussner, I. (2008). Divinyl ether synthesis in garlic bulbs. Journal of Experimental Botany, 59(4), 907–915.
58. Eschen-Lippold, L., Rothe, G., Stumpe, M., Göbel, C., Feussner, I., & Rosahl, S. (2007). Reduction of divinyl ether-containing polyunsaturated fatty acids in transgenic potato plants. Phytochemistry, 68(6), 797–801.
59. Grechkin, A. N., Mukhtarova, L. S., Latypova, L. R., Gogolev, Y., Toporkova, Y. Y., & Hamberg, M. (2008). Tomato CYP74C3 is a multifunctional enzyme not only synthesizing allene oxide but also catalyzing its hydrolysis and cyclization. ChemBioChem, 9(15), 2498–2505.
60. Hamberg, M., Sanz, A., & Castresana, C. (1999). α-Oxidation of fatty acids in higher plants: identification of a pathogen-inducible oxygenase (PIOX) as an α-dioxygenase and biosynthesis of 2-hydroperoxylinolenic acid. Journal of Biological Chemistry, 274(35), 24503–24513.
61. De León, I. P., Sanz, A., Hamberg, M., & Castresana, C. (2002). Involvement of the Arabidopsisα-DOX1 fatty acid dioxygenase in protection against oxidative stress and cell death. The Plant Journal, 29(1), 61–72.
62. Obregón, P., Martín, R., Sanz, A., & Castresana, C. (2001). Activation of defence-related genes during senescence: a correlation between gene expression and cellular damage. Plant Molecular Biology, 46(1), 67–77.
63. Medvedeva, N. V., Mukhtarova, L. S., Mukhitova, F. K., Balandina, A. A., Latypov, S. K., & Grechkin, A. N. (2007). Cyclization of natural allene oxide in aprotic

solvent: formation of the novel oxylipin methyl cis-12-oxo-10-phytoenoate. Chemistry and Physics of Lipids, 148(2), 91–96.

64. Stenzel, I., Hause, B., Miersch, O., Kurz, T., Maucher, H., Weichert, H., Ziegler, J., Feussner, I. and Wasternack, C., 2003. Jasmonate biosynthesis and the allene oxide cyclase family of Arabidopsis thaliana. Plant Molecular Biology, 51(6), 895–911.
65. Kohlmann, M., Bachmann, A., Weichert, H., Kolbe, A., Balkenhohl, T., Wasternack, C., & Feussner, I. (1999). Formation of lipoxygenase-pathway-derived aldehydes in barley leaves upon methyl jasmonate treatment. European Journal of Biochemistry, 260(3), 885–895.
66. Royo, J., León, J., Vancanneyt, G., Albar, J.P., Rosahl, S., Ortego, F., Castañera, P. and Sánchez-Serrano, J.J., 1999. Antisense-mediated depletion of a potato lipoxygenase reduces wound induction of proteinase inhibitors and increases weight gain of insect pests. Proceedings of the National Academy of Sciences, 96(3), 1146–1151.

3 Transcriptional Regulation of Phyto-Oxylipins Signaling Pathway

Temidayo Oluyomi Elufisan[1], *Omotayo Opemipo Oyedara*[2], *and Oluwabusayo Odunola Oluyide*[3]
[1]Centro de Biotecnologia Genomica, Instituto Politecnico Nacional, Blvd de Maestro, S/N Col. Narciso Mendosa, Esq Elias Pina, C.P. 88710, Reynosa, Tamaulipas, Mexico
[2]Departamento de Microbiología e Inmunología, Facultad de Ciencias Biológicas, Universidad Autónoma de Nuevo León, San Nicolás de los Garza, Nuevo León, 66455, Mexico
[3]School of Basic medical sciences, Department of Biomedical Engineering College of Health Sciences and Technology, PMB 316 Epe road, Ijero Ekiti

CONTENTS

DOI: 10.1201/9781003316558-3

3.1 INTRODUCTION

The word phyto-oxylipin is commonly used to refer to the products obtained from the oxidation of plant-derived polyunsaturated fatty acids substrates (i.e., the production of oxygenated product of polyunsaturated fatty acid) [1]. The oxidation process for the generation of the oxygenated product of polyunsaturated fatty acid can be enzymatic or non-enzymatic. The non-enzymatic term means it occurred spontaneously. Oxylipin referred to the oxygenated polyunsaturated fatty acid derivatives derived from plant tissue. The most common polyunsaturated fatty acids in higher plants are the linoleic acid (C18:2 $\Delta^{9,12}$), and α -linolenic acid (C18:3 $\Delta^{9,12,15}$). In lower plants, like algae, bryophytes, and pteridophytes other polyunsaturated fatty acids such as linolenic acid (C18:3 $\Delta^{6,9,12}$), arachidonic acid (C20:4 $\Delta^{5,8,11,14}$), eicosapentaenoic acid (20:5 $\Delta^{5,8,11,14,17}$) and docosahexaenoic acid (C22:6 $\Delta^{4,7,10,13,16,19}$) are widely distributed [1–6].

3.2 NON-ENZYMATIC AND ENZYMATIC BIOSYNTHESIS OF OXYLIPIN

The synthesis of oxylipin can take place in two ways, it can either be a non-enzymatic process involving the auto-oxidation of polyunsaturated fatty acid or an enzymatic process involving the activities of different enzymes. The non-enzymatic synthesis of oxylipin is associated with the direct attack of polyunsaturated fatty acid by reactive oxygen molecules. These reactive oxygen molecules are formed when energy generated from the exposure of bio-sensitizer such as chlorophyll to light are transferred to oxygen in the ground state. The energy acquired by the oxygen molecule converts it from the ground state to the excited state making it highly reactive, which is about 1500 higher than the ground state [7]. In this state the oxygen molecule combines with a membrane bound lipid forming a hydroperoxide, which could be toxic for the membrane by disrupting the membrane fluidity while at the same time possess the tendency to alter the functioning of essential cellular components such as DNA, beta carotene, cholesterol, histidine, methionine, and cysteine. It usually achieved this by interacting with the essential amino acids in the cell [8]. To eliminate the toxicity associated with the direct interaction of reactive oxygen with polyunsaturated fatty acids, the cell has an oxidant-antioxidant balance system which often helps to eliminate or detoxify superoxide that are formed from the reaction between reactive oxygen and polyunsaturated fatty acids. In plants, the oxidant-antioxidant balance system usually involves the activities of two main enzymes, which are superoxide dismutase and ascorbate peroxidase. These enzymes ensure that the free radicals formed from the oxygenation of lipids are readily detoxified. For example, ascorbate peroxidase detoxifies the oxidized tocopherol by converting it back to vitamin E. It conducted this process through the addition of glutathione obtained from the oxidation of reduced glutathione.

The non-enzymatic synthesis of oxylipin is an auto-oxidation process which involved the addition of molecular oxygen in the excited state to a polyunsaturated fatty acid. In this process the molecular oxygen function as a biradical agent with two unpaired electrons in the ground state. The oxidation process is a progressive

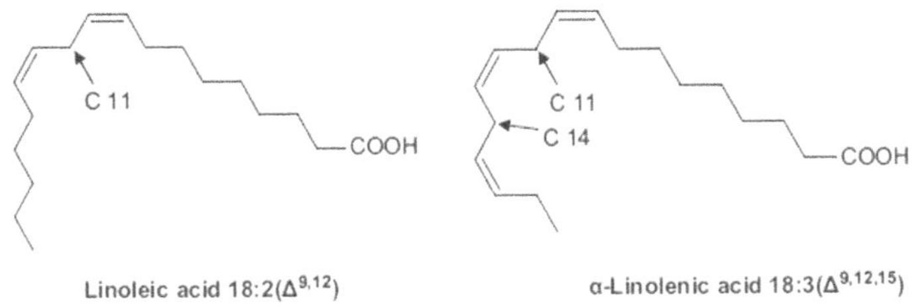

FIGURE 3.1 Structural formular for Linoleic acid ($C_{18:2}\Delta^{9,12}$) and alpha linolenic acid ($C_{18:3}\Delta^{9,12,15}$).

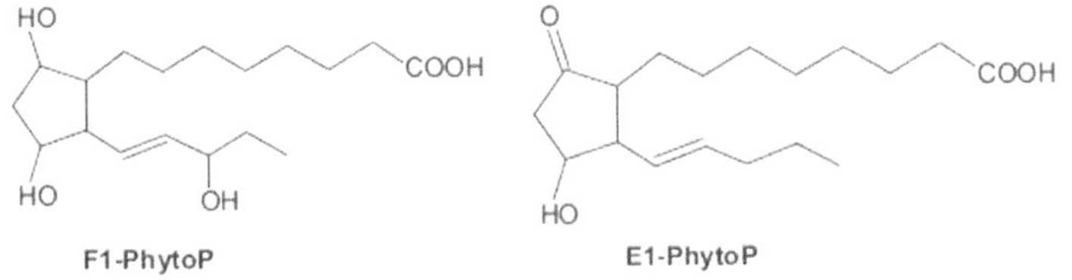

FIGURE 3.2 Structural image of F1- PhytoP and E1 PhytoP.

free-radical chain mechanism involving three steps which may overlap depending on the cell [8]. The oxidation rate depends on the level of saturation of the carbon-carbon chain in the fatty acid. The more unsaturated the carbon chain the faster the oxidation process. For example, the oxidation reaction with simple C18 chain length fatty acid esters 18:2 ($\Delta^{9,12}$) will proceed 40 times faster than with 18:1(Δ^{9}) and α -18:3 ($\Delta^{9,12,15}$) is 2.4 more reactive than 18:2 (Δ 9,12). The factor that determines the rate of auto-oxidation in plants is not limited to the level of unsaturation of the c-c chain, it includes other factors such as (1) the number and position of bis-allylic position present, (2) presence of an acyl group on the fatty acid, (3) presence of a metal ion, and (4) the number and position of methylene carbon. The substrate for the synthesis of oxylipin in plants via the non-enzymatic pathway is linoleic acid (LA, 18:2(n-6): where x:y(z) is a fatty acid containing x carbons and y double bonds in position z counting from the methyl end), α-linolenic acid (ALA, 18:3(n-3)) or roughanic acid (16:3(n-3)) (Figure 3.1) [9].

Once the radical oxygen attacked the linoleic acid in plants a racemic mixture of peroxy fatty acids is formed that are later esterified to complex lipids [10]. In some cases, this may result in the formation of a prostaglandin-like compound, if the fatty acid has at least three double bonds. The oxidation of α-linolenic acid often results in the formation of phytoprostanes commonly referred to as PhytoP. PhytoP are readily detected in vivo either as E PhytoP or F PhytoP (Figure 3.2). In addition to PhytoP, other non-enzymatic products may be formed as a result of the intramolecular radical chain rearrangement of the unstable bicyclic endoperoxide with prostaglandin G ring system [1]. This reduction and rearrangement is responsible for the formation of A 1 -, B 1 -, D 1 -, E 1 -, F 1, L 1 and J 1 -type PhytoP with degradation of the G 1 -type to Malondialdehyde [11–14].

The enzymatic synthesis of oxylipin is a process catalyzed by lipoxygenase (LOX) leading to the formation of hydroperoxide from polyunsaturated fatty acids such as linoleic acid [9]. The formation of hydroperoxides marks the first step in the formation of oxylipin, more enzyme catalyzed reactions can take place leading to the formation of more complex oxylipins such as jasmonic acid and other complex phyto-oxylipins like the plant hormone 12-oxo-phytodienoic acid (OPDA) [9].

The synthesis of oxylipin in plants is characterized by the activities of different enzymes, however, the activities of these enzymes depend on the presence of essential fatty acids. The availability of these fatty acids as substrate for the synthesis of oxylipin is commonly influenced by responses to both biotic and abiotic stress factors and the process of development [1, 16, 17]. The first step in the synthesis of oxylipin in plants is the conversion of a polyunsaturated fatty acids into a hydroperoxide by the addition of dioxygen in a regio or stereo specific way to a to a (1Z, 4Z)-pentadiene system of polyunsaturated fatty acids which is catalyzed by the LOX [1]. α-dioxygenase is the second enzyme known to be associated with the formation of oxylipin but detail information on the mechanisms used by this enzyme has not been fully unraveled, however recent studies have shown that α-dioxygenase is homologous to the cyclooxygenases in mammal (COX) [16]. Thus, the most studied enzyme for the formation of oxylipin is the lipooxygenase (LOX). LOX are classified based on their positional specificity for linoleic acid (LA) oxygenation. When the oxygenation occurs at the C-9 hydrocarbon backbone of the fatty acid with 18-carbon atom the LOX is referred to as lineolate 9-LOX, on the other hand, if the oxygenation occurred at the C-13 hydrocarbon backbone of the fatty acid, the LOX is referred to as lineolate 13-LOX.

In *Arabidopsis*, there are two genes encoding the lineolate 9-LOX and four genes encoding the lineolate 13-LOX. The differences in position specificity by the two enzymes often give rise to two types of compounds after oxygenation. These are (9S)-hydroperoxy and the (13S)-hydroperoxy derived oxylipins [9]. The 9-LOX is known to catalyze free fatty acid leading to the formation of a free fatty acid derivatives. A process which usually involves either an acyl-lipid hydrolase reaction or a thiolase leading to the formation of oxylipin. The C-13, however, catalyzes the oxygenation of both free and esterified fatty acids to generate oxylipin. A good example of an oxylipin formed by the activities of 13-LOX are the galactolipids harboring OPDA, commonly found in *Arabidopsis* [18]. Thus, a specific LOX enzyme or specific acyl-lipid hydrolases and thiolase, can initiate the synthesis of oxylipin. The only situation where acyl-lipid hydrolase have been reported for the synthesis of oxylipin is during the synthesis of DAD1 in the stamen filament of *Arabidopsis* [19]. No other study has given conclusive evidence on other acyl-lipid hydrolase catalyzed synthesis of oxylipin. Some of the reasons suggested for the inability to identify other acyl-lipid hydrolase oxylipin synthesis is that the release of free fatty acid is catalyzed by the enzymes that are available in the cell. Also, it is possible that the first metabolic process for the generation of oxylipin took place in the membrane lipid and these oxylipin are later released by the activities of membrane lipases [16]. Lipoxygenases (LOXs; EC 1.13.11.12) are non-heme iron containing oxidoreductases which also lacked sulfur in their constituent but have either iron or manganese as cofactors. They are primarily involved in catalyzing the oxidation of linoleic acid (LA, C18:2ω6), linolenic acid (ALA, C18:3ω3), and arachidonic acid (AA, C20:4ω6), converting it to hydroperoxy octadecadienoic acid (HPOD), hydroperoxy octadecatrienoic acid (HPOT), and hydroperoxy eicosatetraenoic acid (HPOET), respectively [9, 20]. LOXs enzymes are commonly found in mammals, plants, fishes, mosses, bacteria, yeast, fungi, corals, algae, and mushrooms, implying that they are essential in the biological system [21]. They occur in a multi-gene family which is subdivided into 9-LOX and 13-LOX groups [16].

LOXs are classified according to their regiospecificity, size, and linkage of the enzyme with other proteins. Using the regiospecificity, the LOX can be divided to 5-, 8-, 9-, 10-, 12-, 13-, 15-LOXs called classical LOXs. 9- and 13-LOXs in plants, and 5-, 12-, and 15-LOXs in animals constitute major part of the LOX [22]. The LOX pathway in plants differ significantly from what is obtainable in animals because the LOX catalyzing the synthesis of hydroperoxide in plants belong to the LOX subfamilies 9-LOXs and 13-LOXs. Some dual specific LOX which can catalyze the conversion of whatever regiospecific fatty acid is available as substrate, have been reported in plants [23]. In animals, cyclooxygenases (COX) and other families of LOX are known to catalyze the synthesis of oxylipin. Similarly, lipooxygenase are classified as extra plastidial (type 1) and plastidial (type 2); this classification is based on the location where the enzymes exhibit their activities in the plant cell.

The activities of LOX in plants depends on some essential factors which include (1) plant tissue (whether it is stamen or leaves), (2) the intracellular compartment (plastid or cytosol), and (3) LOX substrate's specificity. The two LOX that are associated with the synthesis of oxylipin exhibit different substrate specificity and this often determine how they influence the synthesis of oxylipin.

3.3 9-LOX PATHWAY

9-LOX is a single chain polypeptide with about 741–886 amino acid. In LOX pathway, polyunsaturated fatty acid is converted to compounds such as 9-HPOD, 9-HPOT, and 9-KOT (9S-keto octadecatrienoic acid).

3.3.1 13-LOX Pathway

Like the 9-LOX, 13-LOX is a single non-heme containing polypeptide with an amino acid of approximately 896–941 sequences. 13-LOX are known to primarily catalyzed the conversion of polyunsaturated fatty acids (PUFAs) to 13 HPOT. HPOT is later metabolized to form compounds such as jasmonic acid a signaling compound in plants [21]. 13-LOX are the most commonly found LOX in plants and the product formed from the catalytic activities of 13-LOX are utilized by other enzymes for the complete synthesis of other metabolites [24]. Enzymes that have been identified to use the products of 13-LOX include members of the CYP74 family such as AOS, HPL, DES, and allene oxide cyclase (AOC). These enzymes are closely related to one another [16]. In the 13-LOX pathway in plants, 13-LOX catalyzes the conversion of α linoleic acid to 13 HPO derivatives. These derivatives are in turn converted to other forms of HPL which later undergo analogous reaction in the 13-LOX pathway to produce new oxylipins as shown above. In general, the LOX is made up of two distinct domains which are the N terminus that is about 25–30 kDa in size and the C terminal that is about 55–65KDa in size. There are 160 amino acids in the N-terminal of LOX. The amino acids were formed by two barrels and two anti-parallel plates. The C terminal on the other hand contains 693 amino acid residues, 23 helix, two anti-parallels and an active iron (Fe^{3+}) site. LOX has an active site containing a highly active Fe^{3+} and an inactive site containing Fe^{2+} [25–27].

The way in which LOX catalyzes the conversion of PUFs to hydroperoxide depends on the substrate (i.e., it is substrate's structure specific). Such that the LOX oxygenation of PUF usually give rise to several types of oxylipin or oxylipin intermediate. For example, LOX-1 type is active with a water-soluble substrate, e.g., linoleoyl sulfate, oxidation of linoleic acid gives rise to hydroperoxide like 6 or 13-lipohydroperoxide, while the oxidation reaction of linolenic acid results in 13-hydroperoxide. While LOX-2 acts on esterification substrates to give 9 or 13-hydroperoxide. LOX-2 and LOX-3 are more active toward triglycerides and methyl esters of fatty acids when compared with free fatty acids [28]. The interaction of the LOX with PUFA has been hypothesized to be determined by the orientation of the substrate such that it is possible for LOX to be inserted with the active site to a PUFAs methyl end head leading to linoleate 13-lipoxygenation. In some situations, however, there could be a head-to-tail inversion before the PUFA penetrate the active site of LOX leading to linoleate 9-lipoxygenation [9].

Once hydroperoxide are synthesized by the activities of LOX, they are available as substrate for either allele hydroperoxide lyase (HPL) and allene oxide synthase (AOS) pathways.

3.3.2 Allene Oxide Synthase

Cytochrome P450 enzymes of the CYP741 family play an essential role in the metabolism of oxylipin [29]. Allene oxide synthase (AOS) belongs to this category of enzyme. They do not need molecular oxygen nor NAD(P)H-dependent cytochrome P450 reductases as a cofactor to catalyze the metabolism of oxylipin, but rather they often rearrange their hydroperoxy fatty acid molecules [16]. AOS catalysis of hydroperoxide may sometimes result in the formation of unstable EOT [(13S)-12,13-epoxy-octadecanoic acid] and EHT [(11S)-10,11-epoxy-hexadecatrienoic acid] intermediate. AOS is the most studied member of the CYP741 family enzyme in plants because of its role in the biosynthesis of jasmonic acid. Arabidopsis, the model plant for studying the oxylipin pathway, possesses a single gene for a 13-AOS that has residual hydroperoxide lyase (HPL) activities. Another type of Arabidopsis (Columbia) has a mutation in the HPL gene. However, some plants possess more than one gene encoding AOS. Enzymes of the CYP74 family only share slightly different similarities. It is quite easy for one to be converted to another. For instance, a single-amino-acid exchange led to the conversion of an AOS to a HPL (111, 131) and the conversion of a DES to an AOS. The enzymes of the CYP74 family can be divided into three subfamilies based on the substrate they used. Those that use 9-hydroperoxide derivatives as substrates, those that use13-hydroperoxide derivatives as substrates, and enzymes that use both substrates. CYP74 have been reported in some non-vascular plants and brown algae [16].

3.3.3 Allene Oxide Cyclase

In plants where allene oxide cyclase (AOC) are present, unstable epoxides formed by the activities of AOS are converted to enantiomers of jasmonic acid (the cis-(+)-isomer of OPDA). AOC is highly important for the biosynthesis of jasmonic acid, and it works closely with the product of AOS catalysis [16]. Molecular analysis of AOC crystallized from Arabidopsis showed that it is similar to the enzymes of the lipocalin family. This implies that it may be using the ring opening mechanism followed by conformational changes to elicit its catalytic activities [30]. However, crystallization of other AOC (AOC1 and AOC2) from other plants such as *P. patens* point to the depth of substrate binding cavity as the determining factor for chain length specificity of AOC [31].

3.3.4 12-Oxo-Phytodienoic Acid Reductase3

12-oxo-phytodienoic acid reductase3 is an enzyme which catalyzes the conversion of 12-oxo-phytodienoic acid, an α-linolenic acid-derived intermediate of jasmonic acid biosynthesis, to 3-oxo-2(2′[Z]-pentenyl)-cyclopentane-1-octanoic acid (OPC8). 12-oxo-phytodienoic acid also possesses its own signaling properties and a cyclopentenone ring as its core structure [16]. 12-oxo-phytodienoic acid reductase3 is a flavin dependent oxidoreductase enzyme. Modulating the proportion of OPD reductase has been described to regulate the biosynthesis of jasmonic acid.

In summary, the synthesis of oxylipin involves the activities of several enzymes which include acyl hydrolases which can initiate the formation of hydroperoxide, or the LOX enzymes which are involved in the addition of reactive oxygen to initiate the formation of hydroperoxide. Other enzymes include allene oxide synthase, which converts hydroperoxide to unstable EOT [(13S)-12,13-epoxy-octadecanoic acid] and EHT [(11S)-10,11-epoxy-hexadecatrienoic acid] intermediates, which are later transformed into OPDA by allene oxide cyclase. This intermediate can on its own act as a signaling molecule in plants or can be converted to 3-oxo-2(2′[Z]-pentenyl)-cyclopentane-1-octanoic acid by 12-oxo-phytodienoic acid reductase3. The process in the biosynthesis of oxylipin involving LOX, AOS and AOC usually takes place in the plastid while the second process involving the reduction of OPDA often occurs in the peroxisomes.

3.4 BETA OXIDATION OF THE CARBOXYL SIDE CHAIN

Once jasmonic acid is synthesized, the carboxyl side chain is reduced by a fatty acid beta oxidation machinery in a process known as beta oxidation [32]. This process completes the formation of jasmonic acid. The importance of beta oxidation in the formation of complex jasmonic acid was demonstrated by the reduction in jasmonic acid production in a mutant deficient in complex import protein. Beta oxidation ensures the reduction of the carbon chain in 3-oxo-2(2′[Z]-pentenyl)-cyclopentane-1-octanoic acid (OPC8) to generate jasmonic acid and other jasmonate. The process involves three main enzymes, which synthesizes the jasmonic-COA and a final enzyme that separates the jasmonic acid from jasmonic-COA. The process usually occurs in the peroxisome. These enzymes are acyl-COA oxidase (ACX), the multifunctional protein (containing 2-trans-enoyl-CoA hydratase and l-3-hydroxyacyl-CoA dehydrogenase activities), and 3-ketoacyl-CoA thiolase (KAT). An additional thioesterase activity is also presumably involved in the release of JA from JA-CoA, the product of the final round of β-oxidation [33–35].

3.5 INTRACELLULAR LOCALIZATION

The enzymes (LOX, AOS and AOC) that are involved in the first pathway for the synthesis of oxylipin are located in plastids while those involved in the second pathway for the synthesis of JA are located in the peroxisome. It is therefore pertinent that the JA intermediate be transported from the chloroplast to the peroxisome. The mechanisms involved in the transportation of this oxylipin intermediate have not been fully understood but certain proteins have been identified that may be involved in the transportation process. An ion trapping mechanism that involves the peroxisomal ATP-binding cassette (ABC) transporter PXA1 [also known as COMATOSE (CTS)] has been described to be involved in the transportation of OPDA from the chloroplast to the peroxisome [36]. OPDA may be transported by the fatty acid transporter fax1 from the plastid to the peroxisome [37, 38]. In Arabidopsis, the transportation of oxylipin intermediates is likely to be affected by the activities of the AtACBP6, a member of the acyl-CoA-binding protein family. (+)-7-iso-JA is first transported by an unknown mechanism into the cytosol, where it is conjugated with amino acids, preferentially isoleucine, to form the (+)-7-iso-JA-Ile complex. This process is catalyzed by the jasmonoyl amino acid conjugate synthase (JAR1) [16]. JA-Ile is then transported into the nucleus by ABC transporter JAT1 as indicated in Figure 3.3 below [39]. JAT1 plays a double role: it also exports JA through the plasma membrane. Intercellular transport of JA or JA-Ile may also take place through the activities of the multifunctional glucosinolate transporter GTR1, which also transports gibberellin [40, 41].

3.6 PHYTO-OXYLIPIN AS SIGNALING MOLECULES

Several oxylipins from plants have been identified as signals, each of them helping plants to respond to both biotic and abiotic stresses. Oxylipin signals have been grouped according to the enzyme playing the signaling roles. They include four genes that were associated with 13-LOX signaling, which are present in Arabidopsis. These genes are known to help in the formation of jasmonates in response to abiotic stress such as wound [42]. LOX2 is the form that always provides substrate for general response. LOX3 is expressed in the circumfasicular parenchyma while LOX4 is expressed in phloem related cells. LOX6 helps in early and xylem specific

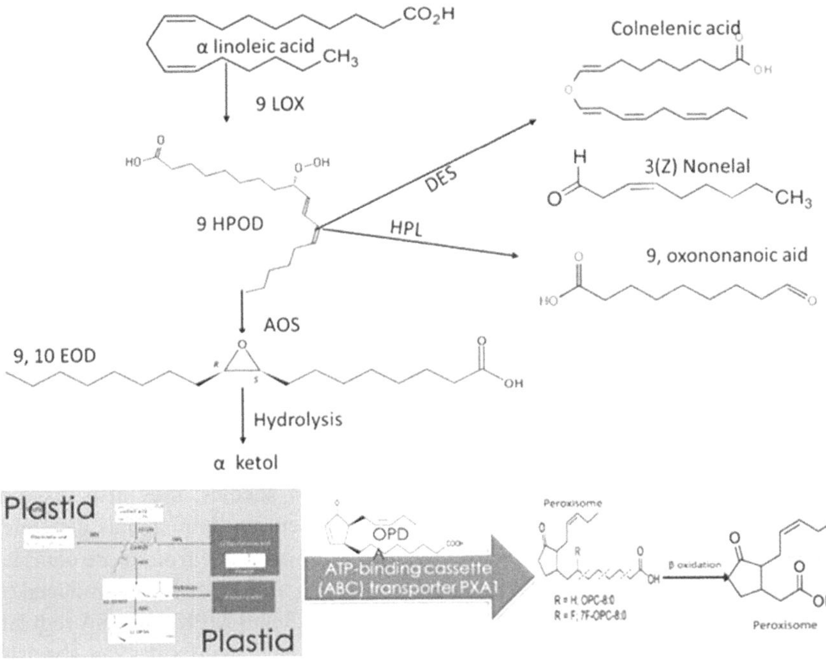

FIGURE 3.3 Synthesis of oxylipins and their intracellular transport. Adapted from Wasternack and Feussner (2018).

responses. LOX2 also takes part in jasmonates pathway at senescence while LOX3 and LOX4 also provide substrate for the jasmonates pathway during stamen and filament production [16]. Within the LOX pathway, intense competition for substrate always occurs between the HPL and AOS branches [43]. The AOS branch mediates direct plant defense responses by forming JA, whereas hexenyl acetate, the dominant HPL product upon wounding in Arabidopsis, mediates indirect defense responses by attracting the natural enemies of plant invaders to their prey through genetic modification of each branch separately [44]. Infested tomato plants also employ (3Z)-hexenol alcohol as a volatile signal to elicit defense responses in unharmed nearby plants [45]. It is possible that HPL-derived volatiles of green leaf can stimulate herbivore eating. *Nicotiana attenuata*'s substrate flow was increased when either AOS or HPL was silenced [46]. Insect-chewing insects suppressed the HPL branch while increasing JA production, according to these studies. In Arabidopsis, a comparable suppression is observed [44]. Using mutant analysis, researchers discovered fascinating interactions between the AOS and HPL branches of rice's genome. Consistent AOS expression in a library led to the discovery of a mutant cea62 that was defective in OsHPL3 but was found to be dramatically overproduced in JA production [45]. It has recently been discovered that the HPL branch retains its ability to block photoinhibition in the presence of strong light. Arabidopsides are also regulated by HPL and compete for hydroperoxyl-fatty-acid-bound lipids with AOS [49].

A number of signals throughout the last decade revealed that OPDA-specific responses were distinct from JA's. There is no evidence to support the hypothesis that the Skp/Cullin/F-box complex (SCF_{COI1})-JAZ coreceptor complex is capable of sensing the OPDA. Despite this, the amount of data supporting OPDA-specific operations has steadily grown [50]. Transcriptomic data [51]; proteomic data and data on seed germination [52]; glutathione conjugation [53]; stomatal closure and improved drought tolerance [54]; the interaction of OPDA with cyclophilin CYP20–3 and its link with sulfur metabolism [55]; and increased defense responses are examples. For *Epipremnum aureum* variegated leaf tissues, OPDA and glutathione levels were nine times higher in the white tissues, ROS were reduced, JA and JA-Ile levels were undetectable, and specific OPDA scavenging gene activity was upregulated compared to the green tissues [56]. Newly discovered cyclopentanones and cyclopentenones generated from 9-LOX were found in infected maize leaves (*Cochliobolus heterostrophus*) with southern leaf blight [57]. Infection necrosis has been dubbed "death acids" because of their ability to kill diseased tissue. Because they inhibit the growth of *Aspergillus* and *Fusarium* species; they also serve as phytoalexins. There are significant differences between oxylipin signals generated by 13-LOX and those generated by 9-LOX. The latter originate from more complex pathways such as the hydroxides produced by 9-LOX, as well as those produced by more simple routes such as CYP74 metabolites. MPK3 and MPK6 and SA regulate stomatal closure in Arabidopsis through LOX1 fatty acid hydroxides, an abscisic-acid-independent mechanism [58]. For the same reason, Arabidopsis appears to use these hydroxides to regulate certain of its defense responses against *P. syringae* and then produce singlet oxygen [59]. The cell-wall-based defense against pathogens is coordinated again, but this time with the help of brassinosteroids [60]. As a result of Phytophthora infection in tobacco, the divinyl ethers may play a direct function as phytoalexins [61]. An even more complicated role in cross-kingdom communication between *Aspergillus* and *Fusarium* species and corn seems to be played by fatty acid hydroxides [52]. Those from the fungus can promote the creation of 9-LOX-derived hydroxides in corn tissue, but both sides here can produce various signatures of fatty acid hydroxides. Infected plant tissue dies as a result of the oxylipins' stimulation of mycotoxins production on the fungus' side [62].

3.6.1 Oxylipins Derived from Ethanolamine

There are bioactive signaling chemicals known as N-Acylethanolamines, which were found in plants more than 60 years ago. Compounds like this one contain an ester of fatty acids and an ethanolamine residue. Arabidopsis has recently been revealed to have the same alteration for LOX-derived hydroxy fatty acids. -linolenic acid hydroxy compounds generated from 9-LOX and 13-LOX were found to inhibit seedling growth [63]. Seedlings' root development was also inhibited by 9-LOX-derived hydroxy derivatives of linoleate that interacted with abscisic acid signals [64]. Oxylipins can be synthesized from unsaturated fatty acids through chemical processes catalyzed by free radicals in addition to enzymes [65]. Oxylipins, like their enzyme-derived cousins, have a signaling function and can activate certain sets of genes. A wide-ranging detoxifying response can be controlled [53].

3.7 TRANSCRIPTIONAL REGULATION OF OXYLIPIN SIGNALING PATHWAY

Jasminate or jasmonic acid is the most studied oxylipin signal in plants. The detailed studies on this oxylipin have been used to elucidate the pathway involved in the oxylipin signal system in plants. The jasmonates signaling pathway consists of an array of functional systems which regulate the transcription of the JA responsive genes. This includes the Coronatine Insensitive 1 (COI1), which perceived the bio-active jasmonoyl-L-isoleucine enhancing its degradation of the JAZ repressor [66, 67]. The JA-Ile complex is responsible for plant's resistance to a wide range of plant consumers like pathogenic bacteria and fungi as well as insect and mammalian plant feeders [68, 69]. The discovery of the JAZ protein influenced the understanding of how the biosynthesis of JA-Ile is associated with the transcriptional activation of the jasmonates' responses. The JA-Ile, a major hormone in vascular tissue that often generates specific and yet functionally diverse response to environmental signals [66]. The importance of this hormone makes it the basis for understanding the transcriptional regulation of the oxylipin signaling pathway.

3.8 THE CORE JASMONATES SIGNALING PATHWAY

The core jasmonates signaling pathway is made of interwoven functional modules that control the transcriptional response of genes to hormones [66, 67]. The most studied jasmonates-Ile dependent transcriptional factor is the basic helix loop (BHLH) protein MYC2 and its contemporaries, such as the MYC3 and MYC4 in Arabidopsis. These BHLH will bind to the G box motifs to regulate the expression of a large portion of jasmonate-responsive genes [68, 70–72]. The first step in the jasmonates signaling pathway is the repression of the MYC transcriptional factors. The repression is achieved by the activities of some groups of JAZ protein. These proteins are members of the protein with a well conserved TIF(F/Y) motifs that are commonly found within the ZIM (zinc finger protein expressed in the inflorescence meristem) domain [66]. These groups of JAZ proteins differ from other TIF domain protein because they have approximately 27 amino acids multifunctional jas motifs that are located near the C-terminus. There are interspecies variations in the number of JAZ genes that are present in different plants. These variations are responsible for the functional diversity and redundancy in evolving gene families. In Arabidopsis, for example there are 13 JAZ genes. These genes are known as the JAZ1—JAZ13. The JAZ gene in Arabidopsis are grouped into five phyllo groups which have been identified as group I–V [73]. All five groups are present in angiosperm but only JAS1 is commonly expressed in monocots [74]. JAZ protein always elicits the repression of the MYC transcription factor through a negative feedback mechanism. Once the concentration of the JA-Ile conjugation has reached a level below the threshold, the jas motif will form an extended α helix which will bind to the JAZ-interacting domain near the N terminus of the MYC transcriptional factor. The binding of the jas motif to the JAZ-interacting domain (JID) prevents the MYC from binding to the activator-interacting domain (ACID) of the MED 25 in the mediator complex. MED 25 of the mediator complex is a conserved evolutionary protein complex that always binds the DNA-RNA transcriptional factor to the RNA polymerase. In doing this, MED 25 always ensures the integration of transcription with cellular signals. Once JAZ-ZIM has bound the MYC, lower cellular signals are detected resulting in the accumulation of jasmonates which will be required for the destruction of the JAZ-MYC complex. In some plants the jas motif are absent, in such plants, jasmonates responsive genes are repressed through the help of a cryptic interaction domain present in them [75]. Another mechanism through which JAZ proteins also attenuate the MYC transcriptional factor is through the help of the TOPLESS (TPL) scaffolding protein. This protein inhibits gene expression by interacting with a histone modifying enzyme like histone decarboxylase (HAD) and the mediator complex [76, 77]. The TPL and TPL-related protein mediates the repression of the MYC transcriptional factor by directly interacting with ethylene-response amphiphilic repression motif (EAR) of the transcriptional repressors [78]. The TIFY(ZIM) domain of the JAZ protein usually indirectly use the TPL or TPR protein through the EAR motif containing novel interactor of JAZ (NINJA) adaptor protein [77]. These mechanisms of repression are not limited to the jasmonate system. It has been reported in many transcriptional complexes [66].

3.8.1 Transcriptional Activation of the Jasmonates Signaling System

The next step in the transcription of the jasmonates signaling pathway which enhances signal transduction is the transcriptional activation of jasmonate signaling system. In this step there is a proteolytic destruction of the jasmonates pathway repressor leading to the conversion of the JAZ bound MYC to a transcriptional activator [66]. This process usually begins with the formation of a hormone-based coreceptor complex involving JA-Ile, JAZ, and the F-box protein CORONATINE INSENSITIVE1 (COI1). The coronate insensitive 1 is a part of the SKP1–CUL1–F-box protein (SCF) E3 ubiquitin ligase complex (SCF^{COI1}) that often specifically relates with the JAZ substrate protein when JA-Ile complex is present. The structure of the COI1-JAZ coreceptor complex makes it possible for it to bind to the JAZ-Ile ligand pocket [79–81]. The jas motif of the COI1 is a bipartite and with a conserved degron (ELPIARR in JAZ1) at the N terminus forms a loop at the terminal that binds the JA-Ile in the ligand pocket resulting in the formation of a stable COI1-JA-Ile ternary complex. The C terminus of the jas motif ensures the appropriate of the JAZ peptide to the surface of the COI1. This JAZ protein attached to SCF will then be degraded by 26S proteosome in a hormone dependent reaction [66].

The concept of the degradation of the JAZ protein attached to SCF by 26S proteosome was justified by the ability of a JAZ protein with mutated degron to remain stable in the presence of JA-Ile and to repress MYC's activity [42].

COI1 on its own usually undergoes multiple levels of regulation in the presence of inositol polyphosphate cofactor [82–84] and regulated proteolysis [85]. The JA-Ile induced SCFCOI1-proteasome system destruction of the JAZ provides ways to dissociate the corepressor modules like NINJA-TPL from the promoters of MYC target genes, leading to the recruitment of the transcriptional coactivators. The biochemical and structural analysis of the JAZ degradation showed that JAZ degradation allowed the JID and TAD to permit the binding of MED 25 and the activities of the RNA polymerase II through the mediator complex leading to the activation of the transcriptional state [66]. The idea of a hormone-based transcriptional activation has been proven to be correct by several structural, biochemical, and genetic studies. An important aspect of this model is the structural changes being undergone by the jas motif such that it could make direct contact with the COI1 JA-Ile and MYC. Structural changes have been reported in the jas moif when the MYC-JAZ is in the resting state compared to when there is transcriptional activation of COI1_JAZ complex [84]. These structural changes act as a switch to activate the MYC activity. As a result of this, there is usually a rapid response to the structure changes leading to the quick expression of the main target in less than 15 minutes, in response to the increased JA-Ile levels [85, 86, 87].

3.9 CONCLUSION

Phyto-oxylipins always act as signaling molecules in the plant to help it to resist many harsh conditions including the activities of humans, insects, or other animals. The signaling activity of phyto-oxylipins depends on their expression. There are several mechanisms that are involved in transcription and expression of phyto-oxylipin signaling. The signaling system of oxylipins is controlled by an array of functional systems that regulate the transcription of JA responsive genes. The most studied oxylipin signaling system is that of jasmonic acid, and the signaling system consists of a CORONATINE INSENSITIVE 1 (COI1) which often interacts with jasmonyl isoleucin to achieve the degradation of JAZ repressor hence resulting in the expression of jasmonic acid. The signaling pathway contains several functional modules that are interacting with one another to ensure the expression and regulation of jasmonic acid. The modules include transcriptional factors of the basic helix protein such as the MYC4, NYC2 and MYC3. Others include the TIF(F/Y) motif commonly found in the ZIM domain and the MED 25 which often interact to ensure the expression of jasmonic acid. Another important protein is the TOPLESS scaffolding protein. This protein ensures the expression of COI 1 which in turn regulates the expression of jasmonic acid.

REFERENCES

1. Griffiths G (2015) Biosynthesis and analysis of plant oxylipins. Free Radic. Res. 49:565–582.
2. Lang I, Hodac L, Friedl T, Feussner I (2011) Fatty acid profiles and their distribution patterns in microalgae: A comprehensive analysis of more than 2000 strains from the SAG culture collection. BMC Plant Biol 11. https://doi.org/10.1186/1471-2229-11-124
3. Wolff RL, Christie WW, Pédrono F, Marpeau AM (1999) Arachidonic, eicosapentaenoic, and biosynthetically related fatty acids in the seed lipids from a primitive gymnosperm, Agathis robusta. Lipids 34:1083–1097. https://doi.org/10.1007/s11745-999-0460-y
4. You J, Zhao X, Suo Y, et al. (2007) Determination of long-chain fatty acids in bryophyte plants extracts by HPLC with fluorescence detection and identification with MS.

J Chromatogr B Anal Technol Biomed Life Sci 848:283–291. https://doi.org/10.1016/j.jchromb.2006.10.025
5. Croisier E, Rempt M, Pohnert G (2010) Survey of volatile oxylipins and their biosynthetic precursors in bryophytes. Phytochemistry 71:574–580. https://doi.org/10.1016/j.phytochem.2009.12.004
6. Bai XW, Song CH, You JM, et al. (2010) Determination of fatty acids (C1-C10) from bryophytes and pteridophytes. Chromatographia 71:1125–1129. https://doi.org/10.1365/s10337-010-1552-7
7. Girotti AW (1998) Lipid hydroperoxide generation, turnover, and effector action in biological systems. J. Lipid Res. 39:1529–1542.
8. Diplock AT (1985) Free radicals in biology and medicine. Biochem Soc Trans 13:976–976. https://doi.org/10.1042/bst0130976
9. Andreou A, Brodhun F, Feussner I (2009) Biosynthesis of oxylipins in non-mammals. Prog Lipid Res 48:148–170. https://doi.org/10.1016/j.plipres.2009.02.002
10. Leverentz MK, Wagstaff C, Rogers HJ, et al. (2002) Leverentz, M. K., Wagstaff, C., Rogers, H. J., Stead, A. D., Chanasut, U., Silkowski, H., Thomas, B., Weichert, H., Feussner, I., & Griffiths, G. (2002). Characterization of a novel lipoxygenase-independent senescence mechanism in Alstroemeria peruviana. Plant Physiol 130:273–283. https://doi.org/10.1104/pp.000919
11. Imbusch R, Mueller MJ (2000) Analysis of oxidative stress and wound-inducible dinor isoprostanes F1 (Phytoprostanes F1) in plants. Plant Physiol 124:1293–1303. https://doi.org/10.1104/pp.124.3.1293
12. Imbusch R, Mueller MJ (2000) Formation of isoprostane F2-like compounds (phytoprostanes F1) from α-linolenic acid in plants. Free Radic Biol Med 28:720–726. https://doi.org/10.1016/S0891-5849(00)00154-4
13. Krischke M, Loeffler C, Mueller MJ (2003) Biosynthesis of 13,14-dehydro-12-oxo-phytodienoic acid and related cyclopentenones via the phytoprostane D1 pathway. Phytochemistry 62:351–358. https://doi.org/10.1016/S0031-9422(02)00566-6
14. Jahn U, Galano JM, Durand T (2010) A cautionary note on the correct structure assignment of phytoprostanes and the emergence of a new prostane ring system. Prostaglandins Leukot Essent Fat Acids 82:83–86. https://doi.org/10.1016/j.plefa.2009.10.005
15. Schmidt A, Boland W (2007) General strategy for the synthesis of B1 phytoprostanes, dinor isoprostanes, and analogs. J Org Chem 72:1699–1706. https://doi.org/10.1021/jo062359x
16. Wasternack C, Feussner I (2018) The oxylipin pathways: Biochemistry and function. Annu Rev Plant Biol 69:363–386. https://doi.org/10.1146/annurev-arplant-042817-040440
17. Wasternack C (2007) Jasmonates: An update on biosynthesis, signal transduction and action in plant stress response, growth and development. Ann Bot 100:681–697. https://doi.org/10.1093/aob/mcm079
18. Wasternack C, Hause B (2013) Jasmonates: Biosynthesis, perception, signal transduction and action in plant stress response, growth and development. An update to the 2007 review in Annals of Botany. Ann Bot 111:1021–1058. https://doi.org/10.1093/aob/mct067
19. Ishiguro S, Kawai-Oda A, Ueda J, et al. (2001) The defective in anther dehiscence1 gene encodes a novel phospholipase A1 catalyzing the initial step of jasmonic acid biosynthesis, which synchronizes pollen maturation, anther dehiscence, and flower opening in Arabidopsis. Plant Cell 13:2191–2209. https://doi.org/10.1105/tpc.010192

20. Brash AR (1999) Lipoxygenases: Occurrence, functions, catalysis, and acquisition of substrate. J. Biol. Chem. 274:23679–23682.
21. Joo YC, Oh DK (2012) Lipoxygenases: Potential starting biocatalysts for the synthesis of signaling compounds. Biotechnol Adv 30:1524–1532. https://doi.org/10.1016/j.biotechadv.2012.04.004
22. Viswanath KK, Varakumar P, Pamuru RR, et al. (2020) Plant lipoxygenases and their role in plant physiology. J Plant Biol 63:83–95. https://doi.org/10.1007/s12374-020-09241-x
23. Hughes RK, West SI, Hornostaj AR, et al. (2001) Probing a novel potato lipoxygenase with dual positional specificity reveals primary determinants of substrate binding and requirements for a surface hydrophobic loop and has implications for the role of lipoxygenases in tubers. Biochem J 353:345–355. https://doi.org/10.1042/bj3530345
24. Brash AR (2009) Mechanistic aspects of CYP74 allene oxide synthases and related cytochrome P450 enzymes. Phytochemistry 70:1522–1531.
25. Aanangi R, Kotapati KV, Palaka BK, et al. (2016) Purification and characterization of lipoxygenase from mung bean (Vigna radiata L.) germinating seedlings. 3 Biotech 6. https://doi.org/10.1007/s13205-016-0427-5
26. Shi Y, Mandal R, Singh A, Pratap Singh A (2020) Legume lipoxygenase: Strategies for application in food industry. Legum. Sci. 2.
27. Mitsuda H, Yasumoto K, Yamamoto A, Kusano T (1967) Study on soybean lipoxygenase: Part I. Preparation of crystalline enzyme and assay by polarographic method. Agric Biol Chem 31:115–118. https://doi.org/10.1271/bbb1961.31.115
28. Singh P, Arif Y, Miszczuk E, et al. (2022) Specific roles of lipoxygenases in development and responses to stress in plants. Plants 11:979. https://doi.org/10.3390/plants11070979
29. Schaller A, Stintzi A (2009) Enzymes in jasmonate biosynthesis — Structure, function, regulation. Phytochemistry 70:1532–1538. https://doi.org/10.1016/j.phytochem.2009.07.032
30. Hofmann E, Zerbe P, Schaller F (2006) The crystal structure of Arabidopsis thaliana allene oxide cyclase: Insights into the oxylipin cyclization reaction. Plant Cell 18:3201–3217. https://doi.org/10.1105/tpc.106.043984
31. Neumann P, Brodhun F, Sauer K, et al. (2012) Crystal structures of physcomitrella patens AOC1 and AOC2: Insights into the enzyme mechanism and differences in substrate specificity. Plant Physiol 160:1251–1266. https://doi.org/10.1104/pp.112.205138
32. Hu J, Baker A, Bartel B, et al. (2012) Plant peroxisomes: Biogenesis and function. Plant Cell 24:2279–2303. https://doi.org/10.1105/TPC.112.096586
33. Shockey JM, Fulda MS, Browse JA (2002) Arabidopsis contains nine long-chain acyl-coenzyme A synthetase genes that participate in fatty acid and glycerolipid metabolism. Plant Physiol 129:1710–1722. https://doi.org/10.1104/pp.003269
34. Reumann S, Ma C, Lemke S, Babujee L (2004) AraPerox. A database of putative arabidopsis proteins from plant peroxisomes. Plant Physiol 136:2587–2608. https://doi.org/10.1104/pp.104.043695
35. Tilton GB, Shockey JM, Browse J (2004) Biochemical and Molecular Characterization of ACH2, an Acyl-CoA Thioesterase from Arabidopsis thaliana. J Biol Chem 279:7487–7494. https://doi.org/10.1074/jbc.M309532200.
36. Theodoulou FL, Job K, Slocombe SP, et al. (2005) Jasmonic acid levels are reduced in COMATOSE ATP-binding cassette transporter mutants. implications for transport of jasmonate precursors into peroxisomes. Plant Physiol 137:835–840. https://doi.org/10.1104/PP.105.059352

37. Li N, Gügel IL, Giavalisco P, et al. (2015) FAX1, a Novel membrane protein mediating plastid fatty acid export. PLoS Biol 13:e1002053. https://doi.org/10.1371/journal.pbio.1002053
38. Nguyen CT, Martinoia E, Farmer EE (2017) Emerging jasmonate transporters. Mol Plant 10:659–661. https://doi.org/10.1016/j.molp.2017.03.007
39. Li Q, Zheng J, Li S, et al. (2017) Transporter-mediated nuclear entry of jasmonoyl-isoleucine is essential for jasmonate signaling. Mol Plant 10:695–708. https://doi.org/10.1016/j.molp.2017.01.010
40. Ishimaru Y, Oikawa T, Suzuki T, et al. (2017) GTR1 is a jasmonic acid and jasmonoyl-L-isoleucine transporter in Arabidopsis thaliana. Biosci Biotechnol Biochem 81:249–255. https://doi.org/10.1080/09168451.2016.1246174
41. Saito H, Oikawa T, Hamamoto S, et al. (2015) The jasmonate-responsive GTR1 transporter is required for gibberellin-mediated stamen development in Arabidopsis. Nat Commun 6:1–11. https://doi.org/10.1038/ncomms7095
42. Wasternack C, Song S (2017) Jasmonates: Biosynthesis, metabolism, and signaling by proteins activating and repressing transcription. J Exp Bot 68:1303–1321. https://doi.org/10.1093/jxb/erw443
43. Matsui K (2006) Green leaf volatiles: hydroperoxide lyase pathway of oxylipin metabolism. Curr Opin Plant Biol 9:274–280. https://doi.org/10.1016/j.pbi.2006.03.002
44. Chehab EW, Kaspi R, Savchenko T, et al. (2008) Distinct roles of jasmonates and aldehydes in plant-defense responses. PLoS One 3:e1904. https://doi.org/10.1371/journal.pone.0001904
45. Sugimoto K, Matsui K, Iijima Y, et al. (2014) Intake and transformation to a glycoside of (Z)-3-hexenol from infested neighbors reveals a mode of plant odor reception and defense. Proc Natl Acad Sci U S A 111:7144–7149. https://doi.org/10.1073/pnas.1320660111
46. Halitschke R, Ziegler J, Keinänen M, Baldwin IT (2004) Silencing of hydroperoxide lyase and allene oxide synthase reveals substrate and defense signaling crosstalk in Nicotiana attenuata. Plant J 40:35–46. https://doi.org/10.1111/j.1365-313X.2004.02185.x
47. Savchenko T, Pearse IS, Ignatia L, et al. (2013) Insect herbivores selectively suppress the HPL branch of the oxylipin pathway in host plants. Plant J 73:653–662. https://doi.org/10.1111/tpj.12064
48. Liu X, Li F, Tang J, et al. (2012) Activation of the jasmonic acid pathway by depletion of the hydroperoxide lyase OsHPL3 reveals crosstalk between the HPL and AOS branches of the oxylipin pathway in rice. PLoS One 7:e50089. https://doi.org/10.1371/JOURNAL.PONE.0050089
49. Nilsson AK, Fahlberg P, Johansson ON, et al. (2016) The activity of hydroperoxide lyase 1 regulates accumulation of galactolipids containing 12-oxo-phytodienoic acid in Arabidopsis. J Exp Bot 67:5133–5144. https://doi.org/10.1093/JXB/ERW278
50. Wasternack C, Strnad M (2016) Jasmonate signaling in plant stress responses and development—active and inactive compounds. N Biotechnol 33:604–613. https://doi.org/10.1016/j.nbt.2015.11.001
51. Taki N, Sasaki-Sekimoto Y, Obayashi T, et al. (2005) 12-Oxo-phytodienoic acid triggers expression of a distinct set of genes and plays a role in wound-induced gene expression in Arabidopsis. Plant Physiol 139:1268–1283. https://doi.org/10.1104/pp.105.067058
52. Christensen SA, Kolomiets M V. (2011) The lipid language of plant-fungal interactions. Fungal Genet Biol 48:4–14. https://doi.org/10.1016/j.fgb.2010.05.005

53. Mueller S, Hilbert B, Dueckershoff K, et al. (2008) General detoxification and stress responses are mediated by oxidized lipids through TGA transcription factors in arabidopsis. Plant Cell 20:768–785. https://doi.org/10.1105/tpc.107.054809
54. Savchenko T, Kolla VA, Wang CQ, et al. (2014) Functional convergence of oxylipin and abscisic acid pathways controls stomatal closure in response to drought. Plant Physiol 164:1151–1160. https://doi.org/10.1104/pp.113.234310
55. Park SW, Li W, Viehhauser A, et al. (2013) Cyclophilin 20–3 relays a 12-oxo-phytodienoic acid signal during stress responsive regulation of cellular redox homeostasis. Proc Natl Acad Sci USA 110:9559–9564. https://doi.org/10.1073/pnas.1218872110
56. Sun YH, Hung CY, Qiu J, et al. (2017) Accumulation of high OPDA level correlates with reduced ROS and elevated GSH benefiting white cell survival in variegated leaves. Sci Rep 7:1–16. https://doi.org/10.1038/srep44158
57. Christensen SA, Huffaker A, Kaplan F, et al. (2015) Maize death acids, 9-lipoxygenase-derived cyclopente(a)nones, display activity as cytotoxic phytoalexins and transcriptional mediators. Proc Natl Acad Sci U S A 112:11407–11412. https://doi.org/10.1073/pnas.1511131112
58. Montillet JL, Leonhardt N, Mondy S, et al. (2013) An abscisic acid-independent oxylipin pathway controls stomatal closure and immune defense in Arabidopsis. PLoS Biol 11:e1001513. https://doi.org/10.1371/journal.pbio.1001513
59. Lõpez MA, Vicente J, Kulasekaran S, et al. (2011) Antagonistic role of 9-lipoxygenase-derived oxylipins and ethylene in the control of oxidative stress, lipid peroxidation and plant defence. Plant J 67:447–458. https://doi.org/10.1111/j.1365-313X.2011.04608.x
60. Marcos R, Izquierdo Y, Vellosillo T, et al. (2015) 9-Lipoxygenase-derived oxylipins activate brassinosteroid signaling to promote cell wall-based defense and limit pathogen infection. Plant Physiol 169:2324–2334. https://doi.org/10.1104/pp.15.00992
61. Fammartino A, Cardinale F, Göbel C, et al. (2007) Characterization of a divinyl ether biosynthetic pathway specifically associated with pathogenesis in tobacco. Plant Physiol 143:378–388. https://doi.org/10.1104/pp.106.087304
62. Brodhagen M, Tsitsigiannis DI, Hornung E, et al. (2008) Reciprocal oxylipin-mediated cross-talk in the Aspergillus-seed pathosystem. Mol Microbiol 67:378–391. https://doi.org/10.1111/j.1365-2958.2007.06045.x
63. Keereetaweep J, Blancaflor EB, Hornung E, et al. (2013) Ethanolamide oxylipins of linolenic acid can negatively regulate Arabidopsis seedling development. Plant Cell 25:3824–3840. https://doi.org/10.1105/tpc.113.119024
64. Keereetaweep J, Blancaflor EB, Hornung E, et al. (2015) Lipoxygenase-derived 9-hydro(pero)xides of linoleoylethanolamide interact with ABA signaling to arrest root development during Arabidopsis seedling establishment. Plant J 82:315–327. https://doi.org/10.1111/tpj.12821
65. Frankel EN (1980) Lipid oxidation. Prog Lipid Res 19:1–22. https://doi.org/10.1016/0163-7827(80)90006–5
66. Howe GA, Major IT, Koo AJ (2018) Modularity in jasmonate signaling for multistress resilience. Annu Rev Plant Biol 69:387–415. https://doi.org/10.1146/annurev-arplant-042817-040047
67. Li C, Xu M, Cai X, et al. (2022) Jasmonate signaling pathway modulates plant defense, growth, and their trade-offs. Int J Mol Sci 23:3945. https://doi.org/10.3390/ijms23073945
68. Campos ML, Kang JH, Howe GA (2014) Jasmonate-triggered plant immunity. J Chem Ecol 40:657–675. https://doi.org/10.1007/s10886-014-0468-3

69. Machado RA, McClure M, Hervé MR, et al. (2016) Benefits of jasmonate-dependent defenses against vertebrate herbivores in nature. Elife 5. https://doi.org/10.7554/elife.13720
70. Chini A, Fonseca S, Fernández G, et al. (2007) The JAZ family of repressors is the missing link in jasmonate signalling. Nat 2007– 4487154 448:666–671. https://doi.org/10.1038/nature06006
71. Kazan K, Manners JM (2013) MYC2: The master in action. Mol Plant 6:686–703. https://doi.org/10.1093/MP/SSS128
72. Fernández-Calvo P, Chini A, Fernández-Barbero G, et al. (2011) The Arabidopsis bHLH transcription factors MYC3 and MYC4 are targets of JAZ repressors and act additively with MYC2 in the activation of jasmonate responses. Plant Cell 23:701–715. https://doi.org/10.1105/TPC.110.080788
73. Thireault C, Shyu C, Yoshida Y, et al. (2015) Repression of jasmonate signaling by a non-TIFY JAZ protein in Arabidopsis. Plant J 82:669–679. https://doi.org/10.1111/tpj.12841
74. Bai Y, Meng Y, Huang D, et al. (2011) Origin and evolutionary analysis of the plant-specific TIFY transcription factor family. Genomics 98:128–136. https://doi.org/10.1016/J.YGENO.2011.05.002
75. Zhang F, Ke J, Zhang L, et al. (2017) Structural insights into alternative splicing-mediated desensitization of jasmonate signaling. Proc Natl Acad Sci U S A 114:1720–1725. https://doi.org/10.1073/pnas.1616938114
76. Ke J, Ma H, Gu X, et al. (2015) Structural basis for recognition of diverse transcriptional repressors by the TOPLESS family of corepressors. Sci Adv 1. https://doi.org/10.1126/sciadv.1500107
77. Pauwels L, Barbero GF, Geerinck J, et al. (2010) NINJA connects the co-repressor TOPLESS to jasmonate signalling. Nature 464:788–791. https://doi.org/10.1038/nature08854
78. Martin-Arevalillo R, Nanao MH, Larrieu A, et al. (2017) Structure of the Arabidopsis TOPLESS corepressor provides insight into the evolution of transcriptional repression. Proc Natl Acad Sci USA 114:8107–8112. https://doi.org/10.1073/pnas.1703054114
79. Xie DX, Feys BF, James S, et al. (1998) COI1: an Arabidopsis gene required for jasmonate-regulated defense and fertility. Science 280:1091–1094. https://doi.org/10.1126/SCIENCE.280.5366.1091
80. Thines B, Katsir L, Melotto M, et al. (2007) JAZ repressor proteins are targets of the SCF(COI1) complex during jasmonate signalling. Nature 448:661–665. https://doi.org/10.1038/NATURE05960
81. Katsir L, Schilmiller AL, Staswick PE, et al. (2008) COI1 is a critical component of a receptor for jasmonate and the bacterial virulence factor coronatine. Proc Natl Acad Sci USA 105:7100–7105. https://doi.org/10.1073/PNAS.0802332105/SUPPL_FILE/0802332105SI.PDF
82. Mosblech A, Thurow C, Gatz C, et al. (2011) Jasmonic acid perception by COI1 involves inositol polyphosphates in Arabidopsis thaliana. Plant J 65:949–957. https://doi.org/10.1111/j.1365-313X.2011.04480.x
83. Laha D, Johnen P, Azevedo C, et al. (2015) VIH2 regulates the synthesis of inositol pyrophosphate InsP8 and jasmonate-dependent defenses in arabidopsis. Plant Cell 27:1082–1097. https://doi.org/10.1105/tpc.114.135160
84. Sheard LB, Tan X, Mao H, et al. (2010) Jasmonate perception by inositol-phosphate-potentiated COI1-JAZ co-receptor. Nature 468:400–407. https://doi.org/10.1038/nature09430

85. Takeuchi M, Hamana K, Hiraishi A (2001) Proposal of the genus Sphingomonas sensu stricto and three new genera, Sphingobium, Novosphingobium and Sphingopyxis, on the basis of phylogenetic and chemotaxonomic analyses. Int J Syst Evol Microbiol 51:1405–1417. https://doi.org/10.1099/00207713-51-4-1405
86. Hoo SC, Koo AJK, Gao X, et al. (2008) Regulation and function of arabidopsis JASMONATE ZIM-domain genes in response to wounding and herbivory. Plant Physiol 146:952–964. https://doi.org/10.1104/pp.107.115691
87. Glauser G, Grata E, Dubugnon L, et al. (2008) Spatial and temporal dynamics of jasmonate synthesis and accumulation in Arabidopsis in response to wounding. J Biol Chem 283:16400–16407. https://doi.org/10.1074/jbc.M801760200

4 Key Enzymes of Oxylipins Pathway

Tamana Khan[1], Labiba Riyaz Shah[1], Sabba Khan[1], Shahjahan Rashid[2], Rizwan Rashid[1], and Baseerat Afroza[1]
Email: Khantamana96@gmail.com
[1]Division of Vegetable Science; Faculty of Horticulture, Sher e Kashmir University of Agricultural Sciences and Technology of Kashmir, Shalimar, Jammu and Kashmir, India
[2]Division of Plant Pathology; Faculty of Horticulture, Sher e Kashmir University of Agricultural Sciences and Technology of Kashmir, Shalimar, Jammu and Kashmir, India

CONTENTS

4.1 INTRODUCTION

The term oxylipins was coined to describe oxygenated compounds derived from fatty acids by at least one monooxygenase or dioxygenase enzyme's activity [1]. Oxylipins are acyclic or cyclic oxidation products formed from fatty acid catabolism that affect a variety of plant defense and developmental pathways [2]. Angiosperms, lichens, seaweeds, microorganisms, and fungus, as well as mammals, are rich in these lipids [3]. Oxylipins play a role in animal, insect, and abiotic stress (such as freeze-thawing) responses, along with pathogen attack. Some plant oxylipins operate immediately by

DOI: 10.1201/9781003316558-4

repelling insect predators, others are sufficiently volatile to warn adjacent plants, yet others may relay cell impairment information over a lengthy span inside the plant to organize a thorough reaction. The jasmonate is particularly important among them, and they are found in all plants. Jasmonic acid (JA) and its methyl ester are found throughout the plant kingdom. Oxylipins and their role have been reported in various plants viz., Arabidopsis [4], potato [4], tomato [5], viciafaba [6] and barley [7]. Oxylipin mechanisms in plants and animals appear to have evolved in distinct ways. The key distinction between them is the oxylipin formation initiating response. Plant oxylipins are made up of linoleic and linolenic acids that have been liberated from their lipid attachments by a variety of acyl hydrolases (lipases). Lipoxygenases play a significant part in the production of practically all plant oxylipins, with cytochrome P450 and pathogen-induced oxygenases playing supporting roles. In plants, oxylipin is synthesized from esterified or free polyunsaturated fatty acids. The liberation of fatty acids from cell membranes by a lipase initiates the formation of oxylipin. The following step is an early oxidation reaction involving various enzymes at various points along the fatty acid chain. In the first stage, molecular oxygen oxidizes the free fatty acid, resulting in a hydroperoxy fatty acid. A lipoxygenase (LOX) or -dioxygenase (-DOX) enzyme can catalyze this process. Non-enzymatically, α-DOX compounds break down into carbon dioxide and shorter aldehyde derivatives, or they can be reduced chemically by (i.e.) glutathione or enzymatically by a peroxygenase (PXG). Other enzymes, such as particular members of the Cyp74-family of P450 enzymes: allene oxide synthase, hydroperoxidelyase, and divinyl ether synthase, PXG or epoxyalcohol synthases metabolize the hydroperoxy products generated by LOXs (EAS).

4.2 LIPASES/ACYLHYDROLASES

Lipases are mostly referred to as acylhydrolases that hydrolyze the glyceryl ester bond to fatty acids and glycerol. Also, numerous enzymes that degrade lipids are present that are similar to esterases in structure and function but differ in relation to substrate specificity. Plant lipases break down the ester bonds of lipids of several types, each with its own structure and function. As a result, they play a role in a variety of processes, such as the biosynthesis and breakdown of lipids in membranes and that are stored, as well as the production of signaling molecules such jasmonic acid which is an important phytohormone. Several lipases have been identified in Arabidopsis that provide fatty acid substrate to the oxylipin pathway. DONGEL (DGL) [9] and DEFECTIVE IN ANTHER DEHISCENCE1 (DAD1) [8], which pertain to the phospholipase group, cause the hydrolysis of glycerophospholipids, however, glycolipids can be used as a substrate by both enzymes. These enzymes have a peptide sequence at the N-terminus, a distinctive G-X-S-X-G motif, and a catalytic triad (S, D and H), according to bioinformatic analyses. In a recent attempt, PLA-Iγ was discovered in Arabidopsis as an additional DAD1-like lipase. This enzyme, unlike DAD1 and DGL, is involved in the response to wounds in the early stages of the plant and could also have a role in the release of jasmonates that are preformed from arabidopsides [9]. Furthermore, pPLA-I, a lipase which is found abundantly in potato (patatin-related), has been demonstrated to regulate basal (but not pathogen-induced) jasmonate synthesis [10]. Lipases in plants enhance the output and composition of oil produced in seeds, thus, acting as a substitute to fossil fuels apart from having a role in tissues of vegetative plant parts. Furthermore, there is a significant effect on the composition of fatty acids defining their potential application in terms of health or industry.

4.3 LIPO-OXYGENASES

LOXs are crucial non-heme, non-sulfur-oxidoreductase enzymes in biological systems that synthesize various signaling molecules, C6-volatile compounds and jasmonates, which play an important role in their physiology. Mammals, plants, fish, moss, bacterium, yeast, fungus, reefs, algae, and mushrooms all have lipoxygenases enzymes [11]. These enzymes are involved in the release of free radicals by controlling reaction with molecular oxygen to release mixed products. Lipoxygenases catalyze the conversion of linoleic acid, linolenic acid, and arachidonic acid to hydroperoxyoctadecadienoic acid, hydroperoxyoctadecatrienoic acid, and hydroperoxyeicosatetraenoic acid [12, 3]. By regulating the creation of volatile chemicals and causing aroma generation through oxidation, LOXs operate as a natural flavoring agent for food preparation. A series of discoveries have been made with respect to occurrence and isolation of LOX from plants like *Arabidopsis, rice, maize, grapes, populus, tea, peach, radish, Arabian cotton*, and *chili* [13]. Aside from that, the lipoxygenase enzyme has been linked to carotenoid oxidation and has been discovered to affect batter quality and operate as a flour bleaching agent [14]. Fat oxidase [15], lipid oxidase, unsaturated lipid oxidase, and carotene oxidase [16] are some of the other names for this enzyme.

4.3.1 Classification

The LOX superfamily is classified according to their regiospecifcity within 5-, 8-, 9-, 10-, 12-, 13-, 15-LOXs called classical lipoxygenases and the major enzymes among the classical LOXs found in plants are 9- and 13-lipoxygenases. There is a tailfirst insertion of complex lipids, and membrane lipids into the active site of 13-LOX (methyl-end ahead), whereas a headfirst (carboxy-terminus first) insertion of substrates of 9-LOX is found in its active site [17, 18]. However, a new cyanobacteriallipoxygenase structure suggests that there may be more enzymes where the tail region of the substrate enters first in both circumstances where steric shielding of the reactive intermediate guides the location of molecular oxygen [19]. Lipoxygenase enzymes are additionally classified according to the specificity of one specific amino acid residue in the active site (also known as Coffa-site), resulting in S-specific lipoxygenase (when a residue of alanine is present in the active site) and R-specific lipoxygenase (when an arginine residue occupies the active site) (when the active site has the glycine residue).

4.3.2 Structure

The majority of what we know about LOX structure comes from study on the soluble proteins with a single polypeptide chain found in soybean seeds, LOX-1, -2, -3a, and -3b [20]. LOXs are known to be dioxygenase redox enzymes with an atomic weight of 90–110 kDa having N-terminus comprising of β-barrel domain of 25–30 kDa and C-terminal of around 55–65 kDawith an α-barrel domain. Two antiparallel plates consisting of an active iron (Fe3+) site with 693 AA residues constitute the N-terminal, while two antiparallel -plates consisting of an active iron (Fe3+) site with 160 AA residues create the C-terminal. The active state for LOX is a high-spin oxidized Fe3+, and the inactive state is a reduced high-spin Fe^{2+}. The active iron is coordinated by five AA residues and H_2O molecule being the sixth ligand in liquid oxygen's active site [21–23]. To summarize, plant LOXs are made up of a single polypeptide chain with the catalytic site of the enzyme occupied by the carboxy-terminal domain, which is made up of a non-heme iron atom bound to five amino acids—with three histidines, one asparagines, and the carboxyl group of the carboxy-terminal isoleucine; the amino-terminal region may be involved in membrane or substrate binding. The native LOX substrates for plant cells are linoleic and linolenic acids, which are structurally substrate specific. Following the oxygenation of several LOX substrates, products are produced. The LOX-1 type becomes active in the presence of water-soluble substrates such as linoleylsulphate, where oxidation of linoleic acid produces 13-lipohydroperoxide and oxidation of linolenic acid produces 13-hydroperoxide. LOX-2 reacts with esterification substrates to produce 9 or 13-hydroperoxide. When compared to free fatty acids, the activities of both LOX 1 and 2 are more directed toward triglycerides and methyl esters of fatty acids. Varying plant species have different pH requirements for LOX activity, although a pH range of 4.5 to 8 is considered sufficient. 5.68, 6.25, and 6.15, respectively, are the optimal isoelectric points for LOX-1, LOX-2, and LOX-3 [21, 24–26].

4.3.3 Process of LOX-Mediated Reaction

The process of the lipoxygenases' enzyme reaction has been thoroughly explored using soybean LOX-1, while LOX-2 and -3 have shown qualitatively comparable behavior [27, 28]. As discussed earlier, the single non-heme iron cofactor can be found as Fe^{2+} which is the non-active form of the enzyme catalytically or can exist as Fe^{3+} which is the active form [27, 28]. The reaction begins when the unsaturated fatty acid binds to the Fe^{3+} form of the enzyme's active site. The synthesis of Fe^{2+} and a pentadienyl radical with a delocalized, unpaired electron results from the separation of H^+ from the methylene group at the heart of the 1,4-pentadiene molecule. The hydroperoxy radical is formed when molecular oxygen combines with the pentadienyl radical in a second stage. The enzyme is then restored to its starting state by Fe^{2+} through the reduction of hydroperoxy radical to the hydroperoxy derivative of the fatty acid [28]. Different enzymes metabolize the hydroperoxy derivatives of fatty acids in plants [27, 29] to produce volatile aldehydes and oxoacids, conjugated dienoic acids, methyl jasmonate, and jasmonic acid, which are active members in plant defensive scheme activities [30], including abiotic and biotic stresses. For example, when 13-hydroperoxylinolenic acid is used as a substrate, c/5–3-hexenal and 12-oxo-c/s-9-dodecenoic acid are produced, whereas the 9-hydroperoxy derivative is transformed to a.s-3,ds-6-nonadienal and 9-oxo-nonanoic acid. These chemicals, as well as their metabolites, contribute to the fruit and leaf's distinct flavor and odor.

4.3.4 LOX Pathway

Plant lipoxygenases are divided into two subfamilies based on their regiospecificity: 9-LOXs and 13-LOXs. LOXs having such dual specificities, were also identified in a few cases, depending on the outcomes primarily generated [31]. In a wide spectrum of cells, the lipoxygenases metabolic pathway starts in the plasmalemma and proceeds to the cytoplasm. Molecular oxygen is integrated at the 9 or 13-carbon position of polyunsaturated fatty acids with 18 carbons in the LOX-mediated mechanism in plants (PUFAs).

4.3.5 9-Lipoxygenase Pathway

9-LOX is a non-heme Fe containing enzyme which has a chain of single polypeptide with amino acids ranging between 741–886 [11]. The 9-LOX route (9S-keto octadecatrienoic acid) converts PUFAs to key metabolites as 9-hydroperoxy octadecadienoic acid, 9-hydroperoxy octadecatrienoic acid, and 9-keto octadecatrienoic acid (Figure 4.1). The bulk of the products produced by this system are involved in physiological functions in plants, particularly pathogen defense. Unlike 13-lipoxygenase derived route, 9-LOX-derived stimulus begin in a variety of situations due to a less complex pathway; nonetheless, the resulting oxylipins from 9-lipoxygenases have a structural similarity to the products derived from 13-lipoxygenase but are somehow different [32].

4.3.6 13-Lipoxygenase Pathway

13-lipoxygenase is an iron-containing non-heme polypeptide with a length of 896–941 amino acids [11]. The 13-LOX pathway converts PUFAs to 13-HPOT, which is then metabolized into plant signaling molecules like jasmonates and green leaf volatiles (GLVs) (Figure 4.1). The 13-LOX family contains the majority of the LOXs discovered in plants so far that are involved in the synthesis of jasmonates. Several downstream pathway branches use 13-LOX products; however, the best-characterized enzymes at the moment are members of the CYP74 family, such as allene oxide synthase, hydroperoxide lyase, divinyl ether synthase, and allene oxide cyclase [33], and such enzymes also have a direct interaction with one another [1]. Since the last decade, the number of identified signaling molecules other than jasmonates has steadily increased, with the 13-LOX system remaining the most studied.

4.3.7 Physiological Functions of Plant LOXs

Many cellular components create LOXs, which are involved in a number of activities such as development and growth, root initiation, reaction to abiotic and biotic stresses and damage, fruit development, aging, death of cells, and biosynthesis of jasmonic acid and absiccic acid. LOX's have a very crucial role to play in germination. LOX serve as storage protein that aids in the degradation of lipid bodies that have been stored [28]. Mung bean (Vignaradiata) seedlings have strong LOX activity, which they use as hydroperoxidelyase (HPL) enzymes when they germinate. There

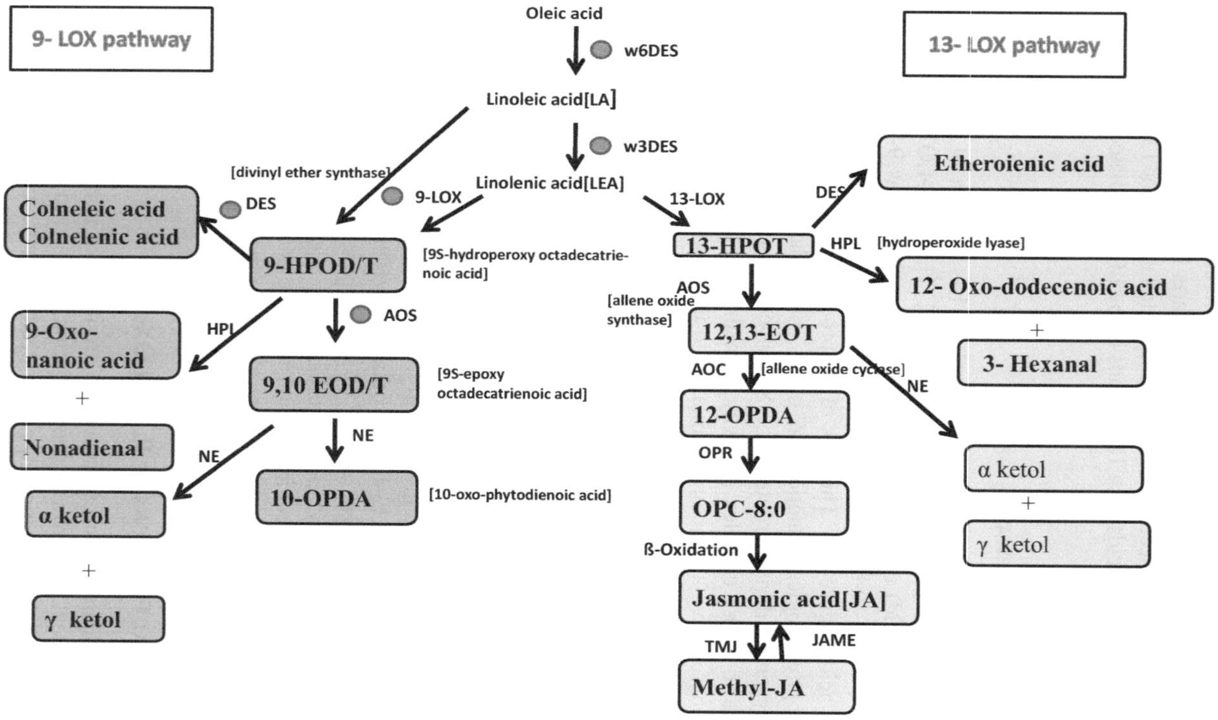

FIGURE 4.1 When 9- Lipoxygenase catalyzes the deoxygenation of ALA, a derivative 9-HPOT is obtained whereas the catalysis of ALA by 13-LOX results in derivative 13-HPOT. It is then transformed into other forms of DES, HPL, and AOS in the 9-LOX pathway and produce oxylipins, especially jasmonic acid as a plant hormone. The principal step of biosynthesis of JA occurs in chloroplast, which is catalyzed by lipoxygenase, allene oxide synthase, and allene oxide cyclase whereas the reactions of OPR and β-oxidation occurs in peroxisomes.

are reports that several novel lipoxygenases are activated during the early seedling growth stages in different plant species such as Pisumsativum, Citrulluslanatus, Phaseolus vulgaris, Lupinus, Eleusinecoracana, Vignaradiata, Daucuscarota, Lensculinaris, Hordeumvulgare, Cucumissativus, Arabidopsis thaliana, Triticum, Papaversomniferum, Phoenix dactylifera, Oryza sativa, and Brassica napus.

LOX encoding genes have been identified in Arabidopsis (6 genes), rice (14 genes), grapes (18 genes), Populus (21 genes), and chili (8 genes) [34]. AtLOX1 is

TABLE 4.1
Genes expressing LOX in Arabidopsis and rice

Crop	Gene Locus	Gene Function	Total Amino Acids
Arabidopsis thaliana	AT1G55020	conferring resistance to pathogens	859
Arabidopsis thaliana	AT3G45140	biosynthesis of JA	896
Arabidopsis thaliana	AT1G17420	flower development, catalyze the oxygenation of fatty acids	919
Arabidopsis thaliana	AT1G72520	flower development, 13-lipoxygenase induced by abiotic stresses, triggers defense responses	926
Arabidopsis thaliana	AT3G22400	defense responses	886
Arabidopsis thaliana	AT1G67560	biosynthesis of JA, PLAT/LH2 domain-containing lipoxygenase family protein	917
Oryza sativa	LOC_Os11g36719	lipoxygenase, putative, expressed	869
Oryza sativa	LOC_Os12g37260	lipoxygenase 2.1, chloroplast precursor, putative, expressed	923
Oryza sativa	LOC_Os12g37320	lipoxygenase 2.2, chloroplast precursor, putative, expressed	359
Oryza sativa	LOC_Os02g10120	lipoxygenase, putative, expressed	927
Oryza sativa	LOC_Os02g19790	lipoxygenase 4, putative, expressed	297
Oryza sativa	LOC_Os03g08220	lipoxygenase protein, putative, expressed	919
Oryza sativa	LOC_Os03g49260	lipoxygenase, putative, expressed	868
Oryza sativa	LOC_Os03g49380	lipoxygenase, putative, expressed	878
Oryza sativa	LOC_Os03g52860	lipoxygenase, putative, expressed	871
Oryza sativa	LOC_Os04g37430	lipoxygenase protein, putative, expressed	798
Oryza sativa	LOC_Os05g23880	lipoxygenase, putative, expressed	848
Oryza sativa	LOC_Os06g04420	lipoxygenase 4, putative	126
Oryza sativa	LOC_Os08g39840	lipoxygenase, chloroplast precursor, putative, expressed	925
Oryza sativa	LOC_Os08g39850	lipoxygenase, chloroplast precursor, putative, expressed	942

involved in pathogen defense in Arabidopsis plant leaves [35], AtLOX2 in JA biosynthesis [36], AtLOX3 and AtLOX4 in flower development and male fertility regulation [37], AtLOX5 in defense response and lateral root development [38], and AtLOX6 in JA biosynthesis and is generally expressed in roots [39]. In Arabidopsis and rice, genes expressing LOX are represented in Table 4.1 [34–39, 40].

When plants are exposed to UV radiation, severe temperatures, oxygen and water shortages, insects, and disease attacks, they are compelled to express the LOX gene. Leone, Melillo, and Bleve-Zacheo [30] discovered that LOX plays a role in parasite defense. LOX activity has been found to be elevated in a variety of plant–pathogen systems. Maximum LOX activity has been found to be performed by necrotic tissues. When plants are infected, some noxious metabolites, along with others, which act as signaling units to activate defense mechanisms, are released. Major oxylipins such as 12-oxo-phytodienoic acid produced by 13-lipoxygenases, 10-oxo-phytodienoic acid, a constitutional isomer of 12-oxo-phytodienoic acid, and 10-oxo-11-phytoenoic acid produced by 9-lipoxygenases lipoxygenases have a key part in plant defense against biting–chewing herbivores [41]. When herbivores consume lipoxygenases, they trigger an oxidative attack against them, causing direct as well as indirect harm to the herbivores, besides triggering plant defense responses [42]. Increased LOX transcript levels were reported from different plant species during pathogen attack like in *Solanum lycopersicum* by *Myzuseuphorbias*, in tobacco by *M. nicotianae* and tobacco hornworm, while in cabbage by caterpillars (cabbage white butterfly, large cabbage white, and cabbage moth), *Tetranychusurticae* (Tetranychusurticae), and locusts. The 9-LOX route is important in pathogen defense [43], and its role in *Arabidopsis thaliana* against *Pseudomonas syringe* epv. Syringae was studied, and it was discovered that the 9-HOT promotes modifications of the plant cell wall to prevent pathogen attack [44]. Plant cells near the infection site die quickly as a result of the hypersensitive reaction (HR). This prevents the pathogen from spreading further and causing damage to plant cells. As a result, lipoxygenases products, particularly 9-LOX products, play an important part in this process. The formation of oxylipin-reactive electrophile species (RES) in tobacco leaves was used to investigate the HR [45].

Plant studies to assess the role of lipoxygenases at the time of abiotic stress have been limited. Ca LOX1 reduces H2O2 accumulation, lipid peroxidation, and increases expression of stress-responsive genes during certain stress conditions like osmotic, high salinity, and drought stress [46]. Overexpression of Dk LOX1, Dk LOX3, and Dk LOX4 in *A. thaliana* enhances ripening and senescence via regulating lipid peroxidation and stress regulatory genes, as well as promoting abiotic and osmotic stress tolerance [47].

Various free radicals produced in wounds, such as reactive oxygen species (ROS), lipid-derived carbonyl, and malondialdehyde, may exacerbate membrane damage, resulting in "hypersensitive response (HR)" cell death. LOX induces the rapid production of wound hormones such C6-aldehydes in plants during wounding or herbicide damage and regulates plant defense by beginning wound and herbivore-induced defense responses. Several Arabidopsis genes were investigated, out of which LOX2 and LOX6 have been discovered to be responsible for the majority of JA synthesis in the leaf and xylem after wounding [48].

A surge in LOX activity has been identified as an indicator of aging tissues of the plants in a number of investigations. Lipoxygenase functioning levels were high during senescence, resulting in the generation of superoxide radicals which resulted in upsurge of lipid peroxidation levels. According to research, LOX has a critical regulation of peroxidation of lipids and plays a role in membrane degradation throughout aging [49]. Apart from senescence, LOX controls the quality and flavor of a variety of climacteric and non-climacteric fruits during ripening [50, 51].

4.4 ALENE OXIDASE SYNTHASE AND HYDROPEROXIDE LYASE

In plants, the CYP74 family of cytochrome P450 enzymes play a key role in the oxylipin metabolizing pathway [52]. AOS, HPL are non-canonical members of this family and belong to CYP74A and CYP74B subgroup, respectively [33]. AOS and HPL differ from canonical cytochrome P450 proteins as both of these do not need O_2 and NADPH oxidoreductase for activity and also have low affinity toward carbon monoxide [53]. Both have moderately conserved amino acid sequences differing primarily in their catalytic residues site and still form similar hydrophobic binding site with substrate. Other member of CYP450 is divinyl ether synthases (DES), belonging to group CYP74D [54]. Crystal structural investigations of guayule and *Arabidopsis thaliana* on AOS, along with site-directed mutagenesis, have revealed important information about AOS and HPL substrate binding and conversion mechanisms [55]. AOS has a typical CYP450 fold, a unique heme-binding site and a 22- Å deep substrate access channel [56]. Furthermore, AOS has an unusual method of membrane binding. In terms of active site residues and its overall topology, AOS from guayule and Arabidopsis are quite similar [57].

When the substrate binds to AOS, hydrogen bond is established by carboxyl group with Thr389 while as hydrophobic interactions occur between aliphatic segments and surrounding side chains of non-polar amino acid. Also, the substrate peroxy group along with heme cofactor and develops useful interaction with the Asn321 catalytic residue. A novel active site capable of controlling the reactivity of an epoxyallylic radical and its cation via interactions with an aromatic pi-system of a conserved Phe residue (Phe137) was detected [55]. Like other enzymes of CYP74, AOS and HPL in proximal Cys loop share a nine-residue insertion that helps in decreasing the donor strength of the thiolate and favors the production of S–Fe (IV)–OH complex, which can then easily participate in electron transfer (AOS) or oxygen rebound (HPL).

Substituting non-polar residues for the amino acids used in these steps as seen in the mutant derivative of AOS (F137L, S155A), ristricts carbocation intermediate from being sufficiently enriched or stabilized at C11 and inhibits the generation of highly reactive hemiacetal [58], which naturally separates into short-chain aldehydes. Therefore, activity of AOS was significantly reduced while transforming the mutant enzyme into an enzyme-like HPL [56]. Evidently, to make sure that 13(S)-HPOT is effectively transformed to allene oxide and not short-chain aldehydes, AOS clips the substrates C11 position in between two pi-systems. The HPL active sites, on the contrary, have evolved to allow radical rearrangement by avoiding aromatic residue (Phe137) strategically positioned at C11 of 13(S)-HPOT [59]. Under biotic and abiotic stress plants produce defensive chemicals that allow them to survive. Several defense-related compounds have been reported, such as jasmonic acid (JA), green leaf volatiles (GLV) (Z-3-hexenal, (Z)-3-hexenol) [60]. The oxygenation of linoleic or α-linolenic acid by lipoxygenases starts this process, leading to the formation of hydroperoxy fatty acids including 9-hydroperoxides (9-HPOD/T) and 13-hydroperoxides (13-HPOD/T) [3]. The hydroperoxy fatty acids produced by LOX are highly reactive and harmful to biological systems of plants and is metabolized by other enzymes of pathway such as AOS, peroxygenase (POX), DES or HPL. The AOS oxidizes 13-HPOT to unstable epoxide, which are cyclized by an allene oxide cyclase (AOC) to the 12-oxo phytodienoic acid (12-OPDA). 12-OPDA is finally converted to JA by 12-oxophytodienoate reductase 3 (OPR3) followed by three β-oxidation cycles. The first part of biosynthesis of JA takes place in plastid, while as OPDA to JA conversion in peroxisomes [3]. Then various metabolic conversions of JA can lead to the formation of different jasmonates. Therefore, it clearly indicates that, in the biosynthesis of jasmonates enzyme AOS is a regulating point [52, 61].

AOS from plants was isolated and characterized first from flaxseed *(Linum usitatissimum)* [62, 63]. Since then, from many other plants, AOS has been found and characterized, for instance *Arabidopsis thaliana* [64], guayule (*Parthenium argentatum*) rubber particles [65], *tulip* (*Tulipa gesneriana cv. Red Apeldoorn*) bulbs [66], corn (*Zea mays* L.) seeds [67] tomato (*Lycopersicon esculentum*) [68], and potato *Solanum tuberosum* [69]. In different monocots and dicots, several AOS genes have been characterized and cloned so far [70, 71]. Different numbers of genes in various plant species code for AOS. For instance, in Arabidopsis a single AOS gene [64], two AOS genes in barley (*Hordeum vulgare*) [72], rice (*Oryza sativa*) [73] and tomato (*Solanum lycopersicum*) [68, 74] and three AOS genes in potato (*S. tuberosum*) [75] has been described. AOS transcripts increase upon insect attack, wounding or methyl jasmonate or ethylene threatment as AOS pathway products play a vital role in plant signaling for defense against pest attack, wounding, and some growth and developmental processes [76].

The HPL enzyme cleaves the fatty acid hydroperoxides between neighboring double-bonded carbon and hydroperoxide carbon resulting in formation of volatile aldehydes and w-oxo acids [77]. HPLs are classified into two subfamilies based on sequence homologies CYP74B and CYP74C. Several HPL enzymes (CYP74B) have specificity to utilize substrate 13-hydroperoxides while some (CYP74C) utilize both 13- and 9-hydroperoxides [78]. The 13-hydroperoxide is metabolized by 13-HPL to 12-oxo-(Z)-9-dodecenoic acid and (Z)-3-hexenal/hexanal and 9- hydroperoxide is metabolized by 9-HPLs to (3Z)-nonenal/(3Z, 6Z)-nonadienal and is 9-oxo-nonanoic acid. Further isomarization of (3Z)-C6- and C9-aldehydes results in the production of (2E) isomers and C12-oxo-acid into 12-oxo-(10E)-dodecenoic acid.

Interestingly, based on structural information, single amino acid substitution resulted in transition of AOS into HPL [79]. The aldehydes as well as their (2E) isomers, corresponding alcohols and esters ((3Z)-hexenyl acetate) produced by HPLs are known as GLVs [77]. GLV act as signaling molecules in plants against stress response to herbivory, insect, and other injuries. Furthermore, they have also been known to have fungicidal and bactericidal activity. Both HPL and AOS compete for the same substrate. In fact, it has been found that inhibiting the HPL branch activates synthesis of jasmonate [53]. HPLs are widely distributed in plants (including moss and probably, algae) [80, 75]. However, whether algae contain HPL has yet to be determined. HPL gene identified so far encodes for protein of 55 kDa [81]. Most HPL enzymes are known to occur as trimers or tetramers with 55–72 kDa subunits. Mostly are membrane bound and some have a chloroplast transit peptide at the N-terminus, whileas others are devoid of transit signals and are believed to be found in microsomes [77].

HPL is a membrane bound enzymes for its extraction and solubilization detergent is required. However, HPL was extracted in buffer from epicotly (etiolated) without detergent in watermelon and sunflower respectively [82, 83]. It indicated that HPL in epicotyl is either loosely bound or soluble, while as in leaves, HPL is bound to membrane and requires higher concentration of detergent for solubilization [83]. To date, HPL crystal structure has not been solved, existing knowledge about HPL structure is based on homology modeling [84] or related AOS structures [56, 55] and other P450 cytochromes [85].

Divinyle ether synthase are enzymes that utilize hydroperoxides of LOX pathway and convert it into divinyle ethers. Unlike other members of the CYP74 family, like AOS and HPLs, these enzymes are less prevalent. DES converts 9-hydroperoxides into colneleic acid and colnelenic acid [86]. Divinyle ethers oxilipins play a vital role in plant defense. The genes for DES over-express during pathogen invasion, viral attack and elicitor treatment [87, 88, 89]. These have been first identified from solanaceous crops. Since then, several DESs have been identified in different plant species: CYP74H1 (*Allium sativum* L.) [75], bulbs and gladiolus roots [90], CYP74B16 (*Linum usitatissimum* L.) [91], aerial parts of the spike moss [92].

4.5 ALLENE OXIDE CYCLASE

Oxylipins are fatty acids that have been oxidized [3]. The oxylipin in plants proceeds at the extent of esterified or unesterified fatty acids (polyunsaturated). The enzyme lipoxygenase (LOX) initiates the formation of phyto-oxlipins by converting fatty acids (polyunsaturated) into their respective hydroperoxides. After being generated from fatty acid, a sequence of reactions catalyzed by allene oxide synthase and allene oxide cyclase convert hydroperoxyoctadecatrienoic acid (HPOT) to cis(+)-12-oxo-phytodienoic acid. However in the absence of AOC, the allylic allene oxide produced by AOS and 13-HPOT (hydroperoxyoctadecatrienoic acid) has a brief half-life in water and is modified to alpha and gamma alkyl group of ketones and alcohols or recurring to produce a racemic mixture of enantiomers of cis(+)- and cis(-)-12-OPDA. In the presence of AOC, the allene oxide is transferred in a pair of reactions with the AOS to the enantiomeric cis(+)-OPDA.

The initial description of allene oxide cyclase came from maize [93], followed by the discovery of the analogue genes in tomato [94], Arabidopsis [95], and barley [96]. While AOC is produced by a sole gene in tomato, it is discovered in four isogenes in *A. thaliana*, which most presumably originated from a single ancestral isoform through gene duplication events.

The AOC is a homotrimeric enzyme that belongs to the lipocalin protein family and has a relative molecular mass of around 20–25 kDa per subunit. Each subunit is mostly made up of an eight-stranded antiparallel barrel realm, the process takes place inside a central hydrophobic cavity or barrel. The section of the protein is particularly firm, and there is no induced fit process when the substrate is bound [97]. One glutamate residue produces a partial charge separation once the subtance is enclosed in the active site, causing the 15-double bond to delocalize. As a result, a positive charge forms between carbon at 13 and carbon at 16, delocalizes, and the epoxy-ring is opened. The oxy-ion (negatively charged) created by hydrogen bonding is stabilized by one distinct water molecule, which is bonded in a polar cavity produced by serine and a asparagines rest. A structural readjustment from the cis to trans geometry circling the carbon at 10 and carbon at 11 bond is required to promote the ring closure that will generate the cyclopentanone molecule. This cis-trans isomerization near the carbon-10 and carbon-11 bond, due to steric limitations within the active site, results in a further l shift of the carbon-8 and carbon-9 bond, which is also moved from the cis- to the trans-geometry.

The allene oxide's tendency to cyclize impulsively in water, generating a mixture of enantiomers (OPDA), indicates that this process has a low energy barrier. As a result, AOC does not require much of an enzyme to reduce this energy. It appears that the spontaneous cyclization reaction is controlled by steric active site determinants and proceeds in a stereoselective manner [98]. The Arabidopsis AOCs have anticipated plastidial target sequence, which makes it easier for the enzymes to enter the chloroplast. Immunocytochemical techniques were used to study the practical import of AOC into the chloroplast [95]. Arabidopsis AOCs have been found to be expressed in all organs of plants, including the root system [99]. This conclusion differs from that of the tomato, where AOC expression is said to be bounded to floral organs and fibrovascular bundles [5]. After deciphering the chemical operation of AOC-catalyzed 12, 13-EOT cyclization, elucidating the functional connectivity of AOS and AOC is one of the most urgent topics. X-ray crystallography was used to establish the form of AOC (isoform) from *Arabidopsis thaliana* [100]. AOC has been shown to form a trimeric quarternary unit in all crystal forms so far [97]. The core 8-stranded antiparallel b-barrel is the most prominent structural feature of AOC. Its cross section is slightly oval, with axes between 14 and 18 A° and walls between 11 and 30 A°. Side chain atoms do not completely fill the barrel, but instead produce an extended cavity (hydrophobic) that extends into the protein. The highest portions of the wall, which have the longest hydrogen bonding network and are thus considered to be the prominent stable areas of the structure, interact with surrounding monomers in the interface of trimer. Allene oxide cyclase (AOC) is a core enzyme in the biosynthesis of jasmonic acid (JA) in plants. It catalyzes the conversion sterotypically of 112,13(S)-epoxy-9(Z),11,15(Z)-octadecatrienoic acid (12,13-EOT) to cis(+)-12-oxophytodienoic acid. The activities of AOC and inflow through the JA biosynthesis pathway may be influenced by its oligomeric structure. In crystallographic studies, AOC exists as a trimer [97], but AOC from dry corn seeds was delineated to exist mostly as a dimer in solution [93]. Allene oxide cyclase was found to be localized in the chloroplast of rice, and its native oligomeric structure was investigated using gel electrophoresis in the absence and presence of a protein-cross linking reagent. The findings show that

AOC is a mixture of multimers (monomers, dimers, and higher order) in solution. At room temperature, AOC prefers to exist as a dimer, but in the presence of SDS, it undergoes temperature-dependent partial denaturation [101]. Several attempts to raise JA levels in *Salvia miltiorrhiza* and wheat, which had been a problem for almost two decades, were achieved efficiently to AOC overexpression, which was accompanied with higher salinity tolerance in wheat [102]. AOC overexpression boosted the production of JA-inducible artemisinin in *Artemisia annua* [103]. It is possible that the intricate regulation of this process, at least in *Arabidopsis*, is because AOC is part of a four-member gene family. Detailed inspection of transgenic lines expressing the GUS reporter gene under the control of distinct AOC promoters revealed largely redundant promoter activities during development, although transcript accumulation demonstrated an organ-specific expression pattern: AOC1, AOC2, and AOC3 promoter activities were found throughout all leaf tissue in fully developed leaves, but AOC4 promoter activity was vascular bundle-specific; only AOC3 and AOC4 had promoter activities in roots; and AOC1 and AOC4 had partially specific promoter activities in flower development [104]. The crystalline structures of AOC1 and AOC2 in *Physcomitrella patens* provide insight into oxylipin cyclization. AOC2 belongs to the lipocalin family and is a trimeric protein. AOC transcript is found in abundance in the flower bud and flower stalk [105].

4.6 12-OXO-PHYTODIENOIC ACID REDUCTASE

Cyclopentenone-containing chemicals are made via oxidation, cyclization, and hydrolysis of lipid-derived molecules in a specific order. The oxidation of the C18 polyunsaturated fatty acid (PUFA) α-linolenic acid (α-LeA) by lipoxygenase (LOX) starts the production of OPDA. Through the action of allene oxide synthase (AOS), the hydroperoxylipid generated enzymatically becomes an epoxide, which is then cyclized by allene oxide cyclase (AOC) to make OPDA. OPDA can be further metabolized to jasmonic acid [106]. An enzyme called as OPDA reductase isoenzyme3 reduces 12S,13S- or to the corresponding cyclopentanone derivative in plants (OPR3). This enzyme is an flavin mononucleotide-dependent oxidoreductase from the early yellow enzyme family, which is known for reducing the double bonds of carbonyls (unsaturated). OPR enzymes have an (α/β) eight-barrel fold, which consists of eight helices around eight parallel -sheets in a cylindrical nature. The FMN-cofactor is noncovalently linked to one of the -barrel ends in the enzyme's center. In the first reaction step, NAD(P)H reduces the FMN-cofactor, which is followed by the release of NAD(P)+. In a second stage, OPDA binds to the enzyme and is reduced to the -C-atom via hydride transfer [107].

From Arabidopsis, the earliest flavin-dependent oxidoreductase transformed cis-(+)-OPDA was isolated and cloned and revealed parallelism to the yeast early yellow enzyme [108]. It was given the name 12-oxophytodienoic acid reductase3 (OPR3) considering it is the only OPR out of the six that can convert the physiologically relevant enantiomer for jasmonic acid production. OPR3 in tomato crystallized as a homodimer, and dimerization resulted in activity reduction [107], implying that OPR3 monomer/dimer balance regulates JA biosynthesis. Furthermore, to its unique role in JA synthesis, OPR3 has been found to play a JA-independent direct role in the growth of primary root under deficiency of phosphate through root tip growth transcriptional inhibition, which includes raillery with the signaling pathways for ethylene and gibberellin [109]. There are families of OPR gene with up to 12 members in maize and rice, some of which are thought to play a role in tassel production (maize) and wound retort (rice). OPDA is prevalent in Arabidopsis vegetative tissues and is involved in the elongation of anther filaments. OPR3 is considered to be found in plastids before being transferred to the peroxisome. Arabidopsis OPR3 is engaged in the penultimate step of JA synthesis, which is followed by three b-oxidation cycles. The crystal structures of OPR3 and OPR1 have shown OPR3's role in JA biosynthesis and offer a possible mechanism for reversible dimerization of OPR3 activity, which requires OPR3 phosphorylation in vivo [105]. Heat shock modulation [110], stomatal conductance control [111], seed dormancy and germination [112], and quick adaption to high light intensity are all regulated by OPDA [113]. Furthermore, the 12-OPDA isoleucine adduct displays bioactivity that is independent of OPDA [114].

4.7 CONCLUSION

Various enzymes having several functions in phyto-oxylipin metabolic processes have been found and characterized in recent decades. The discovery of their structural composition, along with identifying their important research aspects has not only helped in comprehending the catalytic reaction of enzymes but has also highlighted their evolutionary history. Besides, having "traditional" catalytic action (as discussed in this chapter), new enzymes with unique or even additional catalytic activity have been discovered in recent years. It will be critical to investigate these enzymes further in order to completely comprehend the mechanics of oxylipin production. LOXs, in particular, need additional attention in oxylipins generated by plants because of their significant role in plant physiology. Several authors from the past few years have cloned, purified, and characterized several lipoxygenase enzymes in order to understand them better. The discovery of new alleles involved in oxylipin production will add to our understanding of the diversity of oxylipins.

REFERENCES

1. Wasternack C, Feussner I. The oxylipin pathways: biochemistry and function. Annual Review of Plant Biology. 2018 Apr 29;69:363–86.
2. Creelman RA, Mulpuri R. The oxylipin pathway in Arabidopsis. The Arabidopsis Book/American Society of Plant Biologists. 2002;1.
3. Andreou A, Brodhun F, Feussner I. Biosynthesis of oxylipins in non-mammals. Progress in Lipid Research. 2009 May 1;48(3–4):148–70.
4. Weber H, Vick BA, Farmer EE. Dinor-oxo-phytodienoic acid: a new hexadecanoid signal in the jasmonate family. Proceedings of the National Academy of Sciences. 1997 Sep 16;94(19):10473–8.
5. Hause B, Stenzel I, Miersch O, Maucher H, Kramell R, Ziegler J, Wasternack C. Tissue-specific oxylipin signature of tomato flowers: allene oxide cyclase is highly expressed in distinct flower organs and vascular bundles. The Plant Journal. 2000 Oct;24(1):113–26.

6. Gundlach H, Zenk MH. Biological activity and biosynthesis of pentacyclic oxylipins: the linoleic acid pathway. Phytochemistry. 1998 Feb 1;47(4):527–37.
7. Kramell R, Miersch O, Atzorn R, Parthier B, Wasternack C. Octadecanoid-derived alteration of gene expression and the "oxylipin signature" in stressed barley leaves. Implications for different signaling pathways. Plant Physiology. 2000 May;123(1):177–88.
8. Ishiguro S, Kawai-Oda A, Ueda J, Nishida I, Okada K. The DEFECTIVE IN ANTHER DEHISCENCE1 gene encodes a novel phospholipase A1 catalyzing the initial step of jasmonic acid biosynthesis, which synchronizes pollen maturation, anther dehiscence, and flower opening in Arabidopsis. The Plant Cell. 2001 Oct;13(10):2191–209.
9. Ellinger D, Stingl N, Kubigsteltig II, Bals T, Juenger M, Pollmann S, Berger S, Schuenemann D, Mueller MJ. DONGLE and DEFECTIVE IN ANTHER DEHISCENCE1 lipases are not essential for wound-and pathogen-induced jasmonate biosynthesis: redundant lipases contribute to jasmonate formation. Plant Physiology. 2010 May;153(1):114–27.
10. Scherer GF, Ryu SB, Wang X, Matos AR, Heitz T. Patatin-related phospholipase A: nomenclature, subfamilies and functions in plants. Trends in Plant Science. 2010 Dec 1;15(12):693–700.
11. Joo YC, Oh DK. Lipoxygenases: potential starting biocatalysts for the synthesis of signaling compounds. Biotechnology Advances. 2012 Nov 1;30(6):1524–32.
12. Brash AR. Lipoxygenases: occurrence, functions, catalysis, and acquisition of substrate. Journal of Biological Chemistry. 1999 Aug 20;274(34):23679–82.
13. Viswanath KK, Varakumar P, Pamuru RR, Basha SJ, Mehta S, Rao AD. Plant lipoxygenases and their role in plant physiology. Journal of Plant Biology. 2020 Apr;63(2):83–95.
14. Song H, Wang P, Li C, Han S, Lopez-Baltazar J, Zhang X, Wang X. Identification of lipoxygenase (LOX) genes from legumes and their responses in wild type and cultivated peanut upon Aspergillus flavus infection. Scientific Reports. 2016 Oct 12;6(1):1–9.
15. Craig FN. A fat oxidation system in Lupinus albus. Journal of Biological Chemistry. 1936 Jul 1;114(3):727–46.
16. Tauber, H. Unsaturated fat oxidase. J. Am. Chem. Soc. 1940, 62, 2251.
17. Feussner I, Wasternack C. The lipoxygenase pathway. Annual Review of Plant Biology. 2002 Jun;53(1):275–97.
18. Newcomer ME, Brash AR. The structural basis for specificity in lipoxygenase catalysis. Protein Science. 2015 Mar;24(3):298–309.
19. Newie J, Neumann P, Werner M, Mata RA, Ficner R, Feussner I. Lipoxygenase 2 from Cyanothece sp. controls dioxygen insertion by steric shielding and substrate fixation. Scientific Reports. 2017 May 18;7(1):1–2.
20. Axelrod B, Cheesbrough TM, Laakso S. 53. Lipoxygenase from soybeans: EC 1.13. 11.12 Linoleate: oxygen oxidoreductase. In *Methods in Enzymology* 1981 Jan 1 (Vol. 71, pp. 441–451). Academic Press.
21. Shi Y, Mandal R, Singh A, Pratap Singh A. Legume lipoxygenase: Strategies for application in food industry. Legume Science. 2020 Sep;2(3):e44.
22. Aanangi R, Kotapati KV, Palaka BK, Kedam T, Kanika ND, Ampasala DR. Purification and characterization of lipoxygenase from mung bean (Vigna radiata L.) germinating seedlings. 3 Biotech. 2016 Jun;6(1):1–8.
23. Mitsuda H, Yasumoto K, Yamamoto A, Kusano T. Study on Soybean Lipoxygenase: Part I. Preparation of Crystalline Enzyme and Assay by Polarographic Method. Agricultural and Biological Chemistry. 1967 Jan 1;31(1):115–8.

24. Murphy, PA. Soybean proteins. In *Soybeans: Chemistry, Production, Processing, and Utilization*; Johnson LA, White PJ, Galloway R, Eds, AOCS Press: Urbana, IL, USA, 2008; pp. 229–267.
25. Offenbacher, AR, Holman, TR. Fatty acid allosteric regulation of C-H activation in plant and animal lipoxygenases. Molecules 2020, 25, 3374.
26. Casey, R. Lipoxygenases. In *Seed Proteins*; Shewry PR, Casey R, Eds, Springer: Dordrecht, The Netherlands, 1999; pp. 685–708.
27. Gardner HW. Recent investigations into the lipoxygenase pathway of plants. Biochimica et Biophysica Acta (BBA)-Lipids and Lipid Metabolism. 1991 Jul 30;1084(3):221–39.
28. Siedow JN. Plant lipoxygenase: structure and function. Annual Review of Plant Biology. 1991 Jun;42(1):145–88.
29. Hamberg M. Pathways in the biosynthesis of oxylipins in plants. J Lipid Mediat. 1993;6:375–84.
30. Leone A, Melillo MT, Bleve-Zacheo T. Lipoxygenase in pea roots subjected to biotic stress. Plant Science. 2001 Sep 1;161(4):703–17.
31. Hughes RK, West SI, Hornostaj AR, Lawson DM, Fairhurst SA, Sanchez RO, Hough P, Robinson BH, Casey R. Probing a novel potato lipoxygenase with dual positional specificity reveals primary determinants of substrate binding and requirements for a surface hydrophobic loop and has implications for the role of lipoxygenases in tubers. Biochemical Journal. 2001 Jan 15;353(2):345–55.
32. Howe GA, Schilmiller AL. Oxylipin metabolism in response to stress. Current Opinion in Plant Biology. 2002 Jun 1;5(3):230–6.
33. Brash AR. Mechanistic aspects of CYP74 allene oxide synthases and related cytochrome P450 enzymes. Phytochemistry. 2009 Sep 1;70(13–14):1522–31.
34. Meng Y, Liang Y, Liao B, He W, Liu Q, Shen X, Xu J, Chen S. Genome-wide identification, characterization and expression analysis of lipoxygenase gene family in Artemisia annua L. Plants (Basel) 2022;11:655.
35. Melan MA, Dong X, Endara ME, Davis KR, Ausubel FM, Peterman TK. An Arabidopsis thaliana lipoxygenase gene can be induced by pathogens, abscisic acid, and methyl jasmonate. Plant Physiol. 1993;101:441–450.
36. Bell E, Creelman RA, Mullet JE. A chloroplast lipoxygenase is required for wound-induced jasmonic acid accumulation in Arabidopsis. Proc. Natl. Acad. Sci. USA 1995; 92:8675–8679.
37. Vellosillo T, Martínez M, López MA, Vicente J, Cascón T, Dolan L, Hamberg M, Castresana C. Oxylipins produced by the 9-lipoxygenase pathway in Arabidopsis regulate lateral root development and defense responses through a specific signaling cascade. Plant Cell 2007;19:831–846.
38. Caldelari D, Wang G, Farmer EE, Dong X. Arabidopsis lox3 lox4 double mutants are male sterile and defective in global proliferative arrest. Plant Mol. Biol. 2010;75:25–33.
39. Santomauro F, Donato R, Pini G, Sacco C, Ascrizzi R, Bilia A. Liquid and vapor-phase activity of Artemisia annua essential oil against pathogenic Malassezia spp. Planta Med. 2017;84:160–167.
40. Marla SS, Singh VK. LOX genes in blast fungus (Magnaporthe grisea) resistance in rice. Funct. Integr. Genom. 2012;12:265–275.
41. Crozier A. Biosynthesis of hormones and elicitor molecules. In *Biochemistry and Molecular Biology of Plants*; Buchanan BB, Gruissem W, Jones RL, Eds. 2002. Wiley.
42. Kaur KD, Jha A, Sabikhi L, Singh AK. Significance of coarse cereals in health and nutrition: a review. Journal of Food Science and Technology. 2014 Aug;51(8):1429–41.

43. Park YS, Kunze S, Ni X, Feussner I, Kolomiets MV. Comparative molecular and biochemical characterization of segmentally duplicated 9-lipoxygenase genes ZmLOX4 and ZmLOX5 of maize. Planta. 2010 May;231(6):1425–37.
44. Vellosillo T, Aguilera V, Marcos R, Bartsch M, Vicente J, Cascón T, Hamberg M, Castresana C. Defense activated by 9-lipoxygenase-derived oxylipins requires specific mitochondrial proteins. Plant Physiology. 2013 Feb;161(2):617–27.
45. Davoine C, Falletti O, Douki T, Iacazio G, Ennar N, Montillet JL, Triantaphylidès C (2006) Adducts of oxylipin electrophiles to glutathione refect a 13 specifcity of the downstream lipoxygenase pathway in the tobacco hypersensitive response. Plant Physiol 140:1484–1493.
46. Lim CW, Han SW, Hwang IS, Kim DS, Hwang BK, Lee SC. The pepper lipoxygenase CaLOX1 plays a role in osmotic, drought and high salinity stress response. Plant and Cell Physiology. 2015 May 1;56(5):930–42.
47. Hou Y, Meng K, Han Y, Ban Q, Wang B, Suo J, Lv J, Rao J. The persimmon 9-lipoxygenase gene DkLOX3 plays positive roles in both promoting senescence and enhancing tolerance to abiotic stress. Frontiers in Plant Science. 2015 Dec 10;6:1073.
48. Chauvin A, Caldelari D, Wolfender JL, Farmer EE. Four 13-lipoxygenases contribute to rapid jasmonate synthesis in wounded Arabidopsis thaliana leaves: a role for lipoxygenase 6 in responses to long-distance wound signals. New Phytologist. 2013 Jan;197(2):566–75.
49. Schommer C, Palatnik JF, Aggarwal P, Chételat A, Cubas P, Farmer EE, Nath U, Weigel D. Control of jasmonate biosynthesis and senescence by miR319 targets. PLoS Biology. 2008 Sep;6(9):e230.
50. Del Ángel-Coronel OA, León-García E, Vela-Gutiérrez G, Rojas-Reyes JO, Gómez-Lim MÁ, García HS. Lipoxygenase activity associated to fruit ripening and senescence in chayote (Sechium edule Jacq. Sw. cv.“virens levis”). Journal of Food Biochemistry. 2018 Feb;42(1):e12438.
51. Schiller D, Contreras C, Vogt J, Dunemann F, Defilippi BG, Beaudry R, Schwab W. A dual positional specific lipoxygenase functions in the generation of flavor compounds during climacteric ripening of apple. Horticulture Research. 2015 Dec 23;2.
52. Schaller A, Stintzi A. Enzymes in jasmonate biosynthesis–structure, function, regulation. Phytochemistry. 2009 Sep 1;70(13–14):1532–8.
53. Liu X, Li F, Tang J, Wang W, Zhang F, Wang G, Chu J, Yan C, Wang T, Chu C, Li C. Activation of the jasmonic acid pathway by depletion of the hydroperoxide lyase OsHPL3 reveals crosstalk between the HPL and AOS branches of the oxylipin pathway in rice. PLoS One. 2012 Nov 29;7(11):e50089.
54. La Camera S, Gouzerh G, Dhondt S, Hoffmann L, Fritig B, Legrand M, Heitz T. Metabolic reprogramming in plant innate immunity: the contributions of phenylpropanoid and oxylipin pathways. Immunological Reviews. 2004 Apr;198(1):267–84.
55. Lee DS, Nioche P, Hamberg M, Raman CS. Structural insights into the evolutionary paths of oxylipin biosynthetic enzymes. Nature. 2008 Sep;455(7211):363–8.
56. Li L, Chang Z, Pan Z, Fu ZQ, Wang X. Modes of heme binding and substrate access for cytochrome P450 CYP74A revealed by crystal structures of allene oxide synthase. Proceedings of the National Academy of Sciences. 2008 Sep 16;105(37):13883–8.
57. Tyagi C, Singh A, Singh IK. Mechanistic insights into mode of action of rice allene oxide synthase on hydroxyperoxides: An intermediate step in herbivory-induced jasmonate pathway. Computational Biology and Chemistry. 2016 Oct 1;64:227–36.
58. Grechkin AN, Hamberg M. The “heterolytic hydroperoxide lyase” is an isomerase producing a short-lived fatty acid hemiacetal. Biochimica et Biophysica Acta (BBA)-Molecular and Cell Biology of Lipids. 2004 Feb 27;1636(1):47–58.

59. Griffiths G. Biosynthesis and analysis of plant oxylipins. Free Radical Research. 2015 May 4;49(5):565–82.
60. Rustgi S, Springer A, Kang C, Von Wettstein D, Reinbothe C, Reinbothe S, Pollmann S. Allene oxide synthase and hydroperoxide lyase, two non-canonical cytochrome P450s in Arabidopsis thaliana and their different roles in plant defense. International Journal of Molecular Sciences. 2019 Jan;20(12):3064.
61. Farmer EE, Goossens A. Jasmonates: what allene oxide synthase does for plants. Journal of Experimental Botany. 2019 Jun 15;70(13):3373–8.
62. Song WC, Brash AR. Purification of an allene oxide synthase and identification of the enzyme as a cytochrome P-450. Science. 1991 Aug 16;253(5021):781–4.
63. Song WC, Funk CD, Brash AR. Molecular cloning of an allene oxide synthase: a cytochrome P450 specialized for the metabolism of fatty acid hydroperoxides. Proceedings of the National Academy of Sciences. 1993 Sep 15;90(18):8519–23.
64. Laudert D, Pfannschmidt U, Lottspeich F, Holländer-Czytko H, Weiler EW. Cloning, molecular and functional characterization of Arabidopsis thaliana allene oxide synthase (CYP 74), the first enzyme of the octadecanoid pathway to jasmonates. Plant Molecular Biology. 1996 May;31(2):323–35.
65. Pan Z, Durst F, Werck-Reichhart D, Gardner HW, Camara B, Cornish K, Backhaus RA. The major protein of guayule rubber particles is a cytochrome P450: characterization based on cDNA cloning and spectroscopic analysis of the solubilized enzyme and its reaction products. Journal of Biological Chemistry. 1995 Apr 14;270(15):8487–94.
66. Grechkin AN, Mukhtarova LS, Hamberg M. The lipoxygenase pathway in tulip (Tulipa gesneriana): detection of the ketol route. Biochemical Journal. 2000 Dec 1;352(2):501–9.
67. Utsunomiya Y, Nakayama T, Oohira H, Hirota R, Mori T, Kawai F, Ueda T. Purification and inactivation by substrate of an allene oxide synthase (CYP74) from corn (Zea mays L.) seeds. Phytochemistry. 2000 Feb 2;53(3):319–23.
68. Howe GA, Lee GI, Itoh A, Li L, DeRocher AE. Cytochrome P450-dependent metabolism of oxylipins in tomato. Cloning and expression of allene oxide synthase and fatty acid hydroperoxide lyase. Plant Physiology. 2000 Jun;123(2):711–24.
69. Hamberg M. New cyclopentenone fatty acids formed from linoleic and linolenic acids in potato. Lipids. 2000 Apr;35(4):353–63.
70. Chehab EW, Perea JV, Gopalan B, Theg S, Dehesh K. Oxylipin pathway in rice and Arabidopsis. Journal of Integrative Plant Biology. 2007 Jan;49(1):43–51.
71. Mosblech A, Feussner I, Heilmann I. Oxylipins: structurally diverse metabolites from fatty acid oxidation. Plant Physiology and Biochemistry. 2009 Jun 1;47(6):511–7.
72. Maucher H, Hause B, Feussner I, Ziegler J, Wasternack C. Allene oxide synthases of barley (Hordeum vulgare cv. Salome): tissue specific regulation in seedling development. The Plant Journal. 2000 Jan;21(2):199–213.
73. Zeng J, Zhang T, Huangfu J, Li R, Lou Y. Both allene oxide synthases genes are involved in the biosynthesis of herbivore-induced jasmonic acid and herbivore resistance in rice. Plants. 2021 Mar;10(3):442.
74. Sivasankar S, Sheldrick B, Rothstein SJ. Expression of allene oxide synthase determines defense gene activation in tomato. Plant Physiology. 2000 Apr;122(4):1335–42.
75. Stumpe M, Bode J, Göbel C, Wichard T, Schaaf A, Frank W, Frank M, Reski R, Pohnert G, Feussner I. Biosynthesis of C9-aldehydes in the moss Physcomitrella patens. Biochimica et Biophysica Acta (BBA)-Molecular and Cell Biology of Lipids. 2006 Mar 1;1761(3):301–12.
76. Tijet N, Brash AR. Allene oxide synthases and allene oxides. Prostaglandins & Other Lipid Mediators. 2002 Aug 1;68:423–31.

77. Grechkin AN. Hydroperoxide lyase and divinyl ether synthase. Prostaglandins & Other Lipid Mediators. 2002 Aug 1;68:457–70.
78. Julia S, Florian B, Ellen H, Cornelia H, Michael S, Bernd F, Wolfgang F, Ralf R, Ivo F. Biosynthesis of allene oxides in Physcomitrella patens. BMC Plant Biology. 2012.
79. Stolterfoht H, Rinnofner C, Winkler M, Pichler H. Recombinant lipoxygenases and hydroperoxide lyases for the synthesis of green leaf volatiles. Journal of Agricultural and Food Chemistry. 2019 Oct 8;67(49):13367–92.
80. Boonprab K, Matsuia K, Yoshida M, Akakabe Y, Chirapart A, Kajiwara T. C6-aldehyde formation by fatty acid hydroperoxide lyase in the brown alga Laminaria angustata. Zeitschrift Für Naturforschung C. 2003 Apr 1;58(3–4):207–14.
81. Matsui K, Shibutani M, Hase T, Kajiwara T. Bell pepper fruit fatty acid hydroperoxide lyase is a cytochrome P450 (CYP74B). Febs Letters. 1996 Sep 23;394(1):21–4.
82. Vick BA, Zimmerman DC. Lipoxygenase and hydroperoxide lyase in germinating watermelon seedlings. Plant Physiology. 1976 May;57(5):780–8.
83. Itoh A, Vick BA. The purification and characterization of fatty acid hydroperoxide lyase in sunflower. Biochimica et Biophysica Acta (BBA)-Molecular and Cell Biology of Lipids. 1999 Jan 4;1436(3):531–40.
84. Hughes RK, Yousafzai FK, Ashton R, Chechetkin IR, Fairhurst SA, Hamberg M, Casey R. Evidence for communality in the primary determinants of CYP74 catalysis and of structural similarities between CYP74 and classical mammalian P450 enzymes. Proteins: Structure, Function, and Bioinformatics. 2008 Sep;72(4):1199–211.
85. Denisov IG, Makris TM, Sligar SG, Schlichting I. Structure and chemistry of cytochrome P450. Chemical reviews. 2005 Jun 8;105(6):2253–78.
86. Gorina SS, Mukhtarova LS, Iljina TM, Toporkova YY, Grechkin AN. Detection of divinyl ether synthase CYP74H2 biosynthesizing (11Z)-etheroleic and (1′Z)-colnelenic acids in asparagus (Asparagus officinalis L.). Phytochemistry. 2022 Aug 1;200:113212.
87. Göbel C, Feussner I, Schmidt A, Scheel D, Sanchez-Serrano J, Hamberg M, Rosahl S. Oxylipin profiling reveals the preferential stimulation of the 9-lipoxygenase pathway in elicitor-treated potato cells. Journal of Biological Chemistry. 2001 Mar 2;276(9):6267–73.
88. Gullner G, Künstler A, Király L, Pogány M, Tóbiás I. Up-regulated expression of lipoxygenase and divinyl ether synthase genes in pepper leaves inoculated with Tobamoviruses. Physiological and molecular plant pathology. 2010 Sep 1;74(5–6):387–93.
89. Fammartino A, Verdaguer B, Fournier J, Tamietti G, Carbonne F, Esquerré-Tugayé MT, Cardinale F. Coordinated transcriptional regulation of the divinyl ether biosynthetic genes in tobacco by signal molecules related to defense. Plant Physiology and Biochemistry. 2010 Apr 1;48(4):225–31.
90. Ogorodnikova AV, Mukhitova FK, Grechkin AN. Screening of divinyl ether synthase activity in nonphotosynthetic tissue of asparagales. Doklady Biochemistry and Biophysics 2013 Mar 1;449(1):116.
91. Gogolev YV, Gorina SS, Gogoleva NE, Toporkova YY, Chechetkin IR, Grechkin AN. Green leaf divinyl ether synthase: gene detection, molecular cloning and identification of a unique CYP74B subfamily member. Biochimica et Biophysica Acta (BBA)-Molecular and Cell Biology of Lipids. 2012 Feb 1;1821(2):287–94.
92. Ogorodnikova AV, Mukhitova FK, Grechkin AN. Oxylipins in the spikemoss Selaginella martensii: Detection of divinyl ethers, 12-oxophytodienoic acid and related cyclopentenones. Phytochemistry. 2015 Oct 1;118:42–50.

93. Ziegler J, Hamberg M, Miersch O, Parthier B. Purification and characterization of allene oxide cyclase from dry corn seeds. Plant Physiology. 1997 Jun 1;114(2):565–73.
94. Ziegler J, Stenzel I, Hause B, Maucher H, Hamberg M, Grimm R, Ganal M, Wasternack C. Molecular cloning of allene oxide cyclase: the enzyme establishing the stereochemistry of octadecanoids and jasmonates. Journal of Biological Chemistry. 2000 Jun 23;275(25):19132–8.
95. Stenzel I, Hause B, Miersch O, Kurz T, Maucher H, Weichert H, Ziegler J, Feussner I, Wasternack C. Jasmonate biosynthesis and the allene oxide cyclase family of Arabidopsis thaliana. Plant molecular biology. 2003 Apr;51(6):895–911.
96. Maucher H, Stenzel I, Miersch O, Stein N, Prasad M, Zierold U, Schweizer P, Dorer C, Hause B, Wasternack C. The allene oxide cyclase of barley (Hordeum vulgare L.)—cloning and organ-specific expression. Phytochemistry. 2004 Apr 1;65(7):801–11.
97. Hofmann E, Zerbe P, Schaller F. The crystal structure of Arabidopsis thaliana allene oxide cyclase: insights into the oxylipin cyclization reaction. The Plant Cell. 2006 Nov;18(11):3201–17.
98. Schaller F, Zerbe P, Reinbothe S, Reinbothe C, Hofmann E, Pollmann S. The allene oxide cyclase family of Arabidopsis thaliana–localization and cyclization. The FEBS Journal. 2008 May;275(10):2428–41.
99. Delker C, Stenzel I, Hause B, Miersch O, Feussner I, Wasternack C. Jasmonate biosynthesis in Arabidopsis thaliana-enzymes, products, regulation. Plant Biology. 2006 May;8(03):297–306.
100. DeLano, W. L., & Lam, J. W. PyMOL: A communications tool for computational models . In Abstracts of Papers of the American Chemical Society 2005, August;230:U1371–U1372.
101. Yoeun S, Cho K, Han O. Structural evidence for the substrate channeling of rice allene oxide cyclase in biologically analogous Nazarov reaction. Frontiers in Chemistry. 2018 Oct 30;6:500.
102. Gu XC, Chen JF, Xiao Y, Di P, Xuan HJ, Zhou X, Zhang L, Chen WS. Overexpression of allene oxide cyclase promoted tanshinone/phenolic acid production in Salvia miltiorrhiza. Plant Cell Reports. 2012 Dec;31(12):2247–59.
103. Lu X, Zhang F, Shen Q, Jiang W, Pan Q, Lv Z, Yan T, Fu X, Wang Y, Qian H, Tang K. Overexpression of allene oxide cyclase improves the biosynthesis of artemisinin in Artemisia annua L. PLoS One. 2014 Mar 18;9(3):e91741.
104. Stenzel I, Otto M, Delker C, Kirmse N, Schmidt D, Miersch O, Hause B, Wasternack C. Allene Oxide Cyclase (AOC) gene family members of Arabidopsis thaliana: tissue-and organ-specific promoter activities and in vivo heteromerization. Journal of Experimental Botany. 2012 Oct 1;63(17):6125–38.
105. Hunt R, Thomas B, Murphy DJ, Murray D. Growth analysis, individual plants. Encyclopedia of Applied Plant Sciences. 2003;2:579–88.
106. Maynard D, Gröger H, Dierks T, Dietz KJ. The function of the oxylipin 12-oxophytodienoic acid in cell signaling, stress acclimation, and development. Journal of Experimental Botany. 2018 Nov 26;69(22):5341–54.
107. Breithaupt C, Kurzbauer R, Lilie H, Schaller A, Strassner J, Huber R, Macheroux P, Clausen T. Crystal structure of 12-oxophytodienoate reductase 3 from tomato: self-inhibition by dimerization. Proceedings of the National Academy of Sciences. 2006 Sep 26;103(39):14337–42.
108. Schaller F, Weiler EW. Molecular Cloning and Characterization of 12-Oxophytodienoate Reductase, an Enzyme of the Octadecanoid Signaling Pathway fromArabidopsis thaliana: structural and functional relationship to yeast old yellow enzyme. Journal of Biological Chemistry. 1997 Oct 31;272(44):28066–72.

109. Zheng H, Pan X, Deng Y, Wu H, Liu P, Li X. AtOPR3 specifically inhibits primary root growth in Arabidopsis under phosphate deficiency. Scientific reports. 2016 Apr 22;6(1):1–1.
110. Muench M, Hsin CH, Ferber E, Berger S, Mueller MJ. Reactive electrophilic oxylipins trigger a heat stress-like response through HSFA1 transcription factors. Journal of experimental botany. 2016 Nov 1;67(21):6139–48.
111. Meza-Canales ID, Meldau S, Zavala JA, Baldwin IT. Herbivore perception decreases photosynthetic carbon assimilation and reduces stomatal conductance by engaging 12-oxo-phytodienoic acid, mitogen-activated protein kinase 4 and cytokinin perception. Plant, Cell & Environment. 2017 Jul;40(7):1039–56.
112. Dave A, Vaistij FE, Gilday AD, Penfield SD, Graham IA. Regulation of Arabidopsis thaliana seed dormancy and germination by 12-oxo-phytodienoic acid. Journal of Experimental Botany. 2016 Apr 1;67(8):2277–84.
113. Alsharafa K, Vogel MO, Oelze ML, Moore M, Stingl N, König K, Friedman H, Mueller MJ, Dietz KJ. Kinetics of retrograde signalling initiation in the high light response of Arabidopsis thaliana. Philosophical Transactions of the Royal Society B: Biological Sciences. 2014 Apr 19;369(1640):20130424.
114. Arnold MD, Gruber C, Floková K, Miersch O, Strnad M, Novák O, Wasternack C, Hause B. The recently identified isoleucine conjugate of cis-12-oxo-phytodienoic acid is partially active in cis-12-oxo-phytodienoic acid-specific gene expression of Arabidopsis thaliana. PloS One. 2016 Sep 9;11(9):e0162829.

5 Plants Oxylipins Induction and Regulation

Genetic Insights

Abdul Qadir Khan[1], *Ali Muhammad*[2], *Khawaja Shafique Ahmad*[1*], *Ansar Mehmood*[1], *Abdul Hamid*[3,4], *Fahim Nawaz*[5], *and Nazir Suliman*[6]

[1]Department of Botany, University of Poonch Rawalakot, 12350, Azad Jammu and Kashmir, Pakistan

[2]Department of Zoology, University of Poonch Rawalakot, 12350, Azad Jammu and Kashmir, Pakistan

[3]Department of Horticulture, University of Poonch Rawalakot, 12350, Azad Jammu and Kashmir, Pakistan

[4]Vice Chancellor, Women University of Azad Jammu and Kashmir Bagh, Pakistan

[5]Department of Agronomy, MNS, University of Agriculture, Multan, Pakistan

[6]Department of Pharmacy, University of Poonch Rawalakot, 12350, Azad Jammu and Kashmir, Pakistan

*Correspondence: Khawaja Shafique Ahmad, shafiquebot@gmail.com; ahmadks@upr.edu.pk

CONTENTS

DOI: 10.1201/9781003316558-5

5.1 INTRODUCTION

Plant oxylipins are lipid metabolites which are produced when unsaturated fatty acids are oxidized. Plant fatty acids, volatile aldehydes, ketofatty acids, divinyl ethers and the jasmonate are all phyto-oxylipins (JA). Fatty acid hydroperoxides synthesis which can be achieved by the action of enzymes [1] or chemo-oxidationis the first step in oxylipin biosynthesis [2].

5.2 ENZYMATICALLY FORMED OXYLIPINS

The principal catalysts for producing fatty acids hydroperoxides such as linoleate, α-linoleate, and roughanic acids are α-dioxygenase (α-DOX) [3] or lipidoxygenases (LOXs) [4]. There are several different pathways for hydroperoxide conversion initiated by different enzymes such as divinyl ether synthase (DES), hydroperoxide lyases (HPL), allene oxide synthase (AOS), epoxy alcohol synthase (EAS) and peroxygenases (PXG). Oxylipins with reactive epoxid, unsaturated carbonyl, or aldehydes, as well as phytohormones such jasmonic acid, are generated as oxygenated derivatives.

5.3 CHEMICALLY FORMED OXYLIPINS

Chemical membrane lipid peroxidation can be mediated by reactive oxygen species and oxidative stress, as compared to the enzymatic synthesis of pure oxylipin enantiomers [2, 5]. The oxylipins production process, whether enzymatic or chemical, is primarily determined by two factors: (i) LOXs route includes mostly fatty acids hydroperoxides with abundance of one or the other enantiomer [6], (ii) hydroxy fatty acids undergo chemical oxidation that can add molecular oxygen to LA or -leA at C-9 or C-13 generates Position isomers, while the formation of hydroxides of LA and α-LeA is primarily due to reactive oxygen species. Plant tissues contain a high number of oxylipins formed by chemical oxidation as well as enzymatically by LOX [7].

5.4 OCCURRENCE OF OXYLIPINS

Gerwick et al., [9] coined the term oxylipin to characterize oxygenated compounds synthesized by monooxygenase or dioxygenase from fatty acids. Furthermore, to recruit the materialization of oxidized fatty acid end products other enzymes, like hydratases, have been reported [10]. The label oxylipin is nowadays used to describe compounds made chemically from unsaturated fatty acids [11].

Almost every living organism has oxylipins. Prokaryotes like cyanobacteria synthesize just simple oxylipins derived through one or two metabolic paths, but eukaryotes such as mosses, algae as well as angiosperms have complex pathways that result in over 500 distinct compounds [12]. Plants, on the other hand, have made great progress in jasmonate metabolism.

Jasmonate and its derivatives such as methyl ester (JA-Me) were initially originated in fungal species *Lasiodiplodiatheobromae* [13] and were later detected in a wide spectrum of land plants (Meyer et al., 1984). In the same way that spikemosses *Selaginella martensii* and Physcomitrella patens produce 12-oxo-phytodienoic acid [OPDA), a jasmonate precursor but unable to produce JA [14], however *Marchantia polymorpha*, ancient lineage of existing land plants, are unable to produce JA but may synthesize 12-oxo-phytodienoic acid (OPDA) one of the JA precursors [14]. It was reported by Pratiwi et al., [15] that JA, isoleucine jasmonic acid (JA-Ile) and OPDA synthesis can be induced by wound in *Selaginella moellendorffii.*

Furthermore, JA biosynthetic homologs exhibit a diverse distribution pattern, which could reflect the existence and lack of JA in recent evolutionary lineages, due to transfer of gene horizontally from virulent and symbiotic bacteria [16].

In nonvascular land plants, the existence of OPDA but not of JA supports a co-evolution of small-molecular-mass mixtures with divergent signaling characteristics, indicating that these plants emerged from different lineages. In nonvascular terrestrial plants, the absence of JA and the presence of OPDA indicate co-evolution of light weight molecular compounds having divergent signaling characteristics, revealing the diverse origin of plants.

As a component of oomycete pathogens, arachidonic acid (AA) and its oxygenated derivatives, which are absent in angiosperms, interfere strongly with the plant's salicylic acid (SA) and JA pathways, which display AA sensation [17]. According to recent comprehensive analysis, there is an inverse relationship between the presence of JA and AA in nonvascular plants, algae, and lichen, confirming lipid biosynthetic versatility in the kingdom Plantae [18].

5.5 SYNTHESIS OF OXYLIPINS

When polyunsaturated fatty acids such as octadecanoic acid or linoleate are oxidized, they form oxylipins, a category of lipid-derived signaling molecules [19]. Oxylipins a group of lipid-originated signaling compounds are synthesized by the oxidation of polyunsaturated fatty acids (PUFAs) such as octadecanoic acid or linoleate. Lipases, like Dongle (DGL) and in Anther Dehiscence1 (DAD1) from plastidial membrane lipids produce these fatty acids, which are then oxidized by lipoxygenases (LOX) to make hydroperoxides [20] (Figure 5.1).

Within plastid the octadecanoid process that leads to jasmonic acid (JA) in Arabidopsis initiated by means of 13-lipoxygenase (13-LOX) action and convert octadecatrienoic acid to 13-hydroperoxylinolenic acid, which is then transformed to 12-oxo-phytodienoic acid (cis-OPDA). COMATOSE (CTS) is a transporter protein that transports cis-OPDA from the cytosol to the peroxisome [21]. The reduction and activation of cis-OPDA into CoA ester within peroxisomes produces jasmonate, which is then followed by rounds of -oxidation [22]. Along with allen oxide synthase (AOS), hydroperoxide lyases (HPLs) cleave plastidial fatty acid hydroperoxides into hexanaldehyde and green leaf volatiles (GLVs). When HPL is overexpressed, AOS and HPL compete for hydroperoxide substrates, and cis-OPDA and JA levels are lowered [23].

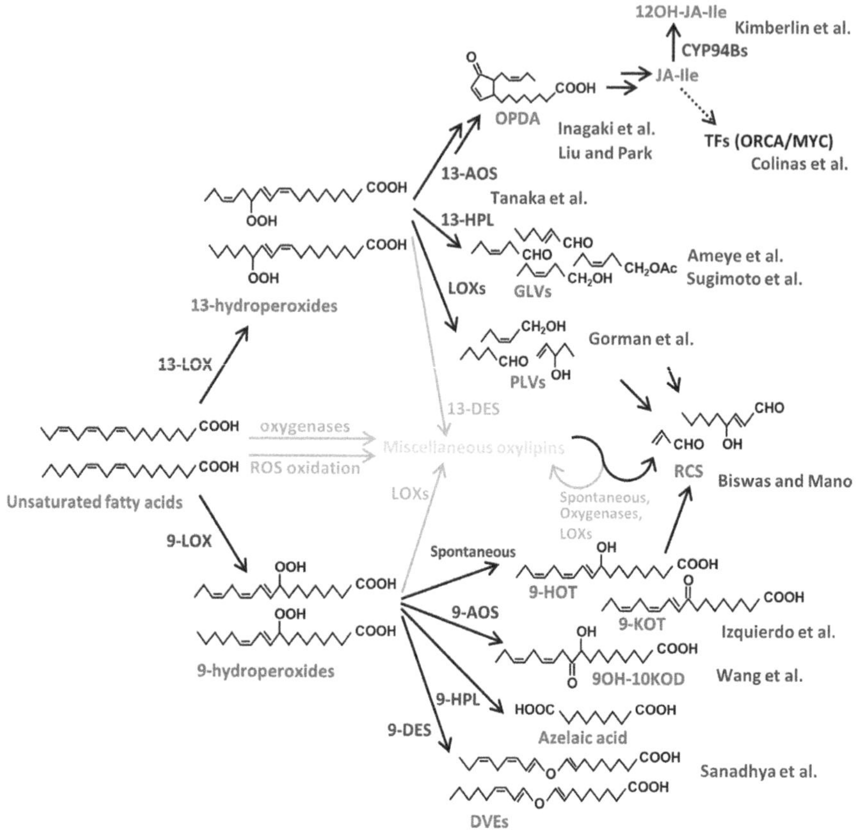

FIGURE 5.1 Various oxylipin biosynthesis pathways in plants. The enzymatic or non-enzymatic oxidation of unsaturated fatty acid's enzymatic or non-enzymatic oxidation, such as linolenic acid and linoleic acid in this diagram, is the first step in the production of plant oxylipins primarily; unsaturated fatty acids like linolenic acid and linoleic are chemically or enzymatically oxidized to initiate oxylipins synthesis. The mechanisms are displayed in blue while compounds involved in this process are indicated as red. The authors' names are displayed in green following the process described by them. AOS, allene-oxide synthase; LOX, lipoxygenase; DVEs divinyl ethers; CYP, cytochrome P450; DES, divinyl ether synthase; HPL, hydroperoxide lyase; RCS, reactive carbonyl species; OPDA, ROS, 12-oxo-phytodienoic acid; reactive oxygen species; JA-Ile, jasmonic acid-isoleucine Conjugate; GLVs, green leaf volatiles; TFs, transcription factors; PLVs, pentyl leaf volatiles; 9OH-10KOD, 9-hydroxy-10keto-octadecadienoic acid [35].

5.6 OXYLIPINS SIGNALING AND BIOSYNTHETIC PATHWAYS

When the unsaturated fatty acids comprising linolenic acids and linoleic acids are oxidized, then the production of phyto-oxylipin begins either enzymatically or non-enzymatically as shown in Figure 5.1. Plant oxylipins are synthesized in a variety of ways. However, we shall examine a few oxylipins synthetic pathways, with a focus on the biosynthesis of jasmonates (JAs).

Jasmonates, also known as defensive phytohormones, are one of the most studied groups of plant oxylipins. The enzyme 13-lipoxygenase (13-LOX) activates jasmonate biosynthesis by converting polyunsaturated fatty acids prevalent in plant membrane lipids to 13-hydroperoxides. 13-allen oxide synthase converts 13-hydroperoxides into 12-oxo-phytodienoic acid (OPDA) and jasmonic acid with the help of allene oxide cyclase, OPDA reductase, and β--oxidation respectively [24].

A cluster of downstream transcription factors regulating translation of certain defense genes are activated by JA [25]. Activation and production of secondary metabolite is one of the defense strategies in plants against various pathogens [26]. Several pharmaceuticals are made from secondary metabolites found in plants. Catharanthus roseus produce monoterpenoid indole alkaloids such as vincristine and vinblastine having anticancer characteristics.

Guo et al., [27] reported that JA signaling dramatically stimulates defense responses without hindering plant development. In order to limit the over expression of defensive mechanism, the active JA is immediately transformed to its lethargic forms by hydroxylation or further process [28]. Liu and Park's latest studies have shown that OPDA promote growth and defense as well as respond against environmental fluctuations. In contrast to vascular plants, mosses do not produce jasmonates and its precursors, rather they synthesize dinor-OPDA and OPDA in response to damage [25]. These mixtures or compounds were discovered to work in mosses via both COI1-independent and COI1-dependent signaling pathways [29].

Additional CYP74 family proteins, 13-hydroperoxide lyase (13-HPL) and 13-divinyl ether synthase (13-DES) create divinyl ethers (DVEs) and green leaf volatiles (GLVs) from 13-hydroperoxides, respectively, in addition to 13-AOS-mediated JA biosynthesis [30]. D'Auria et al., [31] reported that in response to leaf injury, the fast generation of GLVs, known as GLV-burst, is frequently detected in vascular plants, along with leafy-green scent. Tanaka et al., discovered that unlike mosses, all fern species produce GLV-burst. GLVs play a vital role in plants response with their surroundings [32]. Reactive oxygen species (ROS) induction followed by the creation of a range of antioxidative phenylpropanoids, as well as a significant induction of glycosylation processes, were the most significant metabolic modifications discovered. Liavonchanka and Feussner, [33] revealed that as well as the 13-LOX-pathway, another oxylipin synthetic pathway stimulated by 9-LOX is also present in plants that generates 9-hydroperoxides. Using 9-LOX mutants, Wang et al., [34] demonstrated the physiological purpose of several 9-oxylipins. In maize, the 9-LOX mutant was more sensitive to *Fusarium graminearum*-induced *Gibberella* stem rot, implying that 9-oxylipins are involved in pathogen resistance. According to the oxylipin profile and transcriptome analysis, the JA and 9-oxylipin pathways are antagonistically regulated, and JA has an unknown role in increasing sensitivity to this hemi-biotrophic pathogen.

5.7 INDUCTION AND REGULATION OF PHYTO-OXYLIPIN PATHWAYS

Current investigations have revealed that plants have phyto-oxylipin pools of different size, convening an oxylipin mark [36] on a particular cell, tissue, plant, or species.

Upon pathogen attack, injury or cure through signal molecules or elicitors, an abrupt or dramatic change takes place in the configuration of oxidized fatty-acids derivatives, frequently liable to the nature of the strain. For instance, in barley leaves, salicylic acid activates production of hydroxy-fatty-acid derivatives [37], while methyl jasmonate stimulates an addition of aldehydes in the same plants [38]. Moreover, in response to stress circumstances the signs or factors which favor one biosynthetic path over another are disregarded. Conversely, in defining the various phyto-oxylipin profiles, the activities, compartmentalization, and comparative building of the biosynthetic enzymes must retain supreme significance.

In contrast to former findings, in all plants, altered oxylipin biosynthetic enzymes do not constitutively exist. For illustration, for the divinyl ether synthase (CYP74D), the coding gene is lacking from the *Arabidopsis* genome and to date, this stroke of enzyme has been noticed as solitary in *Solanaceae* like tobacco, potato, and tomato. Conversely, the spatial and temporal manifestation of diverse biosynthetic enzymes of oxylipin also seems to exist with ultimate reputation; this is exclusively accurate for the LOX isoforms, which harvest the fatty-acid-derived hydroperoxides that are directed over the diverse divisions of LOX conduit. Stimulation of LOXs by means of pathogen infection, mechanical pressure, or wounding has been described in several kinds of plants. Of these LOXs whose orientations are connected with the jasmonic acid's de novo synthesis in reaction to pest outbreaks or cutting, several certainly create its indispensable antecedent (i.e., 13*S*-hydroperoxylinolenic acid). Hence, insect outbreak simplified vulnerability has been perceived in transgenic plants of potato using condensed stages of these specific LOX isoforms [39] and in linolenic acid deficient Arabidopsis plants [40]. In comparison, the LOX pathway that yields 9-hydroperoxide derivatives has been illustrated in plants confronted by means of elicitors or through pathogens [41]. By this fact, it must be understood that 9- and 13-LOX pathways stop distinctive oxylipins (Figure 5.2).

Moreover, if anyone deliberates that the LOX accountable for the renovation of a resilient tobacco to a vulnerable one (perceive beyond) predominantly catalyzes the 9-hydroperoxide fatty acid formation, it is attractive to determine that the 9-LOX trail essentially plays a hazardous part in conversing conflict [43]. The recognition of the physiological starring role of 9-LOX pathway derivatives has grown considerably only in recent times and it grants a novel and thrilling challenge for the following few years. One more basic factor in the guideline of the phyto-oxylipin pathways lies in the compartmentalization of the diverse biosynthetic enzymes. For instance, at least two CYP74s (AOS and hydroperoxide lyase) are positioned in the spinach plastid's casing with a LOX activity [44]. In total, it was freshly testified than in plastids of tomato, AOS was besieged to the inner covering, while the hydroperoxide lyase exist in the superficial crust of this cover [45], raising queries about the starting point and method of fatty acids discharge that are enzyme's substrates. By numerous lipases, comprising ofacyl hydrolases polyunsaturated fatty acids, phospholipases A and D, galacto-kinases can be unconstrained from membranes.

In comparison to animal structures, in which arachidonic acid is progressive from plasma membranes by phospholipase A2, a first model has been recommended for

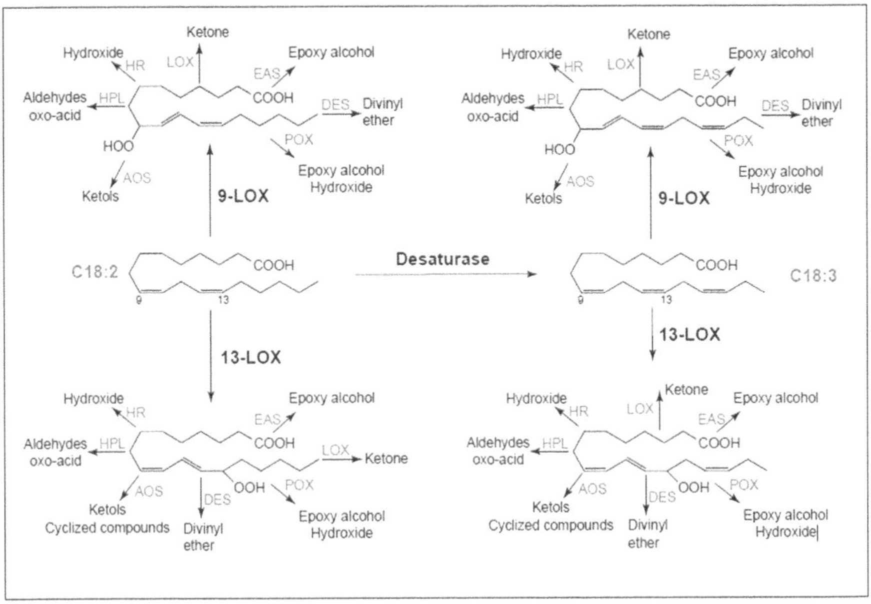

FIGURE 5.2 Linoleic or linolenic acids, which are significant plant's polyunsaturated fatty acids, are the origin of lipoxygenase (LOX) pathways. These fatty acids can be converted into 9- or 13-hydroperoxide derivatives, which are decomposed by epoxy alcohol synthase (EAS), CYP74s, divinyl ether synthase (DES), allene oxide synthase (AOS), hydroperoxide lyase (HPL), LOX otherwise an uncharacterized reductase (HR) depending on LOX mechanism specificity. The existence, qualified quantities, and compartmentalization of enzymes in various biosynthetic paths result in a diversity of pyroxylins produced through different competing processes [7]. As an alternative, 9-LOX-derived fungitoxic compounds such as hydroxylated fatty acids or divinyl ethers readily collect in diseased plants [42].

the release of linolenic acid from plant plasma-lemma by a parallel enzyme. In line with this hypothesis, phospholipase-A activity was established to be persuaded by wounding [46]. Though, it is well-documented that this stress also triggers manifold customs of phospholipase D [47]. Antisense annulment of one isoform led to a partial decline of jasmonic acid accretion in wounded transgenic Arabidopsis, proposing a promising participation of this sort of enzyme in biosynthesis of jasmonic acid [34]. On the other hand, in plasma, the localization of these enzyme actions and the microsomal membranes, advances the interrogation of how the fatty acids that are left on the cell surface might be moved to the plastids to be metabolized into oxylipins.

Next, A1 phospholipase connected to the jasmonic acid establishment, that harmonizes physiological happenings such as anther dehiscence, flower opening, and pollen maturation was set up to be coupled with chloroplasts. Such an enzyme catalyzes the dilapidation of plastidial phosphatidyl choline and might be used in the biosynthesis of jasmonate, which is a signal molecule for plant resistance responses.

In plants, most of the polyunsaturated fatty acids are connected to the galacto-lipids, which are constrained to plastids.

Hence, an alternative would result in the discharge of linoleic acids from galactolipids by a plastidial lipase. In view of this assumption, the cyclic precursor of jasmonic acid has been associated with mono galactosyldiglyceride, and acylhydrolases practiced of hydrolyzing galactolipids are provoked in response to drought, virus attack stress [48]. Though it might appear implausible that all of the phyto-oxylipins consist of plastids, their roots will hang decisively on the nature of stress, isoform of the persuaded LOX and on the fatty acid arrangement of a specific tissue or organ.

5.8 THE ROLE OF PHYTO-OXYLIPINS

Phyto-oxylipins are important chemical compounds that are implicated in plant growth, development, and defense. Recent studies demonstrate that esterified oxylipins, such as linolipins and arabidopsides, have great contribution in defense. These compounds are primarily produced during stressful situations. For instance, in *A. thaliana*, oxylipins production is highest against abiotic and biotic stressors, such as pathogen attack, cold, and wounding [49]. In addition, arabidopsides accumulate not only in injured but also in normal leaves of the infected plant [50]. Furthermore, oxylipins production in *A. thaliana* is influenced by stress condition as more oxidized oxylipins are produced in injury as compared to freezing [49]. In contrast to wild type, A. thaliana lox2–1 mutant is more sensitive to herbivory by *Spodoptera littoralis* larvae because of its lack of arabidopside production [50].

According to a recent study, 24-epibrassinolide (EPB), a plant hormone concerned in plant stress responses, causes enhanced linolipin synthesis in flax leaves [51]. Esterified oxylipins have a development function in plants. Linolipin profiles, for example, vary according to plant development stage. On day 23, in juvenile flax leaves they were not found; nevertheless, production reached an absorption of 71 nmol/g FW by 35 days [52].

5.9 INDIRECT PURPOSES OF ESTERIFIED OXYLIPINS

Oxylipins are supposed to be generated as needed [53]. The discovery of AtPLAI and pPLAIIa, *A. thaliana* phospholipases that can yield free OPDA from oxidized glycolipids supports this idea [54, 55]. Arabidopside concentration is also higher in various mutant forms of A. thaliana which show reduced pPLAIIa expression [56].

Free OPDA can induce a JA-independent response, implying that it could regulate gene expression directly. The ability of OPDA to trigger gene expression results in a number of JA-Ile independent responses [57]. OPDA is implicated in plant defense against fungal infections, drought stress, and insects [58].

5.10 DIRECT FUNCTIONS OF ESTERIFIED OXYLIPINS

Esterified oxylipins were proposed not only to act as a free oxylipins reservoir, but they might also have a direct function. Some of them, such as arabidopside E and

P. syringae, were found to limit pathogen growth in vitro, although the same concentration of free OPDA had no effect on its growth [5]. In addition, arabidopsides G and E reduce *B. cinerea* growth in vitro [59], while its form A exhibits antifungal activities against pathogens including *Sclerotinia sclerotiorum*, *Leptosphaeria maculans*, and *Alternaria brassicicola* [59, 60].

Arabidopside types such as A, B, D, and F can retard the growth of cress roots, implying that plant esterified oxylipins may play a developmental role [61]. They might play a function in senescence as in A. thaliana mutants timely leaf senescence was detected [62]. All of these findings suggest that esterified oxylipins may show a direct part in plant stress responses and developmental processes.

5.11 CONCLUSION

Phyto-oxylipins are important chemical compounds that are implicated in plant growth, development, and defense. These compounds are primarily produced during stressful situations. Oxylipins synthesized by oxidation of polyunsaturated fatty acids are structurally diverse metabolites. They are predominantly produced in response to abiotic and biotic stress such as wound, pathogen attack, or cold. Chemical membrane lipid peroxidation can be mediated by reactive oxygen species and oxidative stress, as compared to the enzymatic synthesis of pure oxylipin enantiomers. One of the oxylipin synthetic pathways includes a lipoxygenase (LOX) pathway that results in jasmonic acid (JA) synthesis. JA synthesis stimulates defense response genes without affecting plant development. Furthermore, oxylipins as being ubiquitous in nature indicates their significant importance in development and defense.

REFERENCES

1. Blée, E., 1998. Phytooxylipins and Plant Defense Reactions. *Progress in Lipid Research*, *37*(1), pp.33–72.
2. Mueller, M.J., 2004. Archetype signals in plants: the phytoprostanes. *Current Opinion in Plant Biology*, *7*(4), pp.441–448.
3. Hamberg, M., de Leon, I.P., Rodriguez, M.J. and Castresana, C., 2005. α-Dioxygenases. *Biochemical and Biophysical Research Communications*, *338*(1), pp.169–174.
4. Feussner, I. and Wasternack, C., 2002. The lipoxygenase pathway. *Annual Review of Plant Biology*, *53*(1), pp.275–297.
5. Andersson, M.X., Hamberg, M., Kourtchenko, O., Brunnstro, Å., McPhail, K.L., Gerwick, W.H., Go, C., Feussner, I. and Ellerstro, M., 2006. Oxylipin profiling of the hypersensitive response in Arabidopsis thaliana: formation of a novel oxo-phytodienoic acid-containing galactolipid, arabidopside E. *Journal of Biological Chemistry*, *281*(42), pp.31528–31537.
6. Schneider, C., Pratt, D.A., Porter, N.A. and Brash, A.R., 2007. Control of oxygenation in lipoxygenase and cyclooxygenase catalysis. *Chemistry & Biology*, *14*(5), pp.473–488.
7. Blée, E., 2002. Impact of phyto-oxylipins in plant defense. *Trends in Plant Science*, *7*(7), pp.315–322.
8. Mosblech, A., Feussner, I. and Heilmann, I., 2009. Oxylipins: structurally diverse metabolites from fatty acid oxidation. *Plant Physiology and Biochemistry*, *47*(6), pp.511–517.

9. Gerwick, W.H., Moghaddam, M. and Hamberg, M., 1991. Oxylipin metabolism in the red alga Gracilariopsislemaneiformis: mechanism of formation of vicinal dihydroxy fatty acids. *Archives of Biochemistry and Biophysics, 290*(2), pp.436–444.
10. Volkov, A., Liavonchanka, A., Kamneva, O., Fiedler, T., Goebel, C., Kreikemeyer, B. and Feussner, I., 2010. Myosin cross-reactive antigen of Streptococcus pyogenes M49 encodes a fatty acid double bond hydratase that plays a role in oleic acid detoxification and bacterial virulence. *Journal of Biological Chemistry, 285*(14), pp.10353–10361.
11. Frankel, E.N., 1980. Lipid oxidation. *Progress in Lipid Research, 19*(1–2), pp.1–22.
12. Andreou, A., Brodhun, F. and Feussner, I., 2009. Biosynthesis of oxylipins in non-mammals. *Progress in Lipid Research, 48*(3–4), pp.148–170.
13. Aldridge, D.C., Galt, S., Giles, D. and Turner, W.B., 1971. Metabolites of Lasiodiplodiatheobromae. *Journal of the Chemical Society C: Organic*, pp.1623–1627.
14. Bowman, J.L., Kohchi, T., Yamato, K.T., Jenkins, J., Shu, S., Ishizaki, K., Yamaoka, S., Nishihama, R., Nakamura, Y., Berger, F. and Adam, C., 2017. Insights into land plant evolution garnered from the Marchantia polymorpha genome. *Cell, 171*(2), pp.287–304.
15. Pratiwi, P., Tanaka, G., Takahashi, T., Xie, X., Yoneyama, K., Matsuura, H. and Takahashi, K., 2017. Identification of jasmonic acid and jasmonoyl-isoleucine, and characterization of AOS, AOC, OPR and JAR1 in the model lycophyte Selaginella moellendorffii. *Plant and Cell Physiology, 58*(4), pp.789–801.
16. Han, G.Z., 2017. Evolution of jasmonate biosynthesis and signaling mechanisms. *Journal of Experimental Botany, 68*(6), pp.1323–1331.
17. Walley, J.W., Kliebenstein, D.J., Bostock, R.M. and Dehesh, K., 2013. Fatty acids and early detection of pathogens. *Current Opinion in Plant Biology, 16*(4), pp.520–526.
18. Gachet, M.S., Schubert, A., Calarco, S., Boccard, J. and Gertsch, J., 2017. Targeted metabolomics shows plasticity in the evolution of signaling lipids and uncovers old and new endocannabinoids in the plant kingdom. *Scientific Reports, 7*(1), pp.1–15.
19. Wasternack, C. and Kombrink, E., 2010. Jasmonates: structural requirements for lipid-derived signals active in plant stress responses and development. *ACS Chemical Biology, 5*(1), pp.63–77.
20. Bell, E., Creelman, R.A. and Mullet, J.E., 1995. A chloroplast lipoxygenase is required for wound-induced jasmonic acid accumulation in Arabidopsis. *Proceedings of the National Academy of Sciences, 92*(19), pp.8675–8679.
21. Theodoulou, F.L., Job, K., Slocombe, S.P., Footitt, S., Holdsworth, M., Baker, A., Larson, T.R. and Graham, I.A., 2005. Jasmonic acid levels are reduced in COMATOSE ATP-binding cassette transporter mutants. Implications for transport of jasmonate precursors into peroxisomes. *Plant Physiology, 137*(3), pp.835–840.
22. Kienow, L., Schneider, K., Bartsch, M., Stuible, H.P., Weng, H., Miersch, O., Wasternack, C. and Kombrink, E., 2008. Jasmonates meet fatty acids: functional analysis of a new acyl-coenzyme A synthetase family from Arabidopsis thaliana. *Journal of Experimental Botany, 59*(2), pp.403–419.
23. Chehab, E.W., Kaspi, R., Savchenko, T., Rowe, H., Negre-Zakharov, F., Kliebenstein, D. and Dehesh, K., 2008. Distinct roles of jasmonates and aldehydes in plant-defense responses. *PloS One, 3*(4), p.e1904.
24. Acosta, I.F. and Farmer, E.E., 2010. Jasmonates. *The Arabidopsis Book/American Society of Plant Biologists, 8.*
25. Yan, Y., Borrego, E. and Kolomiets, M.V., 2013. Jasmonate biosynthesis, perception and function in plant development and stress responses. *Lipid Metabolism. InTech*, pp.393–442.

26. Ding, Y., Northen, T.R., Khalil, A., Huffaker, A. and Schmelz, E.A., 2021. Getting back to the grass roots: harnessing specialized metabolites for improved crop stress resilience. *Current Opinion in Biotechnology*, *70*, pp.174–186.
27. Guo, Q., Major, I.T. and Howe, G.A., 2018. Resolution of growth–defense conflict: mechanistic insights from jasmonate signaling. *Current Opinion in Plant Biology*, *44*, pp.72–81.
28. Koo, A.J., Cooke, T.F. and Howe, G.A., 2011. Cytochrome P450 CYP94B3 mediates catabolism and inactivation of the plant hormone jasmonoyl-L-isoleucine. *Proceedings of the National Academy of Sciences*, *108*(22), pp.9298–9303.
29. Monte, I., Ishida, S., Zamarreno, A.M., Hamberg, M., Franco-Zorrilla, J.M., Garcia-Casado, G., Gouhier-Darimont, C., Reymond, P., Takahashi, K., Garcia-Mina, J.M. and Nishihama, R., 2018. Ligand-receptor co-evolution shaped the jasmonate pathway in land plants. *Nature Chemical Biology*, *14*(5), pp.480–488.
30. Matsui, K., 2006. Green leaf volatiles: hydroperoxide lyase pathway of oxylipin metabolism. *Current Opinion in Plant Biology*, *9*(3), pp.274–280.
31. D'Auria, J.C., Pichersky, E., Schaub, A., Hansel, A. and Gershenzon, J., 2007. Characterization of a BAHD acyltransferase responsible for producing the green leaf volatile (Z)-3-hexen-1-yl acetate in Arabidopsis thaliana. *The Plant Journal*, *49*(2), pp.194–207.
32. Scala, A., Allmann, S., Mirabella, R., Haring, M.A. and Schuurink, R.C., 2013. Green leaf volatiles: a plant's multifunctional weapon against herbivores and pathogens. *International Journal of Molecular Sciences*, *14*(9), pp.17781–17811.
33. Liavonchanka, A. and Feussner, I., 2006. Lipoxygenases: occurrence, functions and catalysis. *Journal of Plant Physiology*, *163*(3), pp.348–357.
34. Wang, C., Zien, C.A., Afitlhile, M., Welti, R., Hildebrand, D.F. and Wang, X., 2000. Involvement of phospholipase D in wound-induced accumulation of jasmonic acid in Arabidopsis. *The Plant Cell*, *12*(11), pp.2237–2246.
35. Sugimoto, Koichi, Silke Allmann, and Michael V. Kolomiets, eds. *Oxylipins: The Front Line of Plant Interactions*. Frontiers Media SA, 2022.
36. Weber, H., Vick, B.A. and Farmer, E.E., 1997. Dinor-oxo-phytodienoic acid: a new hexadecanoid signal in the jasmonate family. *Proceedings of the National Academy of Sciences*, *94*(19), pp.10473–10478.
37. Weichert, H., Stenzel, I., Berndt, E., Wasternack, C. and Feussner, I., 1999. Metabolic profiling of oxylipins upon salicylate treatment in barley leaves—preferential induction of the reductase pathway by salicylate. *FEBS letters*, *464*(3), pp.133–137.
38. Kohlmann, M., Bachmann, A., Weichert, H., Kolbe, A., Balkenhohl, T., Wasternack, C. and Feussner, I., 1999. Formation of lipoxygenase-pathway-derived aldehydes in barley leaves upon methyl jasmonate treatment. *European Journal of Biochemistry*, *260*(3), pp.885–895.
39. Royo, J., León, J., Vancanneyt, G., Albar, J.P., Rosahl, S., Ortego, F., Castañera, P. and Sánchez-Serrano, J.J., 1999. Antisense-mediated depletion of a potato lipoxygenase reduces wound induction of proteinase inhibitors and increases weight gain of insect pests. *Proceedings of the National Academy of Sciences*, *96*(3), pp.1146–1151.
40. McConn, M., Creelman, R.A., Bell, E., Mullet, J.E. and Browse, J., 1997. Jasmonate is essential for insect defense in Arabidopsis. *Proceedings of the National Academy of Sciences*, *94*(10), pp.5473–5477.
41. Rustérucci, C., Montillet, J.L., Agnel, J.P., Battesti, C., Alonso, B., Knoll, A., Bessoule, J.J., Etienne, P., Suty, L., Blein, J.P. and Triantaphylidès, C., 1999. Involvement of lipoxygenase-dependent production of fatty acid hydroperoxides in the development of the hypersensitive cell death induced by cryptogein on tobacco leaves. *Journal of Biological Chemistry*, *274*(51), pp.36446–36455.

42. Göbel, C., Feussner, I., Schmidt, A., Scheel, D., Sanchez-Serrano, J., Hamberg, M. and Rosahl, S., 2001. Oxylipin profiling reveals the preferential stimulation of the 9-lipoxygenase pathway in elicitor-treated potato cells. *Journal of Biological Chemistry, 276*(9), pp.6267–6273.
43. Rancé, I., Fournier, J. and Esquerré-Tugayé, M.T., 1998. The incompatible interaction between Phytophthora parasitica var. nicotianae race 0 and tobacco is suppressed in transgenic plants expressing antisense lipoxygenase sequences. *Proceedings of the National Academy of Sciences, 95*(11), pp.6554–6559.
44. Blée, E. and Joyard, J., 1996. Envelope membranes from spinach chloroplasts are a site of metabolism of fatty acid hydroperoxides. *Plant Physiology, 110*(2), pp.445–454.
45. Froehlich, J.E., Itoh, A. and Howe, G.A., 2001. Tomato allene oxide synthase and fatty acid hydroperoxide lyase, two cytochrome P450s involved in oxylipin metabolism, are targeted to different membranes of chloroplast envelope. *Plant Physiology, 125*(1), pp.306–317.
46. Narváez-Vásquez, J., Florin-Christensen, J. and Ryan, C.A., 1999. Positional specificity of a phospholipase A activity induced by wounding, systemin, and oligosaccharide elicitors in tomato leaves. *The Plant Cell, 11*(11), pp.2249–2260.
47. Wang, X., 2001. Plant phospholipases. *Annual Review of Plant Biology, 52*(1), pp.211–231.
48. Matos, A.R., d'Arcy-Lameta, A., França, M., Pêtres, S., Edelman, L., Kader, J.C., Zuily-Fodil, Y. and Pham-Thi, A.T., 2001. A novel patatin-like gene stimulated by drought stress encodes a galactolipid acyl hydrolase. *Febs Letters, 491*(3), pp.188–192.
49. Vu, H.S., Roston, R., Shiva, S., Hur, M., Wurtele, E.S., Wang, X., Shah, J. and Welti, R., 2015. Modifications of membrane lipids in response to wounding of Arabidopsis thaliana leaves. *Plant Signaling & Behavior, 10*(9), p.e1056422.
50. Glauser, G., Dubugnon, L., Mousavi, S.A., Rudaz, S., Wolfender, J.L. and Farmer, E.E., 2009. Velocity estimates for signal propagation leading to systemic jasmonic acid accumulation in wounded Arabidopsis. *Journal of Biological Chemistry, 284*(50), pp.34506–34513.
51. Lee, J.H., Lee, J., Kim, H., Chae, W.B., Kim, S.J., Lim, Y.P. and Oh, M.H., 2018. Brassinosteroids regulate glucosinolate biosynthesis in Arabidopsis thaliana. *Physiologia Plantarum, 163*(4), pp.450–458.
52. Chechetkin, I.R., Blufard, A.S., Khairutdinov, B.I., Mukhitova, F.K., Gorina, S.S., Yarin, A.Y., Antsygina, L.L. and Grechkin, A.N., 2013. Isolation and structure elucidation of linolipins C and D, complex oxylipins from flax leaves. *Phytochemistry, 96*, pp.110–116.
53. Dave, A. and Graham, I.A., 2012. Oxylipin signaling: a distinct role for the jasmonic acid precursor cis-(+)-12-oxo-phytodienoic acid (cis-OPDA). *Frontiers in Plant Science, 3*, p.42.
54. Yang, W., Devaiah, S.P., Pan, X., Isaac, G., Welti, R. and Wang, X., 2007. AtPLAI is an acyl hydrolase involved in basal jasmonic acid production and Arabidopsis resistance to Botrytis cinerea. *Journal of Biological Chemistry, 282*(25), pp.18116–18128.
55. Yang, W.Y., Zheng, Y., Bahn, S.C., Pan, X.Q., Li, M.Y., Vu, H.S., Roth, M.R., Scheu, B., Welti, R., Hong, Y.Y. and Wang, X.M., 2012. The patatin-containing phospholipase A pPLAIIα modulates oxylipin formation and water loss in Arabidopsis thaliana. *Molecular Plant, 5*(2), pp.452–460.

56. Davoine, C., Abreu, I.N., Khajeh, K., Blomberg, J., Kidd, B.N., Kazan, K., Schenk, P.M., Gerber, L., Nilsson, O., Moritz, T. and Björklund, S., 2017. Functional metabolomics as a tool to analyze Mediator function and structure in plants. *PloS One*, *12*(6), p.e0179640.
57. Wasternack, C. and Strnad, M., 2016. Jasmonate signaling in plant stress responses and development—active and inactive compounds. *New Biotechnol 33*, pp.604–613.
58. Savchenko, T., Kolla, V.A., Wang, C.Q., Nasafi, Z., Hicks, D.R., Phadungchob, B., Chehab, W.E., Brandizzi, F., Froehlich, J. and Dehesh, K., 2014. Functional convergence of oxylipin and abscisic acid pathways controls stomatal closure in response to drought. *Plant Physiology*, *164*(3), pp.1151–1160.
59. Kourtchenko, O., Andersson, M.X., Hamberg, M., Brunnstrom, A., Göbel, C., McPhail, K.L., Gerwick, W.H., Feussner, I. and Ellerström, M., 2007. Oxo-phytodienoic acid-containing galactolipids in Arabidopsis: jasmonate signaling dependence. *Plant Physiology*, *145*(4), pp.1658–1669.
60. Pedras, M.S.C. and To, Q.H., 2017. Defense and signalling metabolites of the crucifer Erucastrumcanariense: Synchronized abiotic induction of phytoalexins and galacto-oxylipins. *Phytochemistry*, *139*, pp.18–24.
61. Nakajyo, H., Hisamatsu, Y., Sekiguchi, M., Goto, N., Hasegawa, K. and Shigemori, H., 2006. Arabidopside F, a new oxylipin from Arabidopsis thaliana. *Heterocycles*, *69*, pp.295–301.
62. Hu, T.H., Lung, S.C., Ye, Z.W. and Chye, M.L., 2018. Depletion of Arabidopsis ACYL-COA-BINDING PROTEIN3 affects fatty acid composition in the phloem. *Frontiers in Plant Science*, *9*, p.2.v.

6 The Role of Oxylipins in Plant Reproduction, Growth, and Development

Babatunde Oluwafemi Adetuyi[1*], *Oluwakemi Semiloore Omowumi*[1], *Banke Ogundipe*[2], *Oluwatosin Adefunke Adetuyi*[3], *Kehinde Abraham Odelade*[1], and *Olubanke Olujoke Ogunlana*[2]
[1]Department of Natural Sciences, Faculty of Pure and Applied Sciences, Precious Cornerstone University, Ibadan
[2]Department of Biochemistry, Covenant University, Ota, Ogun State
[3]Department of Biochemistry, Osun State University, Osogbo, Osun State
*Corresponding author: badetuyi@gmail.com

CONTENTS

DOI: 10.1201/9781003316558-6

6.1 INTRODUCTION

The capacity of plants to endure extreme circumstances and attain matureness will rely upon the capacity to adjust to their current environment. Hence, the plants have fostered a lot of regulatory actions including the age of flagging particles to actuate versatile reactions. These regulatory mechanisms incorporate the following: defense mechanisms to infection, plant development, reproduction, and environmental changes [1]. Over the years, there has been a huge expansion in research of oxylipins for biosynthesis, signal transduction, and digestion. Here, we will zero in on the functions of oxylipins in plant growth, reproduction, and development. Oxylipins, a metabolite of unsaturated fat, are a significant sign of transduction atoms that are associated with inflammation, resistance, vascular, and other physiological and neurotic cycles [2]. Plants need innate defensive mechanisms by the immune system dissimilar to the vertebrates. Thus, plants have developed a proficient defense system against assaults from biotic and natural dangers. Plant oxylipins are known to assume a significant part in these defenses.

6.2 OXYLIPINS

Oxylipins are bioactive lipids produced by oxygenation of poly unsaturated fats produced from chloroplast film by lipases [3]. They play the roles of signaling mediators, development regulators, and endogenous defenders from biotic and abiotic stresses. Oxylipins in plants include plant hormones jasmonic acid, unsaturated fat hydroperoxides, divinyl ethers and 12-oxo phtodienoic acid [4]. They are a developing group of signaling molecules with a role in formative cycles like arrangement of pollen in flowering plants [5]. Oxylipins have a wide scope of natural capacities and many investigations have shown that these signaling molecules assume vital parts in defense processes and plant advancement, but with unclear exact organic roles. They exert their effects through activation of the PPARs or the G coupled protein receptor (GCPRs) [5].

Oxylipins are a gathering of oxygenated regular compounds that are produced using unsaturated fats via dioxygen-subordinate oxidation in at least one step [6]. Cyclooxygenases (COX catalysts), cytochrome P450 epoxygenase, and lipoxygenases (LOX catalysts) all produce oxylipins from polyunsaturated unsaturated fats (PUFAs) [7]. Oxylipins are found in a wide scope of aerobic species, like parasites, plants, and animals. Numerous oxylipins contribute a part in human wellbeing [8, 9]. Commonly, oxylipins are not held in tissues; all things being equal, they are created on request by freeing antecedent unsaturated fats from esterified structures.

Oxylipins derived from plants are a group of lipid metabolites that are synthesized when unsaturated fats are oxidized. Unsaturated fat hydroperoxides, oxo-, hydroxy-, or keto-unsaturated fats, unstable aldehydes, divinyl ethers, or the plant hormones JA are instances of oxylipins delivered by plants [10]. The making of unsaturated fat hydroperoxides, which can happen by enzymatic components or synthetic (auto) oxidation, is the main submitted step in oxylipin biosynthesis [1].

6.3 ENZYMATICALLY PRODUCED OXYLIPINS

A-DOX enzymes (α-dioxygenase) or LOXs, EC 1.13.11.12 (lipoxygenases) create responsive hydroperoxides of the universal unsaturated fats: α-linolenic acid (α-LeA, 18:3), roughanic acid (16:3) [11] or linoleic acid (LA, 18:2: where x:y is an unsaturated fat having x carbons and y double bonds) [12, 83–85]. Elective components for additional hydroperoxide *trans*formation include those started by hydroperoxide lyases (HPL), peroxygenases (PXG), allene oxide synthase (AOS, EC 4.2.1.92), epoxy alcohol synthase (EAS) or divinyl ether synthase (DES). The phytohormone jasmonic acid (JA) is one of the oxygenated subordinates, as are oxylipins with α, β-unsaturated carbonyl, aldehyde functionalities or responsive epoxide [13].

6.4 OXYLIPINS PRODUCED BY SYNTHETIC OXIDATION

In addition to enzymatic change, which produces unadulterated oxylipin enantiomers, oxidative pressure and the development of receptive oxygen species may cause compound film lipid peroxidation [1]. Since the LOXs enzyme speeds up the rate of reactions of either the development of R or S designed hydroperoxides, deciding whether a compound is synthesized through enzymatic reactions or non-enzymatic reactions should be possible in dual ways. First, on account of unsaturated fat hydroperoxides, in view of a higher abundance of either enantiomer, or the perception of a racemic blend, separately, since LOXs enzyme speeds up the rate of reaction of either the arrangement of R or S designed [14]. Alternatively, synthetic oxidation can bring about various positional isomers of hydroxy unsaturated fats, with LOXs embedding sub-atomic oxygen just at C-13 of α-LeA or C-9 of LA, individually, though responsive oxygen species can cause hydroxide arrangement at the tenth carbon (C-10) and the twelfth carbon (C-12) on account of linoleic acid (LA) and furthermore at the fifteenth carbon (C-15) and sixteenth (C-16) on account of α-linolenic acid (α-LeA). Free radicals are especially inclined to oxidizing the most pervasive unsaturated fats, LA and α-LeA, coming about in racemic mixes of peroxy unsaturated fat radicals [1]. The age and aggregation of racemic esterified unsaturated fat hydroperoxides can be set off by such radicals, which can send off a fountain of oxidative cycles. Hydroperoxides of polyunsaturated unsaturated fats (PUFAs) and divalent radicals with beyond what dual double bonds can be additionally oxidized, coming about in bicyclic endoperoxy hydroperoxides which have short half-lives like the phytoprostane PPG1 [1]. Phytoprostanes, which are basically indistinguishable from isoprostanes in vertebrates, are made by different successions of spontaneous occasions. The degrees of phytoprostanes polymerized in the films of certain species of plant are for the most part a significant degree higher than free phytoprostanes [15], and generally phytoprostane levels rise after openness to oxidative stressors like peroxide or when microbes are introduced, or weighty metal treatment [16].

A lot of oxidized lipids delivered during oxidative pressure serves as substrates for protein lipidation and altogether affect the gene expression patterns, proposing that they might go about as oxidant damage mediators. Ketodienes, alkenals, epoxy alcohols, di-and trihydroxy unsaturated fats and ketotrienes are known for most part notable peroxy radicals chemical items [17]. While 4-hydroxy-2-alkenals, for example, 4-hydroxy nonenal are significant oxylipins occupied with protein lipidation in warm blooded animals, phytoprostanes and keto-unsaturated fats give off an impression of being the primary actors in plants [4]. Plants contain phytoprostanes [18] and extracellular utilization of various cyclopentenone phytoprostanes has been displayed to incite defense reactions in plant [19]. It is essential to realize that an incredible measure of oxylipins formed through synthetic oxidation process or non-enzymatic process is seen in the tissues of plant. Nonetheless, it ought to be noticed that a portion of these substances can be delivered enzymatically through LOX pathway [20]. Fundamental degrees of resulted products created from non-enzymatic peroxidation are mostly in a similar reach or over those of the results of enzymatic peroxidation [1].

6.5 DIFFERENT OXYLIPIN PRESENT IN PLANT CELLS

Oxylipins are found in plant cells in two particular structures. These two include non-esterified or free oxylipins and esterified oxylipins.

6.5.1 Free or Non-Esterified Oxylipins

Oxylipins can be found in an assortment of structures in plant cells, according to various examinations. Free oxylipins, which have been found in an assortment of plant systems, present the most essential situation. All through the expansion to liberate oxylipins that can connect with solvent compartments like the plastid stroma, peroxisomal framework or cytosol [21–23], oxylipins have been shown to be polymerized with a wide range of atoms in the cell.

6.5.2 Arabidopsides' Esterified Oxylipins

It is not startling that oxylipins (for example OPDA (12-oxo phytodienoic acid) or dn-OPDA (dinor-OPDA)) are esterified to complex lipids [24]. Arabidopsides are OPDA as well as dn-OPDA-containing subordinates of the plastidial galactolipids digalacto-syldiacylglycerol (DGDG) and the mono galacto-syldiacylglycerol (MGDG), which consists of OPDA, and additionally dn-OPDA rather than greasy acyl moieties. A few arabidopsides (also known as arabidopsides A-G) can be perceived in light of the dispersion of OPDA at one or the other or both sn-1 and sn-2 areas, and new arabidopside species are consistently found [25]. The quick integration of newly created OPDA into plastidial lipids might cause the development of galactolipids which contains OPDA after elicitation or injury. dn-OPDA and OPDA appear to specially bind to galactolipids which upholds this hypothesis. Esterified OPDA that binds to the sn-1 place of phosphatidylglycerol with trans-hexadecenoic acid at the sn-2 position is the main OPDA particle found in the phospholipid division up to this point; this phospholipid is in like manner restrictive to plastids [24]. It is not certain if oxylipins which are bound in plastidial lipids are a capacity type of flagging particles that can be delivered rapidly in case of a pressure. Recent examination recommends that perceptible degrees of arabidopsides are just viewed as in a couple of number of Arabidopsis species [24], inferring that arabidopside pools in many plants are tiny or that the lipids address a one-of-a-kind adaption seen uniquely in a couple of animal species.

6.5.3 Oxylipin-Esters and Forms of Other Oxylipins

Oxylipins can shape esters or forms with carbohydrates, phospholipids, sulfate, ethanolamine, nonpartisan lipids, amino acids, or glutathione. In the impartial phospholipids and lipids of sunflower seeds and cucumber seedlings, the divinyl ether unsaturated fat colneleic acid might be recognized esterified to hydroxyl, phospholipids, keto and hydroperoxy subordinates of one or the other LA or α-LeA can be found [26,27]. The most notable model is jasmonic acid, which can be bound in glycosyl esters and can also exist as methyl ester (MeJA). JA can be hydroxylated at the u-or (u 1)- terminal of its side chain prior to being further sulfated [6], and can also make amide-forms with different amino acids [28]. The form of jasmonic acid and isoleucine (JAIle) has lately been found to be a naturally dynamic type of JA that interfaces with a JA-receptor [29]. One more alteration is glutathionylation, which should be visible in OPDA and (2E)- hexenal, for instance [1].

6.6 OXYLIPIN PRODUCTION

Oxylipins are results of the desaturation interaction of unsaturated fat. Unsaturated fat desaturates (FADS) work with unsaturated fat synthase to shape mono-and polyunsaturated unsaturated fats (MUFAs and PUFAs individually). However, in light of the intensity and short pattern of oxylipins, they are produced de novo and they apply their belongings in an autocrine or paracrine way [30]. PUFAs created de novo in the body from the diet (arachidonic acid, docosahexaenoic acid) or from the desaturation of alpha-linolenic acid (ALA), linoleic acid (LA; omega-6, 18:2) and linolenic (omega-3, 18:3) respectively [31]. Oxylipins are gotten from PUFAs by means of the lipoxygenase, cytochrome P450 and the cyclooxygenase (COX) pathways by cell actuation. Lipoxygenases (LOX) are monomeric proteins with masses of 94–104 kDa, it contains one non-heme iron iota per particle atoms and catalyzes the dioxygenation response of unsaturated fats to relating hydroperoxy subordinates which incorporate leukotrienes, resolvins, lipoxin, maresin [32, 33]. On account of blooming plants, oxylipins are blended from the polyunsaturated C18 family (linoleic and linolenic as they are the most bountiful unsaturated fats in plants) by oxygenation which rates of reaction is accelerated by the enzymes called α-dioxygenases (α-DOXs) or LOXs [34] due to the shortfall of arachidonic acid. The kind of oxylipins produced relies upon the PUFAs oxidized and the catalyst associated with the digestion. The esterification of PUFAs in sn-2 position of glycerophospholipids and put away in the lipid film to give an elevated degree of substrate for the denovo union of oxylipins. The main key stage in the biosynthesis of oxylipins is the oxidative reaction of α-linolenic acid to one or the other 9-or 13-hydroperoxy-octadecatrienoic acids catalyzed by the lipoxygenases (LOX). These mixtures are additionally used by different proteins to produce oxylipins. On initiation of the cell, hydrolysis of PUFAs by cytoplasmic phospholipase A2 happens while the oxygenation of the free PUFAs occur by the 3 classes of catalysts lipoxygenase, cytochrome P450 and COX, and into oxylipins [35]. Lipoxygenase (LOX) speeds up the reaction in the addition of atomic O_2 into unsaturated fat with 1,4-pentadienylfunction; on account of linolenic acid (C18), 9 or 13 also undergo oxidation to form hydroperoxyoctadecadi(tri)enoic acids which can be additionally changed over by LOX to shape ketodienoic unsaturated fats by lack of hydration process. These substrates can be used enzymatically into series of oxylipins by means of the LOX pathway. The diffusion of oxylipins can occur through the plasma membrane while signally the G protein coupled receptors (GPCRs) or enact perixisome proliferator-initiated receptors (PPARs) or ligand actuated record factors [11].

In plants, oxylipin biosynthesis can occur at the degree of either esterified or unesterified polyunsaturated unsaturated fats. To avoid complications, only biosynthesis at the degree of esterified polyunsaturated unsaturated fat will be discussed. The arrival of unsaturated fats from film lipids by the activity of a lipase starts off oxylipin creation. The following response is an underlying oxidation response including various enzymes at various situations along the unsaturated fat backbone. The free unsaturated fat is oxidized by sub-atomic oxygen in the initial step, creating a hydroperoxy unsaturated fat. A lipoxygenase (LOX) or α-dioxygenase (α-DOX) catalyst can catalyze this cycle. The results of α-DOX breakdown non-enzymatically into CO_2 and more limited aldehyde subordinates, or they can be decreased through chemical reaction by glutathione or enzymatic reaction by a PXG (peroxygenase). The hydroperoxy products formed by LOXes, then again, have been demonstrated to be generally steady and are processed by different catalysts like unique individuals from the Cyp74-group of P450 catalysts: hydroperoxide lyase (HPL), epoxyalcohol synthases (EAS), allene oxide synthase (AOS), divinyl ether synthase (DES) or PXG [24].

6.7 FEW ENZYMES ASSOCIATED WITH BIOSYNTHESIS OF OXYLIPINS

6.7.1 Lipases

A few lipases have been recognized in Arabidopsis that give unsaturated fat substrate to the oxylipin pathway. Both DONGEL (DGL) [36] and Defective in Anther Dehiscence1 (DAD1) [37] have been shown to be individuals from the phospholipase family, which fundamentally hydrolyze glycerophospholipids at the sn-1 position; however the two proteins can likewise utilize glycolipids as substrates [36]. A purported patatin-relatedn lipase (pPLA-I) was additionally found to have the ability to control jasmonate synthesis in the absence of pathogens [38].

6.7.2 Alpha-Dioxygenase (A-DOX)

The oxygenation of unsaturated fats at carbon 2 of atom is accelerated or catalyzed by α-DOX by eliminating the proR-hydrogen and embedding sub-atomic oxygen in a stereoselective way, coming about in the separate 2R-hydroperoxy subsidiary

[39]. Curiously, both PGHS-1 and PGHS-2 which are mammalian prostaglandin-synthase isoforms have high homology with α-DOX, and the two compounds share normal synergist highlights [40]. Heme is a co-factor in the two catalysts that is expected for synergist action. It is bound in the two cases by two particular His-deposits on proximal and distal sites of the heme plane. Besides, the two compounds utilize an exceptionally monitored tyrosine buildup for the synergist movement [41, 42].

6.7.3 Lipoxygenase Enzymes (LOX)

While lots of lipoxyenases (LOXes) have been displayed to accelerate dioxygenase reactions (for example bis-oxygenation of unsaturated fats), a couple has been found to catalyze optional transformations of hydroperoxy unsaturated fats, bringing about epoxy-(liquor)- subsidiaries or lyase products [43, 44, 45]. The LOX movement dioxygenase process is described by five distinct basic proteins. These five catalysts incorporate enzyme activation, abstraction of hydrogen, radical reorganization, insertion of oxygen, and reduction of peroxyl radicals. The LOX initiation process is a one-turnover process in which the recently oxidized chemical does not react with hydroperoxide. During catalysis, the Fe redox state cycles between the latent Fe^{2+} - H_2O and the dynamic Fe^{3+}- OH [46, 47]. The production of carbon-centered radical results from the abstraction of bisallylic hydrogen and this is delocalized through the type of electron framework. Therefore, oxygen can be added at two separate focuses on the unsaturated fat spine: [+2] and [-2]. While utilizing LA-linoleic acid as a substrate, where hydrogen abstraction happens at the eleventh carbon (C-11), the two spots for oxygen fuse are C-9 and C-13, bringing about 9-hydroperoxy-and 13-hydroperoxy subordinates, individually [48, 49].

6.7.4 Cyp74 Enzymes

The metabolic pathway for changing over LOX-inferred hydroperoxides has a stretching point that is overwhelmingly catalyzed by compounds from the Cyp74 family, like AOS, HPL, DES, and EAS [11]. The Cyp74 enzyme family is essential for the P450s (cytochrome P450) catalyst superfamily, which contains a cysteine-thiolate-composed heme as a co-factor and has a trademark retention limit of 450 nm on the decrease and CO binding. Mono-oxygenation responses are catalyzed by normal P450s through an instrument that includes oxygen restricting to heme iron, consecutive decrease, protonation of middle person edifices, and water separation [50, 51, 52].

6.7.5 Allene Oxide Cyclase Enzyme

Without AOC, the allylic allene oxide delivered by 13-HPOTE and AOS (see above) has an extremely short time (half-life) in water and is non-enzymatically changed to α- and γ- ketols or cyclized to a racemic combination of both *cis*(+)- and *cis*(-)- 12-oxo phytodienoic acid (OPDA)- enantiomers [53, 54]. The AOC is a homotrimeric chemical with an atomic load of around 20–25 kDa per subunit and has a place with the lipocalin protein family. Every subunit is fundamentally made out of an eight-abandoned enemy of equal-barrel space that shapes a center hydrophobic hole or barrel in which the response happens [55].

The *cis-trans* isomerization at the tenth carbon atom (C-10) and the eleventh carbon atom (C-11) bond, specifically, results in an advanced conformational shift of the eighth carbon atom (C-8) and ninth carbon atom (C-9) bond, which is likewise moved from *cis*-to *trans*-geometry due to steric limitations inside the dynamic site. Following that, Woodward and Hoffmann's standards for cyclization are adhered to [56]. The allene oxide's proclivity for cyclizing suddenly in water, producing an enantiomeric combination of OPDA, shows that this response has a low energy hindrance. Therefore, AOC does not need quite a bit of a catalyst to diminish this energy. It rather appears to be that the unconstrained cyclization response continues in a stereoselective manner that is constrained by steric dynamic site determinants [57].

6.7.6 12-Oxo Phytodienoate Reductases (OPR)

A catalyst known as OPDA reductase isoenzyme 3 reduces *cis*(+)- OPDA, 13S-, or 12S to the appropriate cyclopentanone subordinate in plants (OPR3). This protein is a FMN-subordinate oxido-reductase from the ancient yellow catalyst family, which is known for decreasing the twofold bonds of, α, and β-unsaturated carbonyls. OPR proteins have a (α/β)8-barrel overlap, which comprises of eight helices around eight equal beta-sheets in a tube-shaped structure. The FMN-co-factor is seen as in the compound's middle, where it is non-covalently associated with one of the beta-sheets terminals [57]. Over the co-factor substrate, explicit amino acids are shaping the dynamic site pit of the catalyst, in which the carbonyl-group of the substrate is joined and situated by means of two in number hydrogen bond to a His/His pair. Notwithstanding, His/His pair has been said to be answerable for the initiation of α,β double bond for the movement of hydride to the β- carbon particle of the substrate by its polarization. The decrease of OPDA happens by means of a purported ping-pong bi-bi mechanism: in the initial reaction, the FMN-co-factor is diminished by NAD(P)H which is then followed by the liberation of $NAD(P)^+$. In the second reaction, OPDA is attached to the catalysts and is diminished through hydride move to the β- carbon particle [43].

6.7.7 Peroxygenase (PXG)

Peroxygenase (PXG) is a catalyst which utilizes LOX-determined unsaturated fat hydroperoxides as substrates. This chemical accelerates the decrease of hydroperoxide subordinate to the individual alcohol by moving an O_2 molecule to a substrate which thus will undergo oxidation [58]. Like the individuals from the Cyp74 enzymes, this catalyst is likewise a layer bound in flowering plants and it consists of heme as co-factor driving first to the misconception that peroxygenase additionally has a place with this protein family. Nonetheless, as opposed to Cyp74 catalysts which consist of a thiolate-composed heme, in PXG, heme is bound by means of saved histidine buildup which fills in as the pivotal ligand.

6.8 OXYLIPINS' ROLE IN REPRODUCTION

LOX-determined oxylipins is valuable for different generation cycle like treatment, seed, and root improvement. In a portrayal investigation of a triple mutant of Arabidopsis without linolenic acid, an antecedent for oxylipins; the triple mutant was sterile however delivered fruitful by treatment of the bloom buds with jasmonite acid, a kind of oxylipins [37]. Notwithstanding the role of oxylipin in plant defense, oxylipins likewise seem to assume a part in plant propagation. For instance, exogenous jasmonic acid (JA) diminishes the photosynthetic pace of flowering plants and also it is the reason behind the decrease in bud development [11]. Dicotyledon blossoms or seeds consist of high level of jasmonates which includes amides or amino-acids derivatives, and it has been estimated that a tissue explicit oxylipin mark could control blooming processes in plants. A definitive role of jasmonic acid in blossom advancement is shown through the perception that mutants that surrenders in jasmonic acid biosynthesis/production that have abandon in either bloom improvement or male sterility [37]. Besides, Capella et al., [59] have shown that COI1-subordinate myrosinase movement influences the outflow of bloom explicit myrosinase-restricting protein homologs. A basic necessity for jasmonic acid (JA) however not OPDA in dust advancement was distinguished [60]. A theory has established that JA incorporated in fibers controls the flow or transfer of water in petals and stamens. Recent research on Arabidopsis mutant's damages in the anther dehiscence indicated that DAD1 gene directed JA production is significant for the synchronization of dust development, anther dehiscence and blossom opening [37]. Analysis of Arabidopsis late-blooming mutants fcα-1and cad2–1with imperfections in GSH biosynthesis treated with exogenous GSH or GSH inhibitors uncovered a job for GSH in advancing flowering [61]. Since a portion of the JA lacking or responsiveness mutants have surrenders in blossoming and GSH creation requires JA, it is conceivable that JA-subordinate GSH creation might assume a significant part in plant generation. Concentrates on showing that a significant number of the abiotic stress factors actuate the biosynthesis of a few naturally dynamic oxylipins and advance flowering [24] support the above theory. Notwithstanding, itemized investigations are expected to comprehend how plants incorporate signs exuding from various atoms and prompt a complex physiological reaction like flowering and reproduction.

6.9 OXYLIPINS' ROLE IN PLANT GROWTH AND DEVELOPMENT

Up until the last twenty years, there have been no finished underlying portrayals of plant oxylipins regardless of their reality since a significant stretch of time. The utilization of more established insightful strategies, for example, melanolysis just made the portrayal of the oxylipins part of particles conceivable. According to Wasternack et al, they exhibited that esterified (13S)- hydroxy-(9z,11E)- octadecadienoic acid is framed during cucumber cotyledons germination which further shows that the item is a functioning compound in plant formative cycles [62]. Also, according Miersch and others, they announced the presence of high amounts of esterified oxyipinsa that contains hydroxlinolenic acids (HOD), Ketolinoleic acids (KOT), ketolinoleic acids (KOD) in tomato bloom organs and that the treatment of tomatoes. LOX-determined is ivolved in germination, improvement, and senenscence, and fills in as guard reaction against microbial microorganism, bugs, and wounds. In a review led by Bouarab and others, the presence of LOX-inferred oxylipins and C18 polyunsaturated unsaturated fats was detected. Additionally as indicated by Chechetkin and others, there was no recognition of linolipin atoms in young flax leaves at day 23 of culture however at a later progressive phase, day 35 of culture the grouping of linolipin has reach 71 nmol/g showing that oxylipins could play a part in plant advancement [5].

Plant esterified oxylipins, for example, arabidopsides A, B, D assume a part being developed because of their capacity to repress cress root development as indicated by Zuther et al. [63]. The jobs of oxylipins in plant, for example, moss plant is depicted beneath.

Mosses are flowering plants which grow on land with a somewhat straightforward formative example with rotating haploid gametophyte and diploid sporophyte ages. The gametophyte comprises of two distinguished formative phases which include the adolescent filamentous protonema with chloronema and caulonema sorts of cells, and the grown-up gametophores which are verdant shoots made out of a non-vascular stem with leaves, the conceptive organs, and filamentous rhizoids [5].

The development of chloronema cells with trademark opposite cross dividers and a high thickness of chloroplasts results from the germination of a haploid spore or the division of a protoplast. Caulonemal cells with diagonal cross dividers and thin chloroplasts originate from chloronemal fibers in this manner. New chloronemal or caulonemal cells are formed when caulonemal cells are stretched, resulting in the production of auxiliary chloronemal or caulonemal fibers and buds. Buds become verdant gametophores, which frame the diploid sporophyte age, causing new haploid spores to develop. Unsaturated fat creations in mosses vary depending on the tissue type. While the 16:0 and 20:4 substances are similar in protonemal fibers and verdant gametophores of different moss species, the 18:2 and 18:3 substances are more abundant in gametophores and protonemal tissues, respectively [64]. These metabolic differences are linked to differences in the articulation levels of genes that code for unsaturated fat desaturases [64].

The most abundant unsaturated fats in growing sporophytes of the moss Minimum cuspidotum are 16:0 and 20:4, while 18:2 increases when spores have grown and are ready for dispersal, attaining at comparable quantities as 16:0 [5]. 13-hydroperoxy linoleic acid and 12-HPETE are the most abundant free hydro(per)oxy unsaturated fats found in the protonemal tissues of *P. patens* [65], which can also be used by the chemicals that produce oxylipins with potential jobs in moss improvement. Nonetheless, the specific components of the C18:2, C18.3, and C20:4 routes in various tissues and organs are yet unknown throughout moss development. Because of the high rate of homologous recombination in *P. patens*, specified quality disturbance or single point transformation can be used to investigate qualities encoding proteins involved in unsaturated fat and oxylipin production [66]. Quality interruption has been used to define the *P. patens* qualities encoding Δ6-desaturase, Δ6-elongase, and Δ5-desaturase, confirming their presence in 20:4 and 20:5 productions. Despite the fact that 20:4 and 20:5 ratios are drastically reduced in these mutants, protonema and gametophores of knockout plants do not appear to have changed aggregates, suggesting that 20:4 and 20:5 ratios are excessive, or that remaining measures of these unsaturated fats are adequate for typical turn of events [67–69].

P. patens knockout mutants with genes for oxylipin-producing compounds have also been created. Individual PpAOC1 and PpAOC2 knockout mutants have diminished richness, atypical sporophyte morphology, and impeded sporogenesis [70, 71], (Jiu, et al., 2020; Schultz et al., 2020), but PpHPL, PpAOS1, and PpAOS2 knockout mutants exhibit no formative changes [70]. PpAOC1 and PpAOC2 knockout mutants were unable to acquire twofold, implying that exhaustion of the two proteins is fatal.

As referenced beforehand, just the PpAOS1 mutant is profoundly disabled in OPDA union, albeit the sum created is adequate for ordinary turn of events [71]. OPDA- and J-lacking mutants in *A. thaliana*, as well as mutants in the COI-1 quality, are male sterile, whereas a change in the tomato COI-1 quality renders female sterile plants [72, 73]. As a result, distinct oxylipins contribute to the enhancement of conceptive structures in both greeneries and flowering plants. More research into the many characteristics encoding chemicals involved with the LOX pathways is expected to pique their interest in moss formative cycles. While PpAOC1 and PpAOC2 have similar articulation designs in protonemal and gametophores tissues, PpAOC3 is communicated differently in protonemata tissues, where it could have a clearer role [74].

Ppα-DOX is communicated during improvement in tips of protonemal fibers, with the highest articulation levels in mitotically dynamic undifferentiated apical chloronemal and caulonemal cells, according to recent studies using *P. patens* Ppα-DOX-GUS correspondent lines [75]. Ppα-DOX-GUS is also widely expressed in other mitotically active cells, such as the apical cells of recovering protoplasts. Ppα-DOX-determined oxylipins in undifferentiated apical cells, which are self-recharging foundational microorganisms, need to be investigated further. PGE2, a COX-determined oxylipin in mammals, has beneficial effects on undifferentiation, animate self-recharging, and expansion [76, 77], and Ppα-DOX-inferred oxylipins could have similar effects. Ppα-DOX records accumulate in cells that cause rhizoids and axillary hair development in young buds, suggesting that adjacent indications in these cells contribute to Ppα-DOX articulation. Ppα-DOX is communicated in auxin-producing tissues, including rhizoids and axillary hairs early stage, and axillary hairs and rhizoid in young and grown-up gametophores. Gametophytes and sporophytes of Ppα-DOX mutant are like wild-type plants showing that this protein is not fundamental for legitimate moss advancement. In any case, brooding wild-type tissues with Ppα-DOX-inferred oxylipins, or overexpressing Ppα-DOX, change *P. patens* improvement prompting more modest moss settlements with less protonemal tissues [75]. The Ppα-DOX determined aldehyde, heptadecatrienal, is answerable for the diminished protonemal fiber development. Moss states are likewise more modest and have less protonemal tissues when moss tissues are filled within the sight of 13-LOX-inferred oxylipins, including OPDA and methyl jasmonate. OPDA and jasmonate likewise diminish rhizoid length [78], reliably with the development capture of A. thaliana seedlings and roots brooded with these oxylipins [1]. Curiously, the inhibitory impact of OPDA on development, either by OPDA application or by the age of overexpressing MpAOC plants which delivers elevated degrees of OPDA, was likewise seen in the liverwort *M. polymorpha*, recommending a rationed reaction to this oxylipin among bryophytes. Interestingly, JA did not influence *M. polymorpha* development [79], showing that the development inhibitory action of jasmonate is not moderated among greeneries and liverworts.

One potential clarification is simply *M. polymorpha* does not have the downstream parts vital for detecting the presence of JA. Nonetheless, putative orthologs of the jasmonate ZIM-space (JAZ) repressor and the receptor COI have been recognized in *M. polymorpha*. Furthermore, grouping arrangement shows that the limiting locales are all around preserved between COI orthologs of *P. patens* and *M. polymorpha* and *A. thaliana* COI [80]. Further investigations are expected to comprehend the differential reaction to jasmonates between various bryophytes. Mueller et al. [81] have recommended that in blooming plants the restraint of development saw with OPDA is connected with the hindrance of cell cycle movement. Studies in *A. thaliana* have shown that jasmonate decreases both cell number and cell size in roots and leaves [82]. Reliably, protonemal tissues filled within the sight of heptadecatrienal have fibers with more modest caulonemal cells and strange cell divisions [75]. Taking together, this multitude of perceptions demonstrate that like more mind-boggling plants where oxylipins incorporated from various biochemical pathways go about as controllers of advancement, a tweaking component works to direct oxylipins focuses in moss tissues for legitimate turn of events.

6.10 CONCLUSION

Oxylipins can be said to be cosmopolitan plant metabolites because they can be isolated and found in numerous kinds of plants. Oxylipins play the roles of signaling regulators, development regulators, and endogenous defenders from both biotic and abiotic stresses. Oxylipins also have a wide scope of natural capacities and many investigations have shown that these signaling molecules assume vital parts in defense processes and plant advancement, but with unclear exact organic roles. However, it is recommended that more research should be done on the exact biological roles of oxylipins in plant reproduction, growth, and development. This will give full knowledge on the importance of oxylipins in plants.

ABBREVIATIONS

ACXs	acyl-CoA oxidases
AOS	allene oxide synthase
DES	divinylether synthase
dn-OPDA	dinor-OPDA
α-DOX	α-dioxygenase
EAS	epoxy alcoholsynthase
GLVs	green leaf volatiles
HPL	hydroperoxide lyase
JA	jasmonic acid

JA–Ile	jasmonic acid isoleucine conjugate
KAT	3-ketoacyl-CoA thiolase
LA	linoleic acid
α-LeA	α-linolenic acid
LOX	lipoxygenase
MeJA	jasmonic acid methylester
MFP	multifunctional protein
OPC-8	12-oxo phytoenoic acid
OPDA	12-oxophytodienoic acid
PXG	peroxygenase
PUFA	polyunsaturated fatty acid

REFERENCES

1. Viswanath K, Varakumar P, Pamuru R, Basha SJ, Mehta S, & Rao AD. Plant lipoxygenases and their role in plant physiology. *Journal of Plant Biology*. 2020; *63*(2), 83–95.
2. Maynard D, Gröger H, Dierks T, & Dietz KJ. The function of the oxylipin 12-oxophytodienoic acid in cell signaling, stress acclimation, and development. *Journal of Experimental Botany*. 2018;*69*(22), 5341–5354.
3. Cebo M, Dittrich K, Fu X, Manke MC, Emschermann F, Rheinlaender J & Chatterjee M. Platelet ACKR3/CXCR7 favors antiplatelet lipids over an atherothrombotic lipidome and regulates thromboinflammation. *Blood, The Journal of the American Society of Hematology*. 2022; *139*(11), 1722–1742.
4. Vincenti S, Mariani M, Alberti J-C, Jacopini S, Brunini-Bronzini de Caraffa V, Berti L, Maury J. Biocatalytic Synthesis of Natural Green Leaf Volatiles Using the Lipoxygenase Metabolic Pathway. *Catalysts*. 2019;*9*(10), 873. https://doi.org/10.3390/catal9100873
5. Genva M, Andersson, MX, & Fauconnier, ML. Simple liquid chromatography-electrospray ionization ion trap mass spectrometry method for the quantification of galacto-oxylipin arabidopsides in plant samples. *Scientific Reports*. 2020; *10*(1), 1–11.
6. Wang L, Leister D, Guan L, Zheng Y, Schneider K, Lehmann M & Kleine T. The Arabidopsis SAFEGUARD1 suppresses singlet oxygen-induced stress responses by protecting grana margins. *Proceedings of the National Academy of Sciences*. 2020;*117*(12), 6918–6927.
7. Leiria LO, Wang CH, Lynes MD, Yang K, Shamsi F, Sato M & Tseng YH. 12-Lipoxygenase regulates cold adaptation and glucose metabolism by producing the omega-3 lipid 12-HEPE from brown fat. *Cell Metabolism*. 2019;*30*(4), 768–783.
8. Isah, T. Stress and defense responses in plant secondary metabolites production. *Biological Research*. 2019; 52.
9. Novaković L, Guo T, Bacic A, Sampathkumar A, & Johnson K. L. Hitting the wall—Sensing and signaling pathways involved in plant cell wall remodeling in response to abiotic stress. *Plants*. 2018; *7*(4), 89.
10. Vincenti S., Mariani M, Alberti JC, Jacopini S, Brunini-Bronzini de Caraffa V, Berti L, & Maury J. Biocatalytic synthesis of natural green leaf volatiles using the lipoxygenase metabolic pathway. *Catalysts*. 2019; *9*(10), 873.
11. Wasternack C, & Feussner I. The oxylipin pathways: biochemistry and function. *Annual Review of Plant Biology*. 2018; *69*, 363–386.

12. Stolterfoht H, Rinnofner C, Winkler M, & Pichler H. Recombinant lipoxygenases and hydroperoxide lyases for the synthesis of green leaf volatiles. *Journal of Agricultural and Food Chemistry*. 2019; *67*(49), 13367–13392.
13. Yu D, Boughton BA, Hill CB, Feussner I, Roessner U, & Rupasinghe TW. Insights into oxidized lipid modification in barley roots as an adaptation mechanism to salinity stress. *Frontiers in Plant Science. 2020; 11*, 1.
14. Munir N, Hasnain M, Waqif H, Adetuyi BO, Egbuna C, Olisah MC. Gelling Agents, Micro and Nanogels in Food System Applications. *Application of Nanotechnology in Food Science, Processing and Packaging, 2022*, 153–167.
15. Domínguez-Perles R, Abellán Á, León D, Ferreres F, Guy A, Oger C. & Gil-Izquierdo Á. Sorting out the phytoprostane and phytofuran profile in vegetable oils. *Food Research International.*2018;*107*, 619–628.
16. Farooq MA, Niazi AK, Akhtar J, Farooq M, Souri Z, Karimi N, & Rengel Z. Acquiring control: The evolution of ROS-Induced oxidative stress and redox signaling pathways in plant stress responses. *Plant Physiology and Biochemistry.* 2019; *141*, 353–369.
17. James-Okoro PO, Iheagwam FN, Sholeye MI, Umoren IA, Adetuyi BO, Ogundipe AE, Braimah AA, Adekunbi TS, Ogunlana OE, Ogunlana OO. Phytochemical and in vitro antioxidant assessment of Yoyo bitters *World News of Natural Sciences* 2021; *37*, 1–17.
18. Kanagendran A, Chatterjee P, Liu B, Sa, T., Pazouki L, & Niinemets Ü. Foliage inoculation by Burkholderia vietnamiensis CBMB40 antagonizes methyl jasmonate-mediated stress in Eucalyptus grandis. *Journal of Plant Physiology.* 2019; *242*, 153032.
19. Farooq MA, Niazi AK, Akhtar J, Farooq M, Souri Z, Karimi N, & Rengel Z. Acquiring control: The evolution of ROS-Induced oxidative stress and redox signaling pathways in plant stress responses. *Plant Physiology and Biochemistry.* 2019; *141*, 353–369.
20. Pandian BA, Sathishraj R, Djanaguiraman M, Prasad PV, & Jugulam M. Role of cytochrome P450 enzymes in plant stress response. *Antioxidants* 2020; *9*(5), 454.
21. Chini A, Monte I, Zamarreno AM, Hamberg M., Lassueur S., Reymond P & Solano R. An OPR3-independent pathway uses 4, 5-didehydrojasmonate for jasmonate synthesis. *Nature Chemical Biology* 2018; *14*(2), 171–178.
22. Mielke S, & Gasperini D. Interplay between plant cell walls and jasmonate production. *Plant and Cell Physiology.* 2019; *60*(12), 2629–2637.
23. Ali M, & Baek KH. Jasmonic acid signaling pathway in response to abiotic stresses in plants. *International Journal of Molecular Sciences.* 2020; *21*(2), 621.
24. Maynard D, Gröger H, Dierks T, & Dietz KJ. The function of the oxylipin 12-oxophytodienoic acid in cell signaling, stress acclimation, and development. *Journal of Experimental Botany.* 2018; *69*(22), 5341–5354.
25. Genva M, Obounou Akong F, Andersson MX, Deleu M., Lins L, and Fauconnier ML. New insights into the biosynthesis of esterified oxylipins and their involvement in plant defense and developmental mechanisms. *Phytochemistry Reviews.* 2019; *18*(1), 343–358.
26. Estelle D, Laurence L, Marc O, Magali D, & Marie-Laure F. Linolenic fatty acid hydroperoxide acts as biocide on plant pathogenic bacteria: biophysical investigation of the mode of action. *Bioorganic Chemistry.* 2020; *100*, 103877.
27. Horn PJ, Chapman KD, & Ischebeck, T. Isolation of Lipid Droplets for Protein and Lipid Analysis. In *Plant Lipids* (pp. 295–320). Humana, New York, NY. 2021.
28. Verma M, Mishra J, & Arora NK. Plant growth-promoting rhizobacteria: diversity and applications. In *Environmental Biotechnology: for Sustainable Future* (pp. 129–173). Springer, Singapore. 2019.

29. Adetuyi BO, Adebisi OA, Adetuyi OA, Ogunlana OO, Pere-Ebi T, Chukwuebuka E, Chukwuemelie ZU, Johra K, Obinna CU, Ficus exasperata Attenuates Acetaminophen-Induced Hepatic Damage via NF-κB Signaling Mechanism in Experimental Rat Model *BioMed Research International* 2022 https://doi.org/10.1155/2022/6032511.
30. Adetuyi BO, Okeowo TO, Adetuyi OA, Adebisi OA, Ogunlana OO, Oretade OJ, Najat M, Amany MB, Nermeen NW, Gaber EB. Ganoderma lucidum from red mushroom attenuates formaldehyde- induced liver damage in experimental male rat model. *Biology* 2020, *9*(10), 313.
31. Adetuyi BO, Adebisi OA, Awoyelu EH, Adetuyi OA, Ogunlana OO. Phytochemical and Toxicological effect of Ethanol extract of Heliotropium indicum on Liver of Male Albino Rats. *Letters in Applied NanoBioscience (LIANB)* 2020, *10*(2), 2085–2095.
32. Gabbs M, Leng S., Devassy JG, Monirujjaman M, and Aukema HM. Advances in our understanding of oxylipins derived from dietary PUFAs. *Advances in Nutrition.* 2015; *6*(5), 513–540.
33. Vincenti S, Mariani M, Alberti JC, Jacopini S, Brunini-Bronzini de Caraffa V, Berti L, & Maury J. Biocatalytic synthesis of natural green leaf volatiles using the lipoxygenase metabolic pathway. *Catalysts.* 2019; *9*(10), 873.
34. Yu D, Boughton BA, Hill CB, Feussner I, Roessner U, & Rupasinghe TW. Insights into oxidized lipid modification in barley roots as an adaptation mechanism to salinity stress. *Frontiers in Plant Science.* 2020; *11*, 1.
35. Ogunlana OO, Adetuyi BO, Adekunbi TS, Adegboye BE, Iheagwam FN, Ogunlana OE. Ruzu bitters ameliorates high–fat diet induced non-alcoholic fatty liver disease in male Wistar rats. *Journal of Pharmacy and Pharmacognosy Research* 2021, *9*(3), 251–26.
36. Siddiqi KS & Husen A. Plant response to jasmonates: current developments and their role in changing environment. *Bulletin of the National Research Centre.* 2019; *43*(1), 1–11.
37. Wang J, Wu D, Wang Y, & Xie D. Jasmonate action in plant defense against insects. *Journal of Experimental Botany.* 2019; *70*(13), 3391–3400.
38. Filkin SY, Lipkin AV, & Fedorov AN. Phospholipase superfamily: structure, functions, and biotechnological applications. *Biochemistry (Moscow).* 2020; *85*(1), 177–195.
39. Stolterfoht H, Rinnofner C, Winkler M, and Pichler H. (2019). Recombinant lipoxygenases and hydroperoxide lyases for the synthesis of green leaf volatiles. *Journal of Agricultural and Food Chemistry, 67*(49), 13367–13392.
40. Hammer AK, Albrecht F, Hahne F, Jordan P, Fraatz MA, Ley J & Buchhaupt M. Biotechnological production of odor-active methyl-branched aldehydes by a novel α-dioxygenase from Crocosphaera subtropica. *Journal of Agricultural and Food Chemistry.* 2020; *68*(38), 10432–10440.
41. Wang B., Wu L, Chen J, Dong L, Chen C, Wen Z & Wang D. W. Metabolism pathways of arachidonic acids: Mechanisms and potential therapeutic targets. *Signal Transduction and Targeted Therapy.* 2021; *6*(1), 1–30.
42. Ogunlana OO, Adetuyi BO, Rotimi M, Esalomi I, Adeyemi A, Akinyemi J, Ogunlana O, Adetuyi O, Adebisi O, Opata E, Baty R, Batiha G. Hypoglycemic Activities of Ethanol Seed Extract of *Hunteria umbellate* (Hallier F.) on Streptozotocin-induced Diabetic Rats. *Clinical Phytoscience* 2021, *7* (1), 1–9.
43. Shi Y, Mandal R, Singh A, & Pratap Singh A. Legume lipoxygenase: Strategies for application in food industry. *Legume Science.* 2020; *2*(3), e44.
44. Adetuyi BO, Omolabi FK, Olajide PA, Oloke JK. Pharmacological, Biochemical and Therapeutic Potential of Milk Thistle (Silymarin): A Review *World News of Natural Sciences* 2021; *37*, 75–91.

45. Guillory A, & Bonhomme S. Phytohormone biosynthesis and signaling pathways of mosses. *Plant Molecular Biology.* 2021; *107*(4), 245–277.
46. Guo H, Verhoek IC, Prins GG, van der Vlag R, van der Wouden PE, van Merkerk R & Dekker FJ. Novel 15-lipoxygenase-1 inhibitor protects macrophages from lipopolysaccharide-induced cytotoxicity. *Journal of Medicinal Chemistry.* 2019; *62*(9), 4624–4637.
47. Singh P, Vandemeulebroucke A, Li J, Schulenburg C, Fortunato G, Kohen A & Cheatum CM. Evolution of the Chemical Step in Enzyme Catalysis. *ACS Catalysis.* 2021; *11*(11), 6726–6732.
48. Adetuyi BO, Toloyai PY, Ojugbeli ET, Oyebanjo OT, Adetuyi OA, Uche CZ, Olisah MC, Adumanya OC, Jude C, Chikwendu JK, Akram M, Awuchi CG, Egbuna C. Neurorestorative Roles of Microgliosis and Astrogliosis in Neuroinflammation and Neurodegeneration. *Scicom Journal of Medical and Applied Medical Sciences* 2021, *1*(1):1–5.
49. Hajeyah AA, Griffiths WJ, Wang Y, Finch AJ, and O'Donnell VB. The biosynthesis of enzymatically oxidized lipids. *Frontiers in Endrocrinology.* 2020; *11*, 910.
50. Pandian BA, Sathishraj R, Djanaguiraman M, Prasad PV, & Jugulam M. Role of cytochrome P450 enzymes in plant stress response. *Antioxidants.* 2020; *9*(5), 454.
51. Raza A, Charagh S, Zahid Z, Mubarik MS, Javed R, Siddiqui MH, & Hasanuzzaman M. Jasmonic acid: a key frontier in conferring abiotic stress tolerance in plants. *Plant Cell Reports*. 2021; *40*(8), 1513–1541.
52. Zhang B, Lewis KM, Abril A, Davydov DR, Vermerris W, Sattler SE, & Kang, C. Structure and function of the cytochrome P450 monooxygenase cinnamate 4-hydroxylase from sorghum bicolor. *Plant Physiology.* 2020; *183*(3), 957–973.
53. Yoon H, Shaw JL, Haigism MC, and Greka A. Lipid metabolism in sickness and in health: Emerging regulators of lipotoxicity. *Molecular Cell.* 2021; *81*(18), 3708–3730.
54. Duan J, Song Y, Zhang X, and Wang C. Effect of -3 polyunsaturated fatty acids-derived bioactive lipids on metabolic disorders. *Frontiers in physiology.* 2021;*12*.
55. Wasternack C, & Strnad M. Jasmonates: news on occurrence, biosynthesis, metabolism and action of an ancient group of signaling compounds. *International journal of molecular sciences.* 2018; *19*(9), 2539.
56. Ji M, Zhao J, Han K, Cui W, Wu X, Chen B & Yan F. Turnip mosaic virus P1 suppresses JA biosynthesis by degrading cpSRP54 that delivers AOCs onto the thylakoid membrane to facilitate viral infection. *PLoS Pathogens.* 2021; *17*(12), e1010108.
57. Shi Q, Wang H, Liu J, Li S, Guo J, Li H & Qin B. Old yellow enzymes: structures and structure-guided engineering for stereocomplementary bioreduction. *Applied Microbiology and Biotechnology*. 2020; *104*(19), 8155–8170.
58. Hobisch M, Holtmann D, de Santos PG, Alcalde M, Hollmann F, & Kara S. Recent developments in the use of peroxygenases–Exploring their high potential in selective oxyfunctionalisations. *Biotechnology Advances.* 2021; *51*, 107615.
59. Capella A, Menossi M, Arruda P, and Benedetti C. COI1 affects myrosinase activity and controls the expression of two flower-specific myrosinase-binding protein homologues in Arabidopsis. *Planta.* 2001;*213*(5), 691–699.
60. Oliw E. H. Fatty acid dioxygenase-cytochrome P450 fusion enzymes of filamentous fungal pathogens. *Fungal Genetics and Biology.* 2021; *157*, 103623.
61. Wongkaew A, Asayama K, Kitaiwa T, Nakamura SI, Kojima K, Stacey G, and Ohkama-Ohtsu N. AtOPT6 protein funtions in long-distance transport of glutathione in Arabidopsis thaliana. *Plant and Cell Physiology*. 2018; *59*(7), 1443–1451.
62. Wasternack C & Feussner I. The oxylipin pathways: biochemistry and function. *Annual Review of Plant Biology.* 2018; *69*, 363–386.

63. Zuther E, Schaarschmidt S, Fischer A, Erban A, Pagter M, Mubeen U & Hincha DK. Molecular signatures associated with increased freezing tolerance due to low temperature memory in Arabidopsis. *Plant, Cell & Environment*. 2019;*42*(3), 854–873.
64. Resemann, H. C., Lewandowska, M., Gömann, J., & Feussner, I. (2019). Membrane lipids, waxes and oxylipins in the moss model organism Physcomitrella patens. *Plant and Cell Physiology*, *60*(6), 1166–1175.
65. Mukhtarova, L. S., Lantsova, N. V., Khairutdinov, B. I., & Grechkin, A. N. (2020). Lipoxygenase pathway in model bryophytes: 12-oxo-9 (13), 15-phytodienoic acid is a predominant oxylipin in Physcomitrella patens. *Phytochemistry*, *180*, 112533.
66. Liakh, I., Pakiet, A., Sledzinski, T., & Mika, A. (2020). Methods of the analysis of oxylipins in biological samples. *Molecules*, *25*(2), 349.
67. Meena, P., Nehra, S., & Trivedi, P. C. (2021). Jasmonic Acid-A Novel Plant Hormone. From Chief Editor's Desk, 100.
68. Shanab, S. M., Hafez, R. M., & Fouad, A. S. (2018). A review on algae and plants as potential source of arachidonic acid. *Journal of advanced research*, *11*, 3–13.
69. Haq, M. I. (2020). Understanding the Implications of Anandamide, an Endocannabinoid in an Early Land Plant, Physcomitrella patens (Doctoral dissertation, East Tennessee State University).
70. Jiu S, Xu Y, Wang J, Wang L, Liu X, Sun W & Zhang C. The cytochrome P450 monooxygenase inventory of grapevine (Vitis vinifera L.): genome-wide identification, evolutionary characterization and expression analysis. *Frontiers in Genetics*. 2020;*11*, 44.
71. Schultz, D., Surabhi, S., Stelling, N., Rothe, M., KoInfekt Study Group, Methling, K., ... & Lalk, M. (2020). 16HBE cell lipid mediator responses to mono and co-infections with respiratory pathogens. *Metabolites*, *10*(3), 113.
72. Ali M & Baek K. H. Jasmonic acid signaling pathway in response to abiotic stresses in plants. *International Journal of Molecular Sciences*. 2020;*21*(2), 621.
73. Wagner D, Przybyla D, op den Camp R, Kim C, Landgraf F, Lee KP, Wursch M, Laloi C, Nater M, Apel K. The genetic basis of singlet oxygen induced stress responses of *Arabidopsis thaliana*. *Science* 2004;*306*, 1183–1185.
74. Kim C, Meskauskiene R, Apel K, Laloi C. No single way to understand singlet oxygen signalling in plants. *EMBO Rep* 2008;*9*, 435–439.
75. Acosta IF, Laparra H, Romero SP, Schmelz E, Hamberg M, Mottinger JP, Moreno MA, Dellaporta SL. Tasselseed1 is a lipoxygenase affecting jasmonic acid signalling in sex determination of maize. *Science*. 2009;*323*(5911), 262–265.
76. Yan Y, Christensen S, Isakeit T, Engelberth J, Meeley R, Hayward A, Neil Emery RJ, Kolomiets MV. Disruption of *OPR7* and *OPR8* reveals the versatile functions of jasmonic acid in maize development and defense. *Plant Cell*. 2012;*24*(4), 1420–1436.
77. Hwang IS, Hwang BK. The pepper 9-lipoxygenase gene CaLOX1 functions in defense and cell death responses to microbial pathogens. *Plant Physiology*. 2010;*152*(2), 948–967.
78. Ponce de Leon I, Sanz A, Hamberg M, Castresana C. Involvement of the *Arabidopsis* 585 -DOX1 fatty acid dioxygenase in protection against oxidative stress and cell death. *Plant Journal*. 2002;*586*(29), 61–72.
79. Hamberg M, Sanz A, Rodríguez MJ, Calvo AP, Castresana C. 2003. Activation of the fatty acid-dioxygenase pathway during bacterial infection of tobacco leaves. Formation of oxylipins protecting against cell death. *Journal of Biological Chemistry*. 2003;*278*, 51796–51805.
80. Rance I, Fournier J, Esquerre-Tugaye MT. The incompatible interaction between *Phytophthora parasitica* var.nicotianae race 0 and tobacco is suppressed in transgenic

plants expressing antisense lipoxygenase sequences. *Proceedings of National Academy Sciences U.S.A.* 1998;*95*, 6554–6559.

81. Ogunlana OO, Adetuyi BO, Esalomi EF, Rotimi MI, Popoola JO, Ogunlana OE, Adetuyi OA. Antidiabetic and Antioxidant Activities of the Twigs of Andrograhis paniculata on Streptozotocin-Induced Diabetic Male Rats. *BioChem* 2021; *1*(3), 238–249.
82. Wasternack C, Jasmonates: an update on biosynthesis,signal transduction and action in plant stress response, growth and development. *Annals of Botany (Lond).* 2007;*100*, 681–697.
83. Hamberg M, PoncedeLeon I, Sanz A, Castresana C. Fatty acid alpha-dioxygenases. *Prostaglandins Other Lipid Mediators.* 2002;*68–69*, 363–374.
84. Adetuyi BO, Odine GO, Olajide PA, Adetuyi OA, Atanda OO, Oloke JK. Nutraceuticals: role in metabolic disease, prevention and treatment, *World News of Natural Sciences* 2022, *42*, 1–27.
85. Mosblech A, Feussner I, Heilmann I. Oxylipins:structurally diverse metabolites from fatty acid oxidation. *Plant Physiology and Biochemistry.* 2009;*47*, 511–517.

7 The Role of Oxylipins in Biotic Stress Resistance

Sadaf Rafiq[1], *Tabinda Wani*[1], *Momin Showkat Bhat*[1], *Ifshan Malik*[2], *and Iqra Farooq*[1]
[1]Division of Floriculture and Landscape Architecture, Sher e Kashmir University of Agricultural Sciences and Technology, Kashmir, India
[2]Division of Basic Sciences and Humanities, Sher e Kashmir University of Agricultural Sciences and Technology, Kashmir, India

CONTENTS

7.1 INTRODUCTION

Jasmonates (JAs) are oxylipins, a class of oxidized lipids generated from α-linolenic acids. (+)-7-iso-jasmonoyl-L-isoleucine (JA-Ile) is the most well-known bioactive JA. The biosynthetic pathway that produces JA-Ile also produces a number of intermediates, such as cis(+)-oxophytodienoic acid (cis-OPDA), as well as secondary metabolites, such as methyl jasmonate and cis-jasmone, all of which have important biological functions, some of which are independent of JA-Ile (2–6). Because the bacterial pathogen *Pseudomonas syringae* can easily create coronatine (COR), a homologue of JA-Ile, it is commonly used in JA research. COR is a pathogen toxin that is employed to deflect plant defense responses, albeit biotic defense is only one of JA's functions.

DOI: 10.1201/9781003316558-7

Due to the sedentary nature, plants must constantly adjust to changes in the environment. Plant hormones mediate reactions to factors such as light, salt, deficiency of nutrients, cold, or water deficit which can be categorized as abiotic factors, as well as living organisms such as pathogens, herbivores, nematodes, or mutualistic symbiotic microbes, categorized as biotic factors. Jasmonic acid (JA) is one of the most well-known plant hormones involved in stress responses. JA also acts as a signal in a variety of developmental processes, including seed germination, root and entire plant growth, stamen formation, and senescence. Jasmonates (JAs) are lipid-derived signaling molecules that include JA and its derivatives. JAs are generated in chloroplast membrane by oxidation of α-linolenic acid. The first isolated JA compound was the methyl ester of jasmonic acid (MeJA) which was detected as an odorant in the flowers of *Jasminum grandiflorum*. It was after two decades when the first physiological processes caused by JA or MeJA were described, such as senescence promotion and growth inhibition. In the late 1980s and early 1990s, the first indication for altered gene expression by JA was described by four groups: (i) JA-induced proteins (JIPs), (ii) induction of vegetative storage proteins (VSPs), (iii) accumulation of alkaloids was detected upon elicitation of plant cell cultures leading to an increase in endogenous JA, and (iv) accumulation of proteinase inhibitors (PIs).

7.2 OXYLIPIN SIGNALING IN PLANT STRESS RESPONSES

Oxylipins are a special class of oxidized fatty acids related to signaling in stress responses and innate immunity in plants. Unlike animals, plants lack intricate protective mechanisms, but they have developed an efficient armory of defense systems against attacks all kinds of stresses. Phyto-oxylipins (POs) play the most important role in these defenses. They function as signal molecules and/or protective substances like antibacterial and wound-healing agents, as well as cutin components (the framework of the cuticle that protects all the aerial parts of a plant from its environment). Plants respond to numerous stimuli in a variety of ways, resulting in tissue damage caused by abiotic or biotic factors. The creation of certain oxylipins, which have a variety of biological activities, is frequently part of these stress reactions. Jasmonic acid and its precursor OPDA (12-oxophytodienoic acid) are formed enzymatically and accumulate in response to stresses such as wounding and pathogen infection [1], whereas hydroxyl fatty acids and phytoprostanes, which are formed non-enzymatically, play signaling roles in plant stress responses such as pathogen infection, heavy metal uptake, and others [2].

JA and its derivatives, called jasmonates, get quickly accumulated in damaged plants as they have a key role in systemic wound signaling [3–6]. Some of the metabolites, such as MeJA, are volatile defense elicitors. Plants may use these compounds for the activation of such wound-related pathways, maybe through a different recognition mechanism than MeJA [7]. Plant defense mechanisms, on the other hand, are controlled not just by jasmonic-acid-transducing pathways, but also by a network of signaling cascades involving either salicylic acid or ethylene. All of these defense pathways have a complicated interaction [8–12]. They can work together or against each other. The discovery of multiple Arabidopsis mutants implies that these pathways share signaling components that can influence crosstalk by positive or negative cross-regulation [13–16].

Oxylipins have antifungal or antimicrobial characteristics that make pathogens weaker and/or kill them. The hydroxy and epoxy derivatives of linoleic acid produced via the peroxygenase route were the first fungi-toxic oxylipins to be identified. The enzymes in the peroxygenase pathway catalyze the epoxidation of fatty acid double bonds (peroxygenase) and subsequent stereo-controlled hydrolysis of these epoxides into their vicinal diols (epoxide hydrolase) in a sequential order [17]. Short-chain aldehydes resulting from the breakdown of fatty-acid hydroperoxides, show potent antimicrobial effects and involvement in plant–insect interactions. The transgenic potato plants recently exhibited the role of such aldehydes in plant defense against sucking insect pests by reducing the fecundity of aphids in vivo [18].

It has also been proven that phytoprostanes play an important role in the activation of genes for stress response, which leads to better protection against oxidative stress in the future [14, 19]. These phytoprostanes are classified into several groups based on their ring and side-chain architectures, and plants manufacture a variety of them [20]. Due to presence of a reactive a,b-unsaturated carbonyl structure, the A1-type (PPA1), deoxy-J1-type phytoprostanes, and OPDA belong to reactive electrophile species (RES) oxylipin subgroup. By attaching to the protein's free thiol groups, RES can alter them directly. Weaker electrophiles like JA and B1-type phytoprostanes do not have this feature (PPB1). However, many experts believe that RES causes a common set of defense genes to be activated [21–23]. (+)-7-iso-jasmonoyl-L-isoleucine (JA-Ile), the biologically active form of JA in *Arabidopsis thaliana* leaves, accumulates quickly (within 5 minutes) in leaves distant to sites that have suffered wounding [24–26]. However, it does not appear that this signaling involves the direct transfer of hormones. Furthermore, other even quicker mechanisms may be involved, such as electrical coupling, reactive oxygen species and Ca^{2+} mediated waves, "trio signaling," and so on [27, 28]. When it comes to chemical structure and geometric isomers, the phyto-oxylipin family is extremely versatile. Regio-isomers of the same oxylipin structure can have different biological effects [29]. The biological activity of a particular oxylipin may show drastic changes with a slight modification in the epoxy or hydroxy groups. Moreover, epimerization may convert the biologically active (+)-7-iso-jasmonoyl-L-isoleucine into the inactive form [30].

7.3 JASMONATE SIGNAL TRANSDUCTION AND REGULATION

Signal transduction of jasmonates involves two proteins: JAZ proteins (JASMONATE-ZIM-DOMAIN proteins) and SCF-COI1 complex (a key component of most jasmonate responses). The hormone is recognized by the protein COI1, the subunit of SCF complex which is a ubiquitin ligase (Figure 7.1 (B)). During the resting state (Figure 7.1 (A)), when there is no production or very less production of jasmonates, the transcription factors bind to the JAZ and hence their function of activating jasmonate-responsive genes is prevented. During the active state (Figure 7.1 (A)), there is a stimulus (wounding, anther maturation, etc.) which causes synthesis of jasmonates. This hormone is consequently perceived by COI1, which results in the

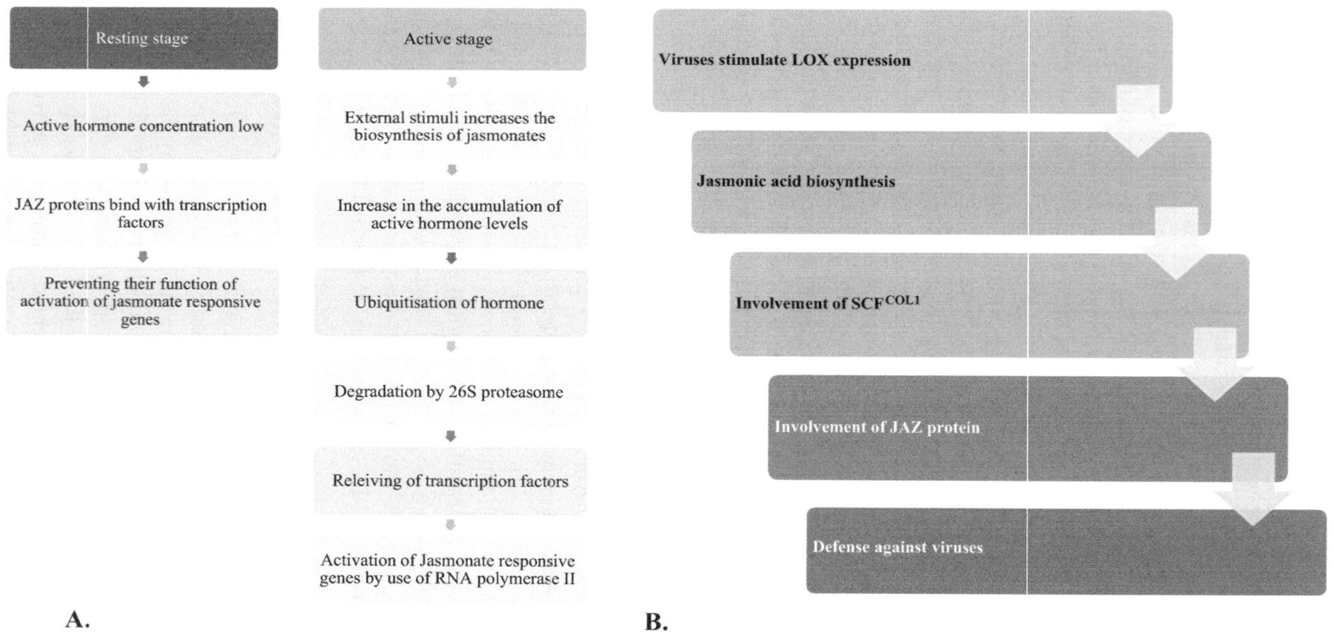

FIGURE 7.1 (A) Model for jasmonate signaling. (B) JA regulated defense against virus.

binding to JAZ proteins to COI1 through their jas motif. Subsequently JAZ proteins undergo ubiquitination and then degradation by the 26S proteasome resulting in the release of transcription factors. These factors activate the transcription by RNA polymerase II which result in the activation of jasmonate-responsive genes.

For a long time, JA and MeJA have been considered the bioactive forms due to their abundance and related physiological effects in the plant body. The existence of the gene (JAR1) that encodes for an enzyme that causes the conjugation of JA to amino acids such as valine, isoleucine, and others, as well as the presence of its corresponding mutant (jar1), clearly demonstrate that JA and MeJA are just the precursors of the isoleucine conjugated jasmonoyl derivative: the actual bioactive molecule (JA-Ile) [30–32]. Nonetheless, several scientists have concluded that JA-Ile is the biologically active component in jasmonic acid signaling [24, 33–34].

According to a vast number of researchers who analyzed the literature, the major signal transduction pathway after jasmonic acid perception converges on basic-helix-loophelix (bHLH) associated transcription factors (TFs) [35–44]. Furthermore, the multifunctional MYC2 is the best studied of these factors. JASMONATE-ZIM-DOMAIN (JAZ) repressors are a class of nuclear proteins that regulate jasmonic acid response under stress. These JAZ repressors cause the co-reception of physiologically active jasmonic acid (JA-Ile) when they bind with the F-box protein COI1 (CORONATINE INSENSITIVE1), which is part of the SCF (Skp-Cullin-F-box) complex [34, 45–46].

Pauwels et al. (47) (2010) proposed a paradigm for understanding the suppression of downstream TFs implicated in JA signaling transcriptional activity. According to this scenario, the JAZ proteins inhibit the activity of bioactive jasmonic acid by utilizing the general co-repressors TOPLESS (TPL) and TPL-related proteins via an association with the adaptor protein Novel Interactor of JAZ (NINJA). JAZ protein degradation, which is mediated by the JA-Ile and SCFCOI1 complexes, contributes in the unblocking of MYC2 [30, 34–38, 40, 42, 47–50]. However, it is worth noting that TPL was originally thought to be a co-repressor of auxin-related response. The ERF (ethylene response factor) associated amphi-philic repressor (EAR) motif seen in such proteins is thought to interact with AUX/IAA repressors [51–53]. Furthermore, JAZ repressors possess a considerable affinity for a number of bHLH TFs, including MYC2, MYC3, MYC4, EGL1 (ENHANCER OF GLABRA3 1), GL3 (GLABRA3), and TT8 (TRANSPARENT TESTA 8) that are implicated in both unique and overlapping jasmonic acid signaling pathways [54–57].

A novel regulatory element in jasmonic acid signaling (JASMONOYL-L-ISOLEUCINE HYDROLASE 1 (JIH1)) that encodes a homeostatic phase in jasmonic acid metabolism is being characterized recently. The JA-Ile burst, which contributes to the regulation of plant defense responses, is diminished when JIH1 is combined with JA-Ile, resulting in inactivation stages such as carboxylation or hydroxylation [58]. The JIH1 silenced lines in *Nicotiana attenuate* had a lower growth level of *Manduca sexta* (the specialist) and *Spodoptera littoralis* (the generalist), collecting larger amounts of JA-Ile derived compounds as a result. Silenced plants also had a larger quantity of herbivore-elicited volatiles, indicating that they were more attractive to natural predators of *M. sexta* eggs.

Vancanneyt et al. [59] recently hypothesized that most plants possess PO pools of varied sizes that impart an oxylipin signature on a particular organelle, tissue, plant, or species after extensive research. Depending on the type of stress (pathogen attack, injury, or treatment with elicitors: signal molecules), the composition of oxylipin derivatives changes dramatically. Glazebrook [60] (2001) investigated the action of salicylic acid on barley leaves and discovered that it acts as a trigger for the nearly exclusive synthesis of hydroxy-fatty-acid derivatives, whereas Foyer [61] (2003) discovered that methyl jasmonate causes aldehyde buildup in these plants. Apart from their unavoidable occurrence, the spatial and temporal expression of many enzymes involved in the production of oxylipins is of paramount relevance. This holds notably true for the LOX isoforms that result in the synthesis of fatty-acid-derived hydroperoxides, transported along the LOX pathway's many branches. In numerous plant species, wounding, mechanical stress, pathogen infection, or pest damage have been found to activate LOXs, which activate the de novo synthesis of jasmonic acid or its precursor (13S-hydroperoxylinolenic acid). Transgenic potato plants with significantly lower amounts of such LOX isoforms, as well as Arabidopsis plants which were deficient in linolenic acid, were more susceptible to insect attacks [62].

7.4 TRANSCRIPTION FACTORS INVOLVED IN DEFENSE

In plants, JAs are important regulators of the balance between defense and growth. Plants are constantly in battle with their surroundings, and their sedentary nature necessitates the finely tuned, well-designed defensive system capable of dealing with a wide range of biotic and abiotic threats. To maintain their survival, plants have developed innate immunity, R-gene-mediated resistance, and systemic acquired resistance. Transcription factors (TFs) are key genetic components that aid in regulation of gene expression and a variety of other physiological processes. They may either increase or repress transcriptional activities depending on the environment. The plant defense system, the role of transcription factors in mediating defensive responses have been discussed hereunder.

7.5 TRANSCRIPTION FACTORS (TFS): MODULATORS OF GENE EXPRESSION

They are regulatory proteins that regulate gene transcription in a mechanistic manner. They control gene expression by acting as an on/off switch, activating and suppressing genes and so regulating their function. These proteins are transcribed and translated in the nucleus and cytoplasm respectively and then they diffuse back in the nucleus for their potential targets in the genomic DNA. Their re-entry into the nucleus is facilitated by nuclear localization regions located in the protein sequences of all TFs. The TFs have specified DNA-binding domains and bind to particular DNA sequences in the promoter region of a gene, termed cis-regulatory elements or TF binding sites (TFBSs). TFBs may be found in the intron region and have regulatory functions. TFBs are important for DNA binding and are used to categorize TFs into different groups or families.

7.6 REGULATORY ROLE OF TFS IN PLANT DEFENSE

TFs are important in innate plant immunity because they regulate genes involved in PTI (Pathogen-associated molecular patterns/PAMP-triggered immunity), ETI (effector triggered immunity), hormone, phytoalexin production and processes. Transcriptional reprogramming is one of the first reactions to pathogen infection and it necessitates large changes in gene expression of plant cells in order to prioritize defense above other metabolic activities including growth and development [63]. According to recent research, a metabolic shift is essential to control the trade-off between growth and immunity and enable adequate resource allocation for plant survival [64]. Many transcription factor groups have been implicated in transcriptional reprogramming. The primary plant TF families that regulate many biological processes, including plant defense, are:

7.6.1 WRKY TFs

WRKY TFs, sometimes known as "Jack-of-all-Trades" TFs, are one of the most numerous TF families in plants [65]. The regulatory role of WRKYs in plant defense has been thoroughly explored, especially in the model plant *Arabidopsis thaliana*, and they have been found to have both destructive and constructive roles in plant defense [66]. PAMP signaling is regulated by the WRKYs, which is associated with mitogen-activated protein kinase (MAPK) signaling pathway [67]. The MAPK cascade is involved in variety of defensive responses, including the detection of PAMPs and ETI [68]. In *Arabidopsis*, for example, WRKY33 has been linked to resistance posed against *Botrytis cinerea* and *Alternaria brassicicola* responsible for causing necrotrophic fungal diseases [69]. ETI is thought to include WRKY TFs interacting with plant R proteins. In the presence of the AVRA10 effector, the mildew resistance locus A10 (MLA10) NB-LRR protein providing powdery mildew resistance, interacts with *Hordeum vulgare* WRKY1 (HvWRKY1) and HvWRKY2 in barley [17]. Both HvWRKY1 and HvWRKY2 suppress the pathogen causing powdery mildew. MLA10 interacts with the above factors (HvWRKY1 and HvWRKY2) to stimulate the defense after infection by *B. graminis* (expressing AVRA10). WRKY52, also known as *Ralstonia solanacearum* 1 (RRS1) in *Arabidopsis* confers resistance to the bacterial disease *Ralstonia solanacearum* [70]. According to map-based cloning and natural variation analysis, RRS1was found to interact with RPS4 for dual resistance to both fungal and bacterial plant pathogens [71].

7.6.2 bHLH TFs

This family of transcription factors was first discovered in mammals and plants in 1989 and yeast in 1990. This is made up of a collection of transcription factors with the "basic helix-loop-helix (bHLH)" domain. This domain is found in proteins that perform a wide range of tasks. The bHLH TF family has roughly 160 members in *Arabidopsis*. However, only a few of them have been thoroughly studied, indicating that while the bHLH may not be directly engaged in plant defense, they may have an indirect relationship through the production of specific metabolites that are necessary under stress. They also interact with the jasmonic acid signaling system, which regulates plant hormonal balance that is important for plant defense [72]. The bHLH mutants were found to be sensitive to JA-inhibited root development and had an increase in JA-induced protection against pathogen infection and insect assault. HBI1, a bHLH TF was found to negatively regulate the genes responsible for plant immunity, reduction in the PAMP-induced growth arrest, mediated the trade-off between growth and PAMP-triggered immunity [73]. Another transcription factor of this group, called ILR3, regulates iron deficiency, glucosinolate biosynthesis, and pathogen responses [74]. MYC2 is one more transcription factor of this group that controls a subset of *Nicotiana attenuate*'s defensive responses [75].

7.6.3 AP2/ERF TFs

This is one more TF family, APETALA2/ethylene response factor (AP2/ERF) which modulates stress responses in plants by participating in secondary metabolite biosynthesis and is specific to plants [76]. The presence of an AP2 DNA-binding domain with 40–70 conserved amino acids distinguishes members of this family [77]. At transcriptional and post-translational levels, it was found that the AP2/ERF TFs control genes are involved in a variety of biological processes, including growth and development, hormone signaling, and stress responses at both the levels of transcription and post translation [78]. Most of the AP2/ERF TFs are found to have a low basal expression that can be activated or lowered by external stress stimuli or hormonal imbalance, according to gene expression profiling [79]. Phosphorylation and other post-translational modifications alter the action and quantity of AP2/ERFs. Phosphorylation has been demonstrated to impact the stability and transactivity of the AP2/ERF protein in several investigations [80]. In Arabidopsis, for example, SNF1-related protein kinases (SnRKs), a positive regulator of the ABA signaling cascade, interacts with and phosphorylates RAV1 to limit its transcription repression activity [81].

ERF is one of the several AP2/ERF subfamilies. The AP2/ERF family has around 145 members in *Arabidopsis thaliana* [79]. About 65 of them have been recognized as ERFs. The involvement of members of the ERF subfamily in plant defense is well-known. The expression of ERF1 in *Arabidopsis* has been demonstrated to improve resistance to numerous necrotrophic fungal infections. [82]. Furthermore, the ERF1 is thought to constitute a link between the JA and ethylene signaling pathways. Members of the ERF subfamily consist of genes that influence disease resisting pathways, according to a thorough assessment of the role of AP2/ERF TFs [83], indicating a key role of this subfamily in the regulation of plant defense responses.

7.6.4 MYB TFs

The MYB transcription factor is one of the biggest and most functionally diversified families found in all eukaryotes. They differ in their structure and are identified by the presence of a conserved MYB domain with two or three faulty repetitions (R1, R2, and R3). MYB TFs have been extensively explored in terms of structure, categorization, and functional diversity [84]. *Zea mays* was the first plant in which

MYB TF were discovered [85]. MYB TFs have now been discovered in a number of other plant species, including *Arabidopsis* [86]. It is one of the most powerful defense tactics of the host plant resistance. The HR response is said to be positively regulated by MYB TFs. AtMYB30 demonstrated a rapid and temporary expression in response to non-virulent infections such as *Xanthomonas campestris* pv *campestris* [87]. According to reports, AtMYB60 and AtMYB96 function through ABA signaling pathway, and AtMYB96-mediated ABA signals induce pathogen resistance responses in *Arabidopsis* through stimulation of salicylic acid (SA) production [88].

Plants generate jasmonic acid (JA) and its cyclopentanone derivatives. Plant growth and defense activities are aided by these multifunctional hormones. JAs protect plants from infections and environmental stressors in addition to their developmental roles. JAs have also been shown to communicate with hormones created by stress to respond swiftly to them [89]. Plant growth, reproduction, flower development, inhibition of growth, ripening of fruits, coiling in tendrils, tuber formation in potato, trichome creation, and fungus arbuscular mycorrhizal association are all affected by them. JA also controls plant fertility and regulates leaf and root morphogenesis in soybeans. Male sterility has been discovered in Arabidopsis mutants lacking JA production. JA also regulates general development of stamen tissue, including gene expression. The biotic stress in plants is induced by various micro- organisms like virus, bacteria, fungi, nematodes, parasites and insect/ pests. Plants create a defensive system in order to defend themselves. Plant defense responses are mediated by main signals such as JA, salicylic acid (SA), brassinosteroids, ethylene, polyamines, and abscisic acid (ABA). Plants generate JA to protect themselves against infection or treatment. Other signaling molecules linked to secondary metabolism have also been discovered [90]. JA pathway directly affects SA synthesis by causing its accumulation and antagonizing the stomatal regulation. They also regulate the defense response against *P. syringae* and various nectrotrophic bacteria (Figure 7.2 (A)). The defense-related genes are activated by salicylic acid, which code for proteins related to pathogenesis. In several plants, a fungal elicitor increased JA synthesis, secondary metabolite biosynthetic gene expression, and metabolite accumulation [91]. It was discovered that inoculating an endophytic fungus into *Atractylodes lancea* activated JA production, which enhanced the amount of oil in the plant [92]. In *A. lancea* plantlets, JA, nitric oxide, hydrogen peroxide, and SA are also known to mediate the signaling pathway [93]. However, JA may operate as a downstream signal of NO, whereas H_2O_2 serves as a link between JA and NO. H_2O_2, SA, and JA have been found to collaborate in fungus-induced volatile oil production in *A. lancea* plantlets. However, it was established that NO mediates fungus-induced volatile oil formation via SA- and H_2O_2-dependent mechanisms [94]. In plant defensive responses, both JA and SA are key signaling chemicals. When an inhibitor interferes with the production of JA, the concentration of SA increases, and vice versa. Anthocyanins and procyanidins have been examined in the presence of methyl jasmonate (MJ), JA, and cis-jasmone [95]. JAs have been used in the form of a solution or vapor [96]. When treated as a solution, JA increased anthocyanin accumulation in *Fagopyrum esculentum* hypocotyls, but when applied as a vapor, it lowered it. In buckwheat seedlings it was found that the production of anthocyanins remained unaffected by JA solution. Because of differences in biochemical activity, MJ functions in both phloem and xylem (96). In another experiment, antioxidant enzymes, ascorbate metabolism, and phenolic compounds were measured in 21-day-old melon (*Cucumis melo*) cells treated with JA at relatively low concentrations (0.5, 5.0, and 10 mol). By creating bioactive chemicals in defense, JA was discovered to activate primary and secondary metabolism in melon cells [97]. Melon cells have increased oxidative enzyme activity as well as ascorbic acid, coumarin, and p-coumaric levels without slowing down their proliferation. Intracellular JA is a signal transducer that acts upstream of H_2O_2 to regulate catalase (CAT), peroxidase (POD), and the development of five isozymes as well as ascorbic- POD detoxification enzymes. It is evident that JA stimulates the formation of secondary metabolites in melon cells, resulting in melon resistance. At 10 mol JA, CAT activity increased by 24%. Plants respond to JA by producing hormones, expressing genes, producing crops, and defending themselves to biotic and abiotic stress [98]. It was found that POD activity was raised after 24 hours to 137% by the action of JA. The existence of five POD isoforms was discovered by enzyme activity. Glutathione reductase (GR), ascorbate peroxidase (APX), and ascorbic oxidase (AOX) all increased. Accordingly, APX aids in the detoxification of H_2O_2 as depicted in the reaction as under:

$$2 \text{ ascorbate} + H_2O_2 \rightarrow 2 \text{ monodehydroascorbate} + 2\, H_2O_2 \text{ ascorbate} + H_2O_2 \rightarrow 2 \text{ monodehydroascorbate} + 2\, H_2O$$

It was found that hydroxylated JA derivatives are more beneficial in potato tuber development, although the process is also influenced by light, temperature, and gibberellic acid [99]. It indicates that JAs indirectly govern tuber development via cross-talk with GA signals [100]. Under stress, reactive oxygen species (ROS) are produced (Figure 7.2 (B)), which harm plants by oxidizing lipids, proteins, and nucleic acids [101]. The antioxidant activity of raspberry fruit is also increased by JA and MJ [102]. In tomato field pots, JAs also boost plant tolerance to pests. They also offer fungus and nematode resistance to culinary plants and vegetables. Plants have been demonstrated to be resistant to herbivores by MJ and cis-jasmone [103]. Different concentrations of JA have been shown to affect marigold plant flower development, height, and weight. The dry weight of the bloom, the height of the plant, and the weight of 1000 seeds are all increased by JA [104]. With increasing JA concentrations, height and weight climbed to their maximum at 150 M JA. With rising JA concentrations over 75 M, the number of flowers grew as well, while carotenoids dropped. Photosynthesis is regulated by JA, but when MJ and JA are combined, plants become more resistant to green mold infection [105]. In the wild type, ozone exposure produced activation of several genes involved in antioxidant metabolism [106]. The induction of antioxidant genes was inhibited in JA-deficient Arabidopsis 12-oxophytodienoate reductase 3 (opr3) mutants.

Although several plants, such as members of the cucurbitaceae family, have been shown to prevent cancer [107], the chemical responsible has only just been discovered [108]. Several human cancer cell lines have been discovered to be resistant to JAs. The activity is caused by JAs interfering with energy metabolism, causing mitochondrial

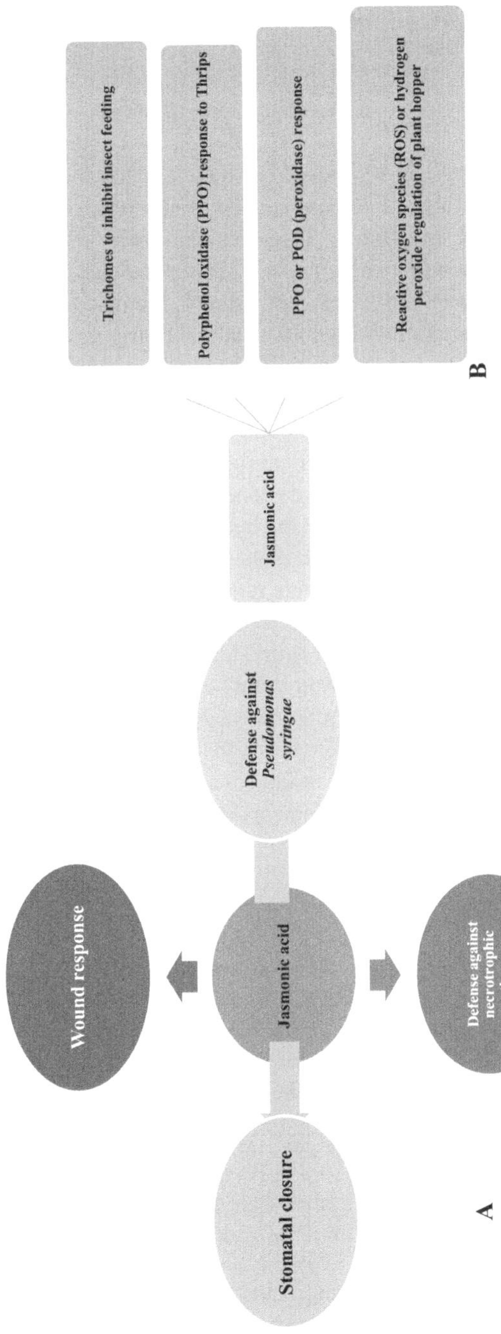

FIGURE 7.2 (A) JA-aided defense against pathogens in Arabidopsis. (B) JA defense against herbivorous insects.

disturbance and the generation of reactive oxygen species (ROS), which causes cell death. In cancer treatment, JA, MJ, and cis-jasmone are quite successful. JA and MJ are abundant in extracts from *Viscum album*, *Jasminum*, *Chloranthus*, *Cymbidium*, *Rosmarinus*, and *Lonicera* plants.

7.7 CONCLUSION

In recent years there has been a lot of research work to study the physiological role of different classes of POs in plant defense and the relationships among them during times of stress: both biotic and abiotic. However, the nature of these POs and the characterization of corresponding enzymes in their biosynthesis is not clear yet and thus needs to be studied more and more. Furthermore, the discovery of the mode of action of these POs at molecular level and how pathogens trigger their biosynthesis is another challenge that needs to be overcome. The processes that underpin molecular crosstalk between different signaling pathways that operate under diverse stress circumstances, as well as the molecular crosstalk itself, remain largely unknown. The role and contribution of various transduction signals in systemic defense response induced in healthy tissues is yet another milestone to be achieved. The volatile stress signals emitted by stress-affected plants on healthy or intact neighboring plants needs a special attention. As research into plant hormone biosynthesis and activity improves, it is becoming obvious that a wide range of metabolites linked to various plant hormones play an important role in plant defense as well as plant–environment interactions. Hydroxylation, methylation, amino acid conjugation and glucosylation, in particular, are important biochemical steps that help phytohormone families diversify their metabolic armament. Modern technologies, analytical approaches and a close collaboration and co-ordination between different classes of plant scientists as well as chemists is the need of the hour to improve our knowledge on POs and discover new regulatory mechanisms and elements thereof which play critical roles in plant stress responses.

REFERENCES

1. Block A, Schmelz E, Jones JB, and Klee HJ. Coronatine and salicylic acid: The battle between Arabidopsis and Pseudomonas for phytohormone control. Molecular Plant Pathology. 2005; 6:79–83.
2. Sattler SE, Mene-Saffrane L, Farmer EE, Krischke M, Mueller MJ, DellaPenna D. Non-enzymatic lipid peroxidation reprograms gene expression and activates defence markers in Arabidopsis tocopherol deficient mutants. Plant Cell. 2006; 18:3706–3720.
3. Howe GA. Plant hormones: metabolic end run to jasmonate. Nature Chemical Biology. 2018; 14:109–110.
4. León Morcillo RJ, Ocampo JA, García Garrido JM. Plant 9-lox oxylipin metabolism in response to arbuscular mycorrhiza. Plant Signaling and Behavior. 2012; 7(12):1584–1588.
5. Lortzing, T and Steppuhn, A. Jasmonate signalling in plants shapes plant–insect interaction ecology. Current Opinion in Insect Science. 2016; 14:32–39.
6. Schilmiller AL and Howe GA. Systemic signaling in the wound response. Current Opinion in Plant Biology. 2005; 8:369–377.

7. Vollenweider S, Weber H, Stolz S, Che´telat A. Farmer EE: Fatty acid ketodienes and fatty acid ketotrienes: Michael addition acceptors that accumulate in wounded and diseased Arabidopsis leaves. Plant Journal. 2000; 24(4):467–476.
8. Kachroo P, Shanklin J, Shah J, Whittle EJ, Klessig DF: A fatty acid desaturase modulates the activation of defence signaling pathways in plants. Proceedings of the National Academy of Sciences of the United States of America. 2001; 98:9448–9453.
9. Straus DS, Glass CK: Cyclopentenone prostaglandins: new insights on biological activities and cellular targets. Medicinal Research Reviews. 2001; 21:185–210.
10. Stelmach BA, Muller A, Hennig P, Gebhardt S, Schubert-Zsilavecz M, Weiler EW. A novel class of oxylipins, sn1–0-(12- oxophytodienoyl)-sn2–0-(hexadecatrienoyl)-monogalactosyl diglyceride, from *Arabidopsis thaliana*. Journal of Biological Chemistry. 2001; 276:12832–12838.
11. Hamberg M. New cyclopentenone fatty acids formed from linoleic and linolenic acids in potato. Lipids. 2000; 35:353–363.
12. Itoh A, Schilmiller AL, McCaig BC, Howe GA. Identification of a jasmonate-regulated allene oxide synthase that metabolizes 9-hydroperoxides of linoleic and linolenic acids. Journal of Biological Chemistry. 2002; 277:46051–46058.
13. Krischke M, Loeffler C, Mueller MJ. Biosynthesis of 13,14-dehydro-12-oxo-phytodienoicacid and related cytopentenones via the phytoprostane D1 pathway. Phytochemistry. 2003; 62:351–358.
14. Thoma I, Loeffler C, Sinha AK, Gupta M, Krischke M, Steffan B, Roitsch T, and Mueller MJ. Cyclopentenone isoprostanes induced by reactive oxygen species trigger defence gene activation and phytoalexin accumulation in plants. Plant Journal. 2003; 34:363–375.
15. Gerwick WH, Moghaddam M, Hamberg M. Oxylipin metabolism in the red alga *Gracilariopsis lemaneiformis*: mechanism of formation of vicinal dihydroxy fatty acids. Archives of Biochemistry and Biophysics. 1991; 290:436–444.
16. Farmer EE. Surface-to-air signals. Nature. 2001; 411:854–856.
17. Seo S, Okamoto M, Seto H, Ishizuka K, Sano H, Ohashi Y. Tobacco MAP kinase: a possible mediator in wound signal transduction pathways. Science. 1995; 270:1988–1992.
18. Van Poecke RM, Posthumus MA, Dicke M. Herbivore-induced volatile production by *Arabidopsis thaliana* leads to attraction of the parasitoid *Cotesia rubecula*: chemical, behavioral and gene-expression analysis. Journal of Chemical Ecology. 2001; 27:1911–1928.
19. Loeffler C, Berger S, Guy A, Durand T, Bringmann G, Dreyer M, von Rad U, Durner J and Mueller M J. B1-phytoprostanes trigger plant defense and detoxification responses. Plant Physiology. 2005; 137(1):328–340.
20. Thoma I, Krischke M, Loeffler C, and Mueller MJ. The isoprostanoid pathway in plants. Chemistry and Physics of Lipids. 2004; 128:135–148.
21. Almeras E, Stolz S, Vollenweider S, Reymond P, Mene-Saffrane L, and Farmer EE. Reactive electrophile species activate defence gene expression in Arabidopsis. Plant Journal. 2003; 34:205–216.
22. Weber H, Che´telat A, Reymond P and Farmer EE. Selective and powerful stress gene expression in Arabidopsis inresponse to malondialdehyde. Plant Journal. 2004; 37:877–888.
23. Farmer, EE and Davoine C. Reactive electrophile species. Current Opinion in Plant Biology. 2007; 10:380–386.
24. Fonseca S, Chico JM, Solano R. The jasmonate pathway: the ligand, the receptor and the core signalling module. Current Opinion in Plant Biology. 2009; 12:539–547.

25. Heyer M, Reichelt M, Mithöfer A. A holistic approach to analyze systemic jasmonate accumulation in individual leaves of Arabidopsis rosettes upon wounding. Frontiers in Plant Science. 2018; 9:1569.
26. Koo AJK, Gao X, Jones AD, Howe GA. A rapid wound signal activates the systemic synthesis of bioactive jasmonates in Arabidopsis. Plant Journal. 2009; 59(6):974–986.
27. Choi W, Hilleary R, Swanson SJ, Kim SH, Gilroy S. Rapid, long-distance electrical and calcium signaling in plants. Annual Review of Plant Biology. 2016; 67:287–310.
28. Choi WG, Miller G, Wallace I, Harper J, Mittler R, Gilroy S. Orchestrating rapid long-distance signalling in plants with $Ca^{2+,}$ ROS and electrical signals. Plant Journal. 2018; 90(4):698–707.
29. Granér G, Hamberg M, Meijer J. Screening of oxylipins for control of oilseed rape (*Brassica napus*) fungal pathogens. Phytochemistry. 2003; 63:89–95.
30. Fonseca S, Chini A, Hamberg M, Adie B, Kramell R, Miersch O, Wasternack C, Solano R. (+)-7-iso-Jasmonoyl-L-Isoleucine is the endogenous bioactive jasmonate. Nature Chemical Biology. 2009; 5:344–350.
31. Staswick PE, Tiryaki I. The oxylipin signal jasmonic acid is activated by an enzyme that conjugates it to isoleucine in Arabidopsis. Plant Cell. 2004; 16:2117–2127.
32. Suza WP, Rowe ML, Hamberg M, Staswick PE. A tomato enzyme synthesizes -7-iso-jasmonoyl-L-isoleucine in wounded leaves. Planta. 2010; 231:717–728.
33. Thines B, Katsir L, Melotto M, Niu Y, Mandaokar A, Liu G, Nomura K, He SY, Howe GA, Browse J. JAZ repressor proteins are targets of the SCF(COI1) complex during jasmonate signalling. Nature. 2007; 448:661–665.
34. Katsir L, Schilmiller AL, Staswick PE, He SY, Howe GA. COI1 is a critical component of a receptor for jasmonate and the bacterial virulence factor coronatin. Proceedings of the National Academy of Sciences of the United States of America. 2008; 105:7100–7105.
35. Balbi V, Devoto A. Jasmonate signalling network in *Arabidopsis thaliana*: crucial regulatory nodes and new physiological scenarios. New Phytologist. 2008; 177:301–318.
36. Chico JM, Chini A, Fonseca S, Solano R. JAZ repressors set the rhythm in jasmonate signaling. Current Opinion in Plant Biology. 2008; 11:486–494.
37. Staswick PE. JAZing up jasmonate signaling. Trends in Plant Science. 2008; 13:66–71.
38. Browse J. Jasmonate passes muster: a receptor and targets for the defence hormone. Annual Reviews in Plant Biology. 2009; 60:183–205.
39. Chini A, Fonseca S, Chico JM, Fernandez-Calvo P, Solano R. The ZIM domain mediates homo- and heteromeric interactions between Arabidopsis JAZ proteins. Plant Journal. 2009; 59(1):77–87.
40. Gfeller A, Dubugnon L, Liechti R, Farmer EE. Jasmonate biochemical pathway. Science Signaling. 2010; 3(109).
41. Pauwels L, Goossens A. The JAZ proteins: a crucial interface in the jasmonate signaling cascade. Plant Cell. 2011; 23:3089–3100.
42. Kazan K, Manners JM. Jasmonate signalling: toward an integrated view. Plant Physiology. 2008; 146:1459–1468.
43. Kazan K, Manners JM. JAZ repressors and the orchestration of phytohormone crosstalk. Trends in Plant Science. 2012; 17:22–31.
44. Wager A and Browse J. Social network: JAZ protein interactions expand our knowledge of jasmonate signalling. Frontiers in Plant Science. 2012; 3:41.
45. Chini A, Fonseca S, Fernandez G, Adie B, Chico JM, Lorenzo O, Garcia-Casado G, Lopez-Vidriero I, Lozano FM, Ponce MR, Micol JL, Solano R. The JAZ family of repressors is the missing link in jasmonate signalling. Nature. 2007; 448:666–671.

46. Yan Y, Stolz S, Chetelat A, Reymond P, Pagni M, Dubugnon L, Farmer EE. A downstream mediator in the growth repression limb of the jasmonate pathway. Plant Cell. 2007; 19:2470–2483.
47. Pauwels L, Barbero GF, Geerinck J, Tilleman S, Grunewald W, Perez AC, Chico JM, Bossche RV, Sewell J, Gil E, Garcia-Casado G, Witters E, Inze D, Long JA, De JaegerG, Solano R, Goossens A. NINJA connects the co-repressor TOPLESS to jasmonate signalling. Nature. 2010; 464:788–791.
48. Chini A, Boter M, Solano R. Plant oxylipins: COI1/JAZs/MYC2 as the core jasmonic acid- signaling module. The FEBS Journal. 2009; 276(17):4682–4692.
49. Chung HS, Niu Y, Browse J, Howe GA. Top hits in contemporary JAZ: an update on jasmonate signaling. Phytochemistry. 2009; 70:1547–1559.
50. Memelink J. Regulation of gene expression by jasmonate hormones. Phytochemistry. 2009; 70:1560–1570.
51. Long JA, Woody S, Poethig S, Meyerowitz EM, Barton MK. Transformation of shoots into roots in Arabidopsis embryos mutant at the TOPLESS locus. Development. 2002; 129:2797–2806.
52. Long JA, Ohno C, Smith ZR, Meyerowitz EM. TOPLESS regulates apical embryonic fate in Arabidopsis. Science. 2006; 312:1520–1523.
53. Szemenyei H, Hannon M, Long JA. TOPLESS mediates auxin dependent transcriptional repression during Arabidopsis embryogenesis. Science. 2008; 319:1384–1386.
54. Cheng Z, Sun L, Qi T, Zhang B, Peng W, Liu Y, Xie D. The bHLH transcription factorMYC3 interacts with the Jasmonate ZIM-domain proteins to mediate jasmonate response in Arabidopsis. Molecular Plant. 2011; 4:279–288.
55. Fernández-Calvo P, Chini A, Fernández-Barbero G, Chico JM, Gimenez-Ibanez S, Geerinck J, Eeckhout D, Schweizer F, Godoy M, Franco-Zorrilla JM, Pauwels L, Witters E, Puga MI, Paz-Ares J, Goossens A, Reymond P, De Jaeger G, Solano R. The Arabidopsis bHLH transcription factors MYC3 and MYC4 are targets of JAZ repressors and act additively with MYC2 in the activation of jasmonate responses. Plant Cell. 2011; 23:701–715.
56. Niu Y, Figueroa P, Browse J. Characterization of JAZ interacting bHLH transcription factors that regulate jasmonate responses in Arabidopsis. Journal of Experimental Botany. 2011; 62:2143–2154.
57. Qi T, Song S, Ren Q, Wu D, Huang H, Chen Y, Fan M, Peng W, Ren C, Xie D. The Jasmonate-ZIM-Domain proteins interact with the WD-Repeat/bHLH/MYB complexes to regulate jasmonate- mediated anthocyanin accumulation and trichome initiation in *Arabidopsis thaliana.* Plant Cell. 2011; 23:1798–1814.
58. Woldemariam MG, Onkokesung N, Baldwin IT, Galis I. Jasmonoyl-L-isoleucine hydrolase 1 (JIH1) regulates jasmonoyl-L-isoleucine levels and attenuates plant defences against herbivores. Plant Journal. 2012; 72:758–767.
59. Vancanneyt G, Sanz C, Farmaki T, Paneque M, Ortego F, Castanera P, Sanchez-Serrano JJ. Hydroperoxide lyase depletion in transgenic potato plants leads to an increase in aphid performance. Proceedings of the National Academy of Sciences of the United States of America. 2001; 98:8139–8144.
60. Glazebrook J. Genes controlling expression of defence responses in Arabidopsis — 2001 status. Current Opinion in Plant Biology. 2001; 4:301–308.
61. Foyer CH. Redox metabolism in plant biotic stress. Current Opinion in Plant Biology. 2003.
62. Gunstone FD, Harwood JL, Padley FB (Eds): The Lipid Handbook. London: Chapman Hall, 1994.

63. Lozano-Durán R, Macho AP, Boutrot F, Segonzac C, Somssich IE, Zipfel C. The transcriptional regulator BZR1 mediates trade-off between plant innate immunity and growth. eLife. 2013; 2:e00983.
64. Imran QM, Lee SU, Mun BG, Hussain A, Asaf S, Lee IJ, Yun BW. WRKYs, the Jack-of-various-Trades, modulate dehydration stress in *Populus davidiana* — A transcriptomic approach. International Journal of Molecular Sciences. 2019; 20(2): 414.
65. Pandey SP and Somssich IE. The role of WRKY transcription factors in plant immunity. Plant Physiology. 2009; 150(4):1648–1655.
66. Asai T, Tena G, Plotnikova J, Willmann MR, Chiu WL, Gomez-Gomez L, Sheen J. MAP kinase signalling cascade in Arabidopsis innate immunity. Nature. 2002; 415(6875):977–983.
67. Meng X and Zhang S. MAPK cascades in plant disease resistance signaling. Annual Review of Phytopathology. 2013; 51:245–266.
68. Zheng Z, Qamar SA, Chen Z, Mengiste T. Arabidopsis WRKY33 transcription factor is required for resistance to necrotrophic fungal pathogens. The Plant Journal. 2006; 48(4):592–605.
69. Shen QH, Saijo Y, Mauch S, Biskup C, Bieri S, Keller B, Schulze-Lefert P. Nuclear activity of MLA immune receptors links isolate-specific and basal disease-resistance responses. Science. 2007; 315(5815):1098–1103.
70. Deslandes L, Olivier J, Theulières F, Hirsch J, Feng DX, Bittner-Eddy P, Marco Y. Resistance to *Ralstonia solanacearum* in *Arabidopsis thaliana* is conferred by the recessive RRS1-R gene, a member of a novel family of resistance genes. Proceedings of the National Academy of Sciences. 2002; 99(4):xd2404–2409.
71. Narusaka M, Kubo Y, Hatakeyama K, Imamura J, Ezura H, Nanasato Y, Narusaka Y. Interfamily transfer of dual NB-LRR genes confers resistance to multiple pathogens. PLoS One. 2013; 8(2):e55954.
72. Goossens J, Mertens J, Goossens A. Role and functioning of bHLH transcription factors in jasmonate signalling. Journal of Experimental Botany. 2017; 68(6):1333–1347.
73. Fan M, Bai MY, Kim JG, Wang T, Oh E, Chen L, Wang ZY. The bHLH transcription factor HBI1 mediates the trade-off between growth and pathogen-associated molecular pattern–triggered immunity in Arabidopsis. The Plant Cell. 2014; 26(2):828–841.
74. Aparicio F and Pallas V. The coat protein of Alfalfa mosaic virus interacts and interferes with the transcriptional activity of the bHLH transcription factor ILR3 promoting salicylic acid-dependent defence signalling response. Molecular Plant Pathology. 2017; 18:173–186.
75. Woldemariam MG, Dinh ST, Oh Y, Gaquerel E, Baldwin IT, Galis I. NaMYC2 transcription factor regulates a subset of plant defence responses in *Nicotiana attenuata*. BMC Plant Biology. 2013; 13(1):1–14.
76. Zhou M and Memelink J. Jasmonate-responsive transcription factors regulating plant secondary metabolism. Biotechnology Advances. 2016; 34(4):441–449.
77. Riechmann JL and Meyerowitz EM. The AP2/EREBP family of plant transcription factors. Biological Chemistry. 1998; 379:633–646.
78. Dietz KJ, Vogel MO, Viehhauser A. AP2/EREBP transcription factors are part of gene regulatory networks and integrate metabolic, hormonal and environmental signals in stress acclimation and retrograde signalling. Protoplasma. 2010; 245(1):3–14.
79. Feng JX, Liu DI, Pan YI, Gong W, Ma LG, Luo JC, Zhu YX. An annotation update via cDNA sequence analysis and comprehensive profiling of developmental, hormonal or environmental responsiveness of the Arabidopsis AP2/EREBP transcription factor gene family. Plant Molecular Biology. 2005; 59(6):853–868.

80. Xie Z, Nolan TM, Jiang H, Yin Y. AP2/ERF transcription factor regulatory networks in hormone and abiotic stress responses in Arabidopsis. Frontiers in Plant Science. 2019; 10:228.
81. Feng CZ, Chen Y, Wang C, Kong YH, Wu WH, Chen YF. Arabidopsis RAV 1 transcription factor, phosphorylated by S n RK 2 kinases, regulates the expression of ABI 3, ABI 4, and ABI 5 during seed germination and early seedling development. The Plant Journal. 2014; 80(4):654–668.
82. Berrocal-Lobo M, Molina A, Solano R. Constitutive expression of ETHYLENE-RESPONSE-FACTOR1 in Arabidopsis confers resistance to several necrotrophic fungi. The Plant Journal. 2002; 29(1):23–32.
83. Gutterson N and Reuber TL. Regulation of disease resistance pathways by AP2/ERF transcription factors. Current Opinion in Plant Biology. 2004; 7(4):465–471.
84. Kanei-Ishii C, Sarai A, Sawazaki T, Nakagoshi H, He DN, Ogata K, Ishii S. The tryptophan cluster: a hypothetical structure of the DNA-binding domain of the myb protooncogene product. Journal of Biological Chemistry. 1990; 265(32):19990–19995.
85. Paz-Ares J, Ghosal D, Wienand U, Peterson PA, Saedler H. The regulatory c1 locus of *Zea mays* encodes a protein with homology to myb proto-oncogene products and with structural similarities to transcriptional activators. The EMBO Journal. 1987; 6(12):3553–3558.
86. Dubos C, Stracke R, Grotewold E, Weisshaar B, Martin C and Lepiniec L. MYB transcription factors in Arabidopsis. Trends in Plant Science. 2010; 15(10):573–581.
87. Daniel PT, Scholz C, Essmann F, Westermann J, Pezzutto, A, Dorken, B. Dendritic cells inhibit CD95/Fas-triggered apoptosis of activated T lymphocytes by a mechanism upstream of caspase-activation. In Blood. 1999; 94(10):688A–688A.
88. Seo PJ and Park CM. MYB96-mediated abscisic acid signals induce pathogen resistance response by promoting salicylic acid biosynthesis in Arabidopsis. New Phytologist. 2010; 186(2):471–483.
89. Du H, Liu H, Xiong L. Endogenous auxin and jasmonic acid levels are differentially modulated by abiotic stresses in rice. Frontiers in Plant Science. 2013; 4:397.
90. Gao FK, Ren CG, Dai CC. Signalling effects of nitric oxide, salicylic acid, and reactive oxygen species on isoeuphpekinensin accumulation in *Euphorbia pekinensis* suspension cells induced by an endophytic fungal elicitor. Journal of Plant Growth Regulation. 2012; 31:490–497.
91. Kunkel BN and Brooks DM. Cross talk between signaling pathways in pathogen defence. Current Opinion in Plant Biology. 2002; 5:325–331.
92. Ren CG, Dai CC. Jasmonic acid is involved in the signaling pathway for fungal endophyte-induced volatile oil accumulation of *Atractylodes lancea* plantlets. BMC Plant Biology. 2012; 12:128.
93. Wang Y, Dai CC, Zhao YW, Peng Y. Fungal endophyte-induced volatile oil accumulation in *Atractylodes lancea* plantlets is mediated by nitric oxide, salicylic acid and hydrogen peroxide. Process Biochemistry. 2011a; 46:730–735.
94. Wang H, Wu Z, Chen Y, Yang C, Shi D. Effects of salt and alkali stresses on growth and ion balance in rice (*Oryza sativa* L.). Plant, Soil and Environment. 2011b; 57:286–294.
95. Horbowicz M, Mioduszewska H, Koczkodaj D, Saniewski M. The effect of cis-jasmone, Jasmonic acid and methyl jasmonate on accumulation of anthocyanins and proanthocynidins in seedlings of common buckwheat (*Fagopyrum esculentum* Moench). Acta Societatis Botanicorum Poloniae. 2009; 78:271–277.
96. Zhang ZP, Baldwin IT. Transport of (2-C-14) jasmonic acid from leaves to roots mimics wound-induced changes in endogenous jasmonic acid pool in *Nicotiana sylvestris*. Planta. 1997; 203:436–441.

97. Nafie E, Hathout T, Mokadem ASA. Jasmonic acid elicits oxidative defence and detoxification systems in *Cucumis melo* L. cells. Brazilian Journal of Plant Physiology. 2011; 23:161–174.
98. Ahmad P, Rasool S, Gul A, Sheikh SA, Akram NA, Ashraf M, Kazi AM, Gucel S. Jasmonates: multifunctional roles in stress tolerance. Frontiers in Plant Science. 2016; 7:813.
99. Lin T, Sharma P, Gonzalez DH, Viola IL, Hannapel DJ. The impact of the long-distance transport of a BEL1-like messenger RNA on development. Plant Physiology. 2013; 161:760–772.
100. Wasternack C, Hause B. Jasmonates: biosynthesis, perception, signal transduction and action in plant stress response, growth and development. An update to the 2007 review in annals of botany. Annals of Botany. 2013; 111:1021–1058.
101. Gill SS and Tuteja N. Reactive oxygen species and antioxidant machinery in abiotic stress tolerance in crop plants. Plant Physiology and Biochemistry. 2010; 48:909–930.
102. Ghasemnezhad M and Javaherdashti M. Effect of methyl jasmonate treatment on antioxidant capacity: internal quality and postharvest life of raspberry fruit. Caspian Journal of Environmental Sciences. 2008; 6:73–78.
103. James DG. Further field evaluation of synthetic herbivore-induced plan volatiles as attractants for beneficial insects. Journal of Chemical Ecology. 2005; 31:481–495.
104. Ataei N, Moradi H, Akbarpour V. Growth parameters and photosynthetic pigments of marigold under stress induced by jasmonic acid. Notulae Scientia Biologicae. 2013; 5(4):513–517.
105. Rohwer CL and Erwin JE. Horticultural applications of jasmonates: A review. Journal of Horticultural Science and Biotechnology. 2008; 83(3):283–304.
106. Sasaki-Sekimoto Y, Taki N, Obayashi T. Coordinated activation of metabolic pathways for antioxidants and defence compounds by jasmonates and their roles in stress tolerance in Arabidopsis. Plant Journal. 2005; 44:653–668.
107. van Poppel G, Verhoeven D, Verhagen H, Goldbohm R. Brassica vegetables and cancer prevention. Epidemiology and mechanisms. Advances in Experimental Medicine and Biology. 1999; 472:159–168.
108. Farooqi AA, Butt G, Razzaq Z. Algae extracts and methyl jasmonate anti-cancer activities in prostate cancer: choreographers of 'the dance macabre'. Cancer Cell International. 2012; 12:50.

8 The Role of Oxylipins in Abiotic Stress Resistance

Navneet Kaur[1], Owais Ali Wani[2], Sweeta Manhas[1], Shilpa Raina[1], Hamayun Shabir[3], Sajad un Nabi[4], and Sheikh Mansoor[1]*
[1]Division of Biochemistry, FBSc, SK-University of Agricultural Sciences & Technology of Jammu, India
[2]Division of Soil Science, SKUAST Kashmir
[3]Division of Horticulture, Sher-e-Kashmir University of Agricultural Sciences and Technology of Kashmir (SKUAST-K), Shalimar, Srinagar, India
[4]ICAR - Central Institute of Temperate Horticulture, Rangreth Srinagar Kashmir

CONTENTS

8.1 INTRODUCTION

Nowadays, a multitude of stresses including biotic and abiotic are imposing the worse effect on plants, thereby deteriorating environment health. The major biotic factors include pathogen infection and herbivore wounding whereas high or low temperature, surplus or deficit water, heavy metals, and salt, along with others, are the primary abiotic factors. As per the estimation of Boyer in the early 1980s, numerous environment factors were observed that halt 70% of crop productivity. In much of research to date, the majority of crop loss has been attributed to mainly abiotic stress. Moreover, Food and Agricutlture Organization data shows that 96.5% of crop land is adversely affected by abiotic stress. In response to these stresses, plants have evolved various physical barriers and morphological adaptations to overcome the adverse effects. The defense mechanisms in plants are chiefly responsible for coping with either pathogen attack or herbivore wounding, for which receive and transfer the signal

DOI: 10.1201/9781003316558-8

to the downstream signal transduction cascade. In respect of the inducible response mechanisms, an interesting class of compounds known as oxylipins plays a key role in abiotic stress resistance. Particularly in plant stress responses, oxidized fatty acids or oxylipins acting as signaling molecules are basically derived from metabolism of polyunsaturated fatty acids.

Despite tremendous progress in the study of a different molecules' response to abiotic stress, relatively little is known as to the function of oxylipins for plant adaption to abiotic challenges [1]. There is a complicated relationship between multiple pathways in plants, which might affect resistance to additional stressors owing to defensive mechanisms due to one stress. Significant overlaps in mechanisms of stress resistance show that oxylipins have wide regulatory effects under many stress circumstances. Many adaptive responses elicited by jasmonate can also offer benefits under abiotic stress circumstances. In general, the regulatory impact of jasmonates may be regarded as a "switching" from "growth mode" to "defense mode" when adapted to adverse conditions, because in many situations, defensive mechanisms are suppressed by growth and photosynthetic inhibition [2, 3]. Some experimental evidence has shown that cyclic oxylipins, phytoprostanes and 12OPDAs participate in the detoxification regulatory process, including genes upregulating coding for enzymes such as cytochrome P450, UDP glucose transportation, ABC transporters, heat shock proteins, and alternative oxidases. Jasmonate regulation is also associated with the biosynthesis of various secondary metabolites including phenylpropanoids, alkaloids, terpenoids and glucosinolates [4, 5]. The defensive role of such metabolites has been reiterated in abiotic environments, therefore several of these molecules may have a protective role [3].

8.2 TISSUE DAMAGE/INJURY

Most abiotic stimuli, such wind, rain, and grass; or biotic forces, such herbivores or pathogenic infections, cause mechanical harm to the tissue of a plant. Plant life is frequently dependent on quick identification and repair of damage to the tissue and the organ needed to avoid water loss and pathogens from entering damaged regions [6, 7]. It is not unexpected that injuries lead to considerable alterations in the profile of gene expression. Literally, the secondary metabolites of allene oxide synthases are the main regulators of the modification of gene expression to mechanical injury [8, 9]. As many genes of jasmonate biosynthesis have positive feedback loops control, initial growth in jasmonate levels increases the expression of jasmonate genes and formation of additional oxylipins leading to signal amplification [1]. There have been several reports recently which describe wounding as a structural element of biotic stress and and have investigated the involvement of jasmonates in this process [10, 11].

Some JA-induced systems can only protect plants from insects and pathogenic substances, whereas others can give benefits across a wide variety of adverse ambient circumstances. Anti-nutrient molecule biosynthesis, which can disrupt and/or inhibit insect nutrition uptake, makes damaged plant tissue unsuitable for micro-organisms and is an example of systems especially designed to address biotic problems [12]. These "antinutrients" are inhibitors of proteinase and certain poisonous secondary methods such as terpenoids, phenypropanoids, or alkaloids that reduce the nutrient value of plant tissue. Not only JA, but its metabolic precursor is controlled for biosynthesis of stress proteins, including proteinase-based inhibitors [13, 14]. The production of jasmonate trichome-dependent forming is an example of processes that improve plant resilience to diverse adverse situations. Trichomas, epidermal sprouts on the surface of several plant organs, defend plants against biotic challenges and under the circumstances of dehydration and UV radiation stress. It should be noted that JA generates "systemic" local responses in distal areas of the plant. The HPL metabolite traumatin, also termed the wound hormone, participates in plant reactions to wounds, as its names suggests [15, 16]. Contrary to JA, there is a growth driving activity of traumatin and its derivatives. The growth enhancing capability requires that these metabolites participate in the cell proliferation in an injured location. In potatoes and tomatoes, the forming of the tumorand in the abscission zone in cotton, traumatin plays a critical role [17]. The strongest inducer of cell proliferation is 12-hydroxy-(2)-dodecenoic acid from the HPL metabolites. This stimulates the increase of soy callus biomass in pea roots and accelerates up the mitotic cycle [17, 18]. However, the range of traumatin-mediated defensive responses and their products is not confined to growth induction. Some HPL metabolites activate the synthesis and production of antioxidants. Prosystemin is a precursor of a polypeptide hormone system that controls different plant responses to wounds and other biotic and abiotic stressors [19, 20].

8.3 DROUGHT AND SALINITY

Plants suffer in situations of water or osmotic stress in soil scarcity or owing to excessive perspiration, as is frequently the case under circumstances of dryness, high temperature or salt of soil [21]. Adaptation of plants to water deficiency is a highly complex process that affects all components of plant life, including biological mechanisms such as perspiration control, plant various metabolic reorganization mediated by gene expression profile alteration, and even plant morphology changes and lifecycles [22, 23]. In these processes the involvement of oxylipins is not thoroughly investigated, and the data available is mostly confined to jasmonate effects. In conjunction with amino acids, the levels of jasmonates, particularly JA, rise in relation to osmotic stress and barley water deprivation [24]. After exposure of plants with osmotically active chemical sorbitol, the amounts of Arabidopsis and free 12OPDA are significantly increasing in leaves [25].

In response to osmotic stress and dryness, jasmonate levels increase in the roots of Arabidopsis. It has been established that LOX6, the activity of one of six lipoxygenases, is needed in order to accumulate jasmonate in roots causing stress [26, 27]. Transient acumulation of JA in soybean leaves represents a rapid reaction to dryness, prior to the accumulation of ABA, a significant drought resistant hormone, high salt, and different temperature concentrations. In many situations, contact with ABA transduction pathways provides JA participation in plant response to osmotic stress and water insufficiency [28]. There have been studies describing anti-jasmonate interactions with ABA. The results of these interactions on the antagonistic nature were based on the hypersensitivity of jasmonate Arabidopsis jasmone to

ABA and the opposite effect of JA and ABA on gene expression in rice plants under conditions of high salt deficiency and water deficits, jasmonate jasmone (jasmonate insensitive 4) [29, 30]. Antagonistic regulation, however, is normal only for the ethylene and JA cooperatively controlled genes. Later investigations showed that interactions between JA and ABA are not necessarily negative. During seed germination 12OPDA cooperates with ABA signaling and causing the buildup of ABI5 (ABA Insensitive 5) proteins that lead to increased polygalacturonase level and a decrease of seed germination, positive interactions between the jasmonates and ABA are found. Stomata closure is an important mechanism to limit transpiration of water in water scarcity situations [31, 32]. ABA is a primary regulator of this process but not the only regulator. ABAs can produce independent stomach closures; however, this action is reported predominantly in response to stress conditions such infection by the bacteria or administration of bacterial peptide flg22, with fatty acids and 9-hydroperoxides [33]. The activation of methyl jasmonate closures was observed in various works. It is only known that the alkalization and the creation of the cell cytosol ROS by NADPH oxidase happens after the jasmonate process, which leads to a reduction in the aperture the molecular processes remain unknown. Results of a few research studies show that the presence of ABA is necessary for maximum action on the stomata. Jasmonate's beneficial impact goes beyond regulating stomata size [34, 35]. The bacterial phytotoxin coronatine, a structural analogue of JA that imitates JA functionally, provides a direct protective effect under situations of water stress. The use of coronatine mitigates the dehydration of wheat in improved plant physiologic, increased tissue water content, reduced radical super oxidants, and the activated antioxidants system [34, 36–38].

The majority of the regulatory actions of jasmonates are undeniably based on the hormone's potential to influence the expression of stress responding genes. JA promotes zinc finger transcription factor ZPT23 in the ornamental petunia plant, a model plant which is being increasingly exploited in modern biology [39, 40]. In response to injuries, colds, droughts, and heavy metals, this gene is also expressed more clearly and demonstrates interaction between diverse channels of signaling, however transgenic plants with ZPT23 over-expressed solely by increased drought resistance. In plants, ZPT23 is the powerful repressor for several genes that determine the strategy for survival under drought stress [41, 42]. The buildup of osmoprotectants such as glycine betaine and proline is one of the processes that protect plants under water deprivation circumstances. The JA-promoted buildup of glycine betaine in pear leaves has been demonstrated to be more prevalent under water deprivation circumstances [43]. Talking about the roles of jasmonates under the conditions of drought and salt stresses, it is important to realize the possession of such compounds in order to restrict the development of plants, activate the detoxification processes, and control the accumulation of secondary metabolites [43, 44].

Expression abiotic stressors, including drought, salt, and low and high temperatures, is activated in Arabidopsis peroxygenase. Since peroxygenase catalyzes 18-carbon cutin monomer production from oleic acid, peroxygenases are essential enzymes in cuticle biosynthesis. An essential protection against water loss is the water-impermeable cuticular layer [45, 46]. The cuticle is not only a passive barrier for water loss prevention, but also acts as the mediator for the transmission of osmotic stress signals. Dehydration always seems to be part of salt stress and has a detrimental effect on plants' ability to absorb water. In addition to the dehydration impact, the presence of excessive salt ion concentrations disrupts the structure of the bran, induces ROS production and photosynthesis suppression, and reduces nutritional absorption [47–49].

8.4 TEMPERATURE

Circadian and seasonal temperature changes are continually occurring on the plant. Temperature influences the geographical distribution and inhibits the utilization of agricultural areas, which is one of the most significant abiotic influences. Low temperatures are the biggest limiting factor in agriculture, which makes it a highly essential work for applied biological sciences to increase plant cold tolerances and freeze tolerances [50, 51].

Cold temperature plant adaptations are followed by profound changes in the profile of gene expression that modify the manifestation of more than 10% of the genes, including transcription factors such as chaperones, antifreeze, enzymes, mRNA proteins, and others. Many studies have shown that transcriptional modifications in plants with lower temperature stress are more adaptable to low temperatures. Only variables influencing major genes can be regarded as the possible modulators of natural resistance mechanisms for practical use due to such complexities as the reaction to adverse environmental circumstances [52–55]. A wide spectrum of oxylipin regulatory actions and considerable evidence that these metabolites are capable of boosting plant adaptation to low temperatures enable us to use oxylipins as a means to improve low temperature plant tolerance [56]. The defense effects of jasmonates at low temperatures have mostly been described in early papers by the capacity of jasmonates to limit photosynthesis and to lead to flavonoid accumulation. Recent findings have revealed that the ICECBF/DREB1, a transcription route that plays a vital role in adapting plants to low temperatures, is regulated by jasmonate. Jasmonate is the main factor in the processing of the transcription. Many investigations have proven persuasively that endogenous jasmonate accumulation and exogenous jasmonate treatment protects plants against damages induced by low temperatures. On several models and agricultural plants, jasmonate accumulation and their protecting function was seen [57]. Works on post-harvest resistance to fruits and vegetables are particularly noteworthy, because in these circumstances, administration of jasmonate is already proving to be a dependable technique of reducing post-harvest losses. Prohydrojasmonate (npropyldihydrojasmonate), a synthetic analogue of jasmonates, is frequently used to treat fruit plants to encourage anthocyanin formation, to enhance sugar content and freezing tolerance. High-temperature exposure also leads, according to some studies, to the accumulation of jasmonate within plant tissues, including 12OPDA, JA, and JA–isoleucine conjugates [57, 58]. Arabidopsis mutant cpr51 (PR1 component expressor) is extremely temperature-tolerant, loses thermo-tolerance upon biosynthesis disruption or signaling. The protective impact of jasmonate is likely to be determined in this circumstance by interaction with salicylic acid components of signal transducer pathways [59]. Interestingly, the variable volatility emissions correspond to the strength of stress [60]. The ecological importance of these volatile emissions remains unknown. The production and emission of volatile HPL metabolites can be an alternative to disposing of harmful metabolic precursors under sub-optimal circumstances of temperature [61–63].

8.5 CONCLUSION AND FUTURE PERSPECTIVES

As already mentioned, both the biological importance of the molecular crosstalk across various kingdoms remains under a shadow. The important portions of this message are in the early hours of decoding. Recent investigations in both pathogenic and host plants have improved our understanding in this field utilizing molecular genetics and biochemical techniques. There has been considerably greater understanding of the quantity, event, biosynthesis, and effect of jasmonates. In addition, the unique signaling features for abiotic stress responses as well as for development were recently reported for various oxylipins, such as hydroxy fatty acids. The equilibrium of active and inactive molecules after synthesis and metabolic conversion supports these signaling characteristics. A better knowledge of the effects of oxylipins in plant stress response and growth will result from transcriptomic, proteomic, metabolomic, and lipidomic techniques, as well as improving spatial and temporal resolution. Identifying novel alleles active in the production of oxylipins will provide fresh insights on oxylipins diversity. Preferential focus will be given to regulatory elements and system biology techniques. In plant stress reactions, for instance, by gathering data from a single stress, two or more shocks, are reflected more in the analysis. The investigation will be able to record cell-specific oxylipin activities via new analytical and cell biological approaches, such as reporters' systems.

REFERENCES

1. Savchenko, T., O. Zastrijnaja, and V. Klimov, *Oxylipins and plant abiotic stress resistance*. Biochemistry (Moscow), 2014. **79**(4): p. 362–375.
2. Reinbothe, C., et al., *Plant oxylipins: role of jasmonic acid during programmed cell death, defence and leaf senescence*. The FEBS Journal, 2009. **276**(17): p. 4666–4681.
3. Chini, A., M. Boter, and R. Solano, *Plant oxylipins: COI1/JAZs/MYC2 as the core jasmonic acid-signalling module*. The FEBS Journal, 2009. **276**(17): p. 4682–4692.
4. Wasternack, C. and M. Strnad, *Jasmonates are signals in the biosynthesis of secondary metabolites—Pathways, transcription factors and applied aspects—A brief review*. New Biotechnology, 2019. **48**: p. 1–11.
5. Erb, M. and D.J. Kliebenstein, *Plant secondary metabolites as defenses, regulators, and primary metabolites: the blurred functional trichotomy*. Plant Physiology, 2020. **184**(1): p. 39–52.
6. Schulze, E.-D., et al., *Interactions Between Plants, Plant Communities and the Abiotic and Biotic Environment*, in *Plant Ecology*. 2019, Springer. p. 689–741.
7. Cheong, Y.H., et al., *Transcriptional profiling reveals novel interactions between wounding, pathogen, abiotic stress, and hormonal responses in Arabidopsis*. Plant Physiology, 2002. **129**(2): p. 661–677.
8. Schulze, E.-D., et al., *General Themes of Molecular Stress Physiology*, in *Plant Ecology*. 2019, Springer. p. 9–55.

9. Farmer, E.E. and C.A. Ryan, *Octadecanoid-redived signals in plants*. Trends in Cell Biology, 1992. **2**(8): p. 236–241.
10. Zhang, G., et al., *Jasmonate-mediated wound signalling promotes plant regeneration*. Nature Plants, 2019. **5**(5): p. 491–497.
11. Yang, T.-H., et al., *Jasmonate precursor biosynthetic enzymes LOX3 and LOX4 control wound-response growth restriction*. Plant Physiology, 2020. **184**(2): p. 1172–1180.
12. Aerts, N., M. Pereira Mendes, and S.C. Van Wees, *Multiple levels of crosstalk in hormone networks regulating plant defense*. The Plant Journal, 2021. **105**(2): p. 489–504.
13. Genva, M., et al., *New insights into the biosynthesis of esterified oxylipins and their involvement in plant defense and developmental mechanisms*. Phytochemistry Reviews, 2019. **18**(1): p. 343–358.
14. Deboever, E., et al., *Plant–pathogen interactions: Underestimated roles of phyto-oxylipins*. Trends in Plant Science, 2020. **25**(1): p. 22–34.
15. David, L., A.C. Harmon, and S. Chen, *Plant immune responses-from guard cells and local responses to systemic defense against bacterial pathogens*. Plant Signaling & Behavior, 2019. **14**(5): p. e1588667.
16. Hilleary, R. and S. Gilroy, *Systemic signaling in response to wounding and pathogens*. Current Opinion in Plant Biology, 2018. **43**: p. 57–62.
17. Thakur, M. and A. Udayashankar, *Lipoxygenases and Their Function in Plant Innate Mechanism*, in *Bioactive Molecules in Plant Defense*. 2019, Springer. p. 133–143.
18. Bae, G. and G. Choi, *Decoding of light signals by plant phytochromes and their interacting proteins*. Annu. Rev. Plant Biol., 2008. **59**: p. 281–311.
19. Ruan, J., et al., *Jasmonic acid signaling pathway in plants*. International Journal of Molecular Sciences, 2019. **20**(10): p. 2479.
20. He, Y., et al., *Relative contribution of LOX10, green leaf volatiles and JA to wound-induced local and systemic oxylipin and hormone signature in Zea mays (maize)*. Phytochemistry, 2020. **174**: p. 112334.
21. Akıncı, Ş. and D.M. Lösel, *Plant water-stress response mechanisms*. Water Stress, 2012: p. 15–42.
22. Kramer, P.J., *Water Stress and Plant Growth 1*. Agronomy Journal, 1963. **55**(1): p. 31–35.
23. Filipović, A., *Water Plant and Soil Relation under Stress Situations*, in *Soil Moisture Importance*. 2020, IntechOpen.
24. Brossa, R., et al., *Interplay between abscisic acid and jasmonic acid and its role in water-oxidative stress in wild-type, ABA-deficient, JA-deficient, and ascorbate-deficient Arabidopsis plants*. Journal of Plant Growth Regulation, 2011. **30**(3): p. 322–333.
25. Viswanath, K.K., et al., *Plant lipoxygenases and their role in plant physiology*. Journal of Plant Biology, 2020. **63**(2): p. 83–95.
26. Grebner, W., et al., *Lipoxygenase6-dependent oxylipin synthesis in roots is required for abiotic and biotic stress resistance of Arabidopsis*. Plant Physiology, 2013. **161**(4): p. 2159–2170.
27. Kinoshita, N., et al., *IAA-Ala Resistant3, an evolutionarily conserved target of miR167, mediates Arabidopsis root architecture changes during high osmotic stress*. The Plant Cell, 2012. **24**(9): p. 3590–3602.
28. Roychoudhury, A., S. Paul, and S. Basu, *Cross-talk between abscisic acid-dependent and abscisic acid-independent pathways during abiotic stress*. Plant Cell Reports, 2013. **32**(7): p. 985–1006.
29. Fujita, Y., et al., *ABA-mediated transcriptional regulation in response to osmotic stress in plants*. Journal of Plant Research, 2011. **124**(4): p. 509–525.

30. de Ollas, C. and I.C. Dodd, *Physiological impacts of ABA–JA interactions under water-limitation*. Plant Molecular Biology, 2016. **91**(6): p. 641–650.
31. Poltronieri, P., et al., *Monitoring the activation of jasmonate biosynthesis genes for selection of chickpea hybrids tolerant to drought stress*. Abiotic Stresses in Crop Plants, 2015.
32. Per, T.S., et al., *Jasmonates in plants under abiotic stresses: Crosstalk with other phytohormones matters*. Environmental and Experimental Botany, 2018. **145**: p. 104–120.
33. Chen, L. and D. Yu, *ABA regulation of plant response to biotic stresses*, in *Abscisic Acid: Metabolism, Transport and Signaling*. 2014, Springer. p. 409–429.
34. Munemasa, S., et al., *Ethylene inhibits methyl jasmonate-induced stomatal closure by modulating guard cell slow-type anion channel activity via the OPEN STOMATA 1/SnRK2. 6 kinase-independent pathway in Arabidopsis*. Plant and Cell Physiology, 2019. **60**(10): p. 2263–2271.
35. Singh, R., et al., *Reactive oxygen species signaling and stomatal movement: current updates and future perspectives*. Redox Biology, 2017. **11**: p. 213–218.
36. Yu, X., et al., *The roles of methyl jasmonate to stress in plants*. Functional Plant Biology, 2019. **46**(3): p. 197–212.
37. Feys, B.J., et al., *Arabidopsis mutants selected for resistance to the phytotoxin coronatine are male sterile, insensitive to methyl jasmonate, and resistant to a bacterial pathogen*. The Plant Cell, 1994. **6**(5): p. 751–759.
38. Sharma, P., et al., *Reactive oxygen species, oxidative damage, and antioxidative defense mechanism in plants under stressful conditions*. Journal of Botany, 2012. **2012**.
39. Lischweski, S., et al., *Jasmonates act positively in adventitious root formation in petunia cuttings*. BMC Plant Biology, 2015. **15**(1): p. 1–10.
40. van der Krol, A.R., et al., *Developmental and wound-, cold-, desiccation-, ultraviolet-B-stress-induced modulations in the expression of the Petunia zinc finger transcription factor geneZPT2–2*. Plant Physiology, 1999. **121**(4): p. 1153–1162.
41. Kubo, K. and H. Takatsuji, *Transgene-dependent incompatibility induced by introduction of the SK2: ZPT2–10 chimeric gene in petunia*. Transgenic Research, 2007. **16**(1): p. 85–97.
42. Arrey-Salas, O., et al., *Comprehensive Genome-Wide Exploration of C2H2 Zinc Finger Family in Grapevine (Vitis vinifera L.): Insights into the Roles in the Pollen Development Regulation*. Genes, 2021. **12**(2): p. 302.
43. Hanif, S., et al., *Biochemically triggered heat and drought stress tolerance in rice by proline application*. Journal of Plant Growth Regulation, 2021. **40**(1): p. 305–312.
44. Suprasanna, P., G. Nikalje, and A. Rai, *Osmolyte accumulation and implications in plant abiotic stress tolerance*, in Iqbal, N., Nazar, R., and Khan, N. A. (Eds.) *Osmolytes and plants acclimation to changing environment: Emerging omics technologies*. 2016, Springer. p. 1–12.
45. Partridge, M. and D.J. Murphy, *Roles of a membrane-bound caleosin and putative peroxygenase in biotic and abiotic stress responses in Arabidopsis*. Plant Physiology and Biochemistry, 2009. **47**(9): p. 796–806.
46. Hanano, A., et al., *Specific caleosin/peroxygenase and lipoxygenase activities are tissue-differentially expressed in date palm (Phoenix dactylifera L.) seedlings and are further induced following exposure to the toxin 2, 3, 7, 8-tetrachlorodibenzo-p-dioxin*. Frontiers in Plant Science, 2017. **7**: p. 2025.
47. Chassot, C. and J. Métraux, *The cuticle as source of signals for plant defense*. Plant Biosystems-An International Journal Dealing with all Aspects of Plant Biology, 2005. **139**(1): p. 28–31.

48. Lim, G.-H., et al., *The plant cuticle regulates apoplastic transport of salicylic acid during systemic acquired resistance*. Science Advances, 2020. **6**(19): p. eaaz0478.
49. Kamtsikakis, A., et al., *Asymmetric water transport in dense leaf cuticles and cuticle-inspired compositionally graded membranes*. Nature Communications, 2021. **12**(1): p. 1–11.
50. Hatfield, J.L., et al., *Climate impacts on agriculture: implications for crop production*. Agronomy Journal, 2011. **103**(2): p. 351–370.
51. Kurukulasuriya, P. and S. Rosenthal, *Climate Change and Agriculture: A Review of Impacts and Adaptations*. 2013. Environment department papers;no. 91. Climate change series. World Bank, Washington, DC. © World Bank. https://openknowledge.worldbank.org/handle/10986/16616 License: CC BY 3.0 IGO.
52. Agarwal, M., et al., *A R2R3 type MYB transcription factor is involved in the cold regulation of CBF genes and in acquired freezing tolerance*. Journal of Biological Chemistry, 2006. **281**(49): p. 37636–37645.
53. Shinozaki, K. and K. Yamaguchi-Shinozaki, *Gene networks involved in drought stress response and tolerance*. Journal of Experimental Botany, 2007. **58**(2): p. 221–227.
54. Yamaguchi-Shinozaki, K. and K. Shinozaki, *Transcriptional regulatory networks in cellular responses and tolerance to dehydration and cold stresses*. Annu. Rev. Plant Biol., 2006. **57**: p. 781–803.
55. Sharma, P., et al., *The role of key transcription factors for cold tolerance in plants*, in *Transcription Factors for Abiotic Stress Tolerance in Plants*. 2020, Elsevier. p. 123–152.
56. Upchurch, R.G., *Fatty acid unsaturation, mobilization, and regulation in the response of plants to stress*. Biotechnology Letters, 2008. **30**(6): p. 967–977.
57. Sharma, M. and A. Laxmi, *Jasmonates: emerging players in controlling temperature stress tolerance*. Frontiers in Plant Science, 2016. **6**: p. 1129.
58. Hu, Y., et al., *Jasmonate regulates leaf senescence and tolerance to cold stress: crosstalk with other phytohormones*. Journal of Experimental Botany, 2017. **68**(6): p. 1361–1369.
59. Glauser, G., et al., *Velocity estimates for signal propagation leading to systemic jasmonic acid accumulation in wounded Arabidopsis*. Journal of Biological Chemistry, 2009. **284**(50): p. 34506–34513.
60. Gorman, Z., et al., *Green leaf volatiles and jasmonic acid enhance susceptibility to anthracnose diseases caused by Colletotrichum graminicola in maize*. Molecular Plant Pathology, 2020. **21**(5): p. 702–715.
61. Wang, K.-D., et al., *Oxylipins other than jasmonic acid are xylem-resident signals regulating systemic resistance induced by Trichoderma virens in maize*. The Plant Cell, 2020. **32**(1): p. 166–185.
62. Oliw, E.H. and M. Hamberg, *An allene oxide and 12-oxophytodienoic acid are key intermediates in jasmonic acid biosynthesis by Fusarium oxysporum*. Journal of Lipid Research, 2017. **58**(8): p. 1670–1680.
63. Mukhtarova, L.S., et al., *Lipoxygenase pathway in model bryophytes: 12-oxo-9 (13), 15-phytodienoic acid is a predominant oxylipin in Physcomitrella patens*. Phytochemistry, 2020. **180**: p. 112533.

9 The Roles of Oxylipin Biosynthesis Genes in Programmed Cell Death

Abdul Mujib G. Yusuf,[1] *and*
Kamoru A. Adedokun[2]
[1]King Saud University, College of Food and Agriculture, Plant Protection Department, Riyadh, Saudi Arabia
[2]King Saud University Medical City, DUH, Oral Pathology Department, Riyadh, Saudi Arabia
Correspondence: yusufabdulmujib@yahoo.com

CONTENTS

9.1 INTRODUCTION

Programmed cell death (PCD) is a form of self-destruction that is intracellularly mediated and is vital in the development and success of both eukaryotes [1], and the prokaryotes [2]. PCD in eukaryotes occurs during the homeostasis of cells and tissue and gives functional defense against destructive environmental stimuli

DOI: 10.1201/9781003316558-9

[3]. Mechanistically, cell death in animals is well understood and has been originally separated into three groups based on morphological description; apoptosis, autophagy, and necrosis [4]. Apoptosis, a name given to PCD by Kerr et al. [5], is the most frequently observed form of PCD [6]. Apoptosis is defined by the reduction of cellular mass, condensation and fragmentation of nuclear material, and other cellular organelle modifications that are enclosed to form an apoptotic body without eliciting an immune response [7]. The PCD signaling pathway [3] involves the release of the mitochondrial intermembrane space (IMS), protein cytochrome c, caspase activation leading to irreversible cell destruction, and activation of endonucleases on DNA at the internucleosomal site, all of which allow the identification of apoptosis [8]. A PCD in plants that encompass all the features of animal apoptosis, however, has not been characterized, thus apoptosis with its proper features does not exist in plant cells [8].

On the other hand, apoptotic-like cell death is a term that indicates PCD in plants and presents similar features to animal apoptosis [9]. Analysis of the plant plasma membrane revealed acute changes in the morphology of the cells, such as blebbing, cell shrinkage, and cytoplasmic condensation indicating programmed cell death, typical of the concerted dismantling of the cellular structure known as apoptosis [10]). Characteristically speaking, the feature of autophagic PCD includes cytoplasm vacuolization then follows a lysosomal activation that leads to the destruction of cell components [8]. Autophagic cell death is different from apoptosis in its morphology [11], but can inhibit or precede it [12], and has also been found in some plants PCD [8]. On the other hand, necrosis is observed morphologically to involve swelling and ultimate destruction of cellular organelles and early loss of plasma membrane integrity [13], as a response to an implicated stressor triggering the actions [3].

PCD in plants comprises a complex matrix of signaling pathways that involve the activities of various molecular signals like the plant hormones, microelements, nucleotides, and reactive oxygen species [14], as well as crosstalk between the various cellular organelles involved in the activation of PCD [15]. In response to an invading plant pathogen, various biochemical events such as the production of reactive oxygen species (ROS), nitric oxide (NO), ionic efflux, phytoalexin and biosynthesis of phytohormones are activated within the localized plant cells [16]. In addition, salicylic acid (SA)-mediated defense system is another response triggered upon stress by biotrophs and oxylipin/ethylene-mediated defense mechanism, and is active in response to necrotrophs [17]. Oxylipins, meanwhile, are metabolites derived from lipid compounds that have been implicated repeatedly in both plant defense and development.

Generally, lipids are important cellular components that provide a structural basis for cell membranes, and energy for metabolism [18], with suggested roles in plant immunity [19]. Derivative molecules of this lipid present signaling functions during plant responses to biotic and abiotic stresses [18]. A diverse range of lipid classes are involved in signaling, these include the lysophospholipid, fatty acid, phosphatidic acid, inositol phosphate, sphingolipid, and oxylipins, among others [20]. There are various types of lipases and esterases that utilize different substrates with different modes of induction when stressed [18]. Genes that encrypt lipoxygenases and kinases also use lipids as substrates [21] and are thus crucial in various plant responses.

Oxylipins are a large family of oxidized polyunsaturated fatty acids that are found in connection with diverse functions throughout the plant and animal kingdoms. Hydroperoxides, hydroxy-fatty acids, oxo-fatty acids, keto-fatty acids, divinyl ethers, volatile aldehydes, or the plant JA are kinds of oxylipins formed in plants [22]. These important active components of plant cells are implicated in plants' physiological activities, such as growth and development, senescence, and defense responses to non-infectious disease agents and infectious disease agents [23]. The lyoxygenase (LOX) pathway, with different branches of multienzymes, produces the majority of the oxylipins. The initial crucial step in oxylipins biosynthesis is the formation of fatty acid hydroperoxides occurring through a series of enzymatic processes [24], or through chemical oxidation [25]. The addition of oxygen to the acyl chain of polyunsaturated fatty acids activates the oxylipin biosynthetic pathway enzymatically, primarily through the action of 9/11-LOX, and reactive hydroperoxide of the fatty acid including linoleic acid, α-linolenic acid, and roughanic acid [23]. And the formation can also occur as a result of the actions of α-dioxygenase (α-DOX) [26]. LOXs are classified into the 9- or 13-LOX, depending on the oxygenation site on the hydrocarbon chain, where the regio- and stereo-specific deoxygenation of polyunsaturated fatty acids (PUFAs) are catalyzed, leading to the generation of either 9-hydroperoxyl and 13- hydroperoxyl derivatives of the substrate respectively [27]), especially in the fatty acid with 18 carbon atoms [28]. Oxylipins biosynthesis is preceded by the availability of the fatty acid substrate which is made available by the plant's responses to biotic and abiotic stress alongside some other plant developmental processes [29].

Other mechanisms leading to the synthesis of oxylipins, such as those activated by a number of enzymes including allene oxide synthase, divinyl ether synthase (DES), hydroperoxide lyases (HPL), peroxygenase (PXG), or epoxy alcohol synthase (EAS), have been studied in recent years. These alternate pathways produce oxygenated derivatives of the phytohormone, Jasmonate (JA) and other oxylipins with reactive epoxide characteristics, as well as α, β—unsaturated carbonyl [30]. Furthermore, nuclear DNA degradation is one of the characteristics of PCD. In a synergistic threat of multiviral-infections, silencing of the JA perception gene COI1 (Coronatine insensitive 1) has shown an accelerated cell death and was associated with increased expression of oxylipin biosynthesis genes and dioxygenase activity [31]. As demonstrated, oxylipin metabolic activity plays an important role in PCD regulation during plant-pathogen interactions. It is worth investigating how oxylipin biosynthesis gene expression performs under different conditions, both challenged and unchallenged. As a result, the various roles of oxylipin biosynthesis genes and their products in PCD are discussed in this chapter.

9.2 CELL DEATH PATHWAY

PCD is a genetically regulated mechanism in plants that removes certain cells in response to environmental stimuli to remove damaged tissues. PCD is a common process in plants that must be strictly maintained in order for them to grow, develop, and interact with their surroundings normally. A number of signaling pathways and cellular processes linked to various forms of plant PCD have been discovered over the last two decades of research. However, the lack of comparable sequences in plants for mammalian genes that control apoptosis, as well as possible functional redundancy, has made identifying genes/pathways that regulate PCD in plants problematic [32]. Furthermore, even though PCD pathways may be context-dependent based on whether the plant is challenged or unchallenged, we look at common regulators of PCD in plants in contrast to our extensive understanding of animal cell death in this section.

Meanwhile, several cell organelles such as lysosome, nucleus, cell membrane, vacuole, and mitochondria play key roles in eukaryotic cell deaths. Cell death in animals is well understood and has been originally divided into three groups based on morphological description: apoptosis, autophagy, and necrosis [4]. Apoptosis, a name given to PCD by Kerr et al. [5], is the most frequently observed form of PCD [6]. Reduction of cellular mass, condensation and fragmentation of nuclear material, and other cellular organelles modifications [4] that are enclosed to form an apoptotic body without triggering an immune response [7], are characteristics of apoptosis. Releases of the mitochondria intermembrane space (IMS), protein cytochrome c, caspase activation leading to irreversible destruction of the cell, and activation of endonucleases on the DNA at the internucleosomal site are all implicated in the PCD signaling pathway [3], which all together enables the identification of apoptosis [8]. In animals, the mitochondrion plays a key role in PCD, serving as a sensor of death signals as well as an initiator of the metabolic steps that lead to the cell's controlled death; however, the role of mitochondria in plant cell death has received less attention [33]. A PCD in plants that encompass all the features of animal apoptosis has not been characterized, thus apoptosis with its proper features does not exist in plant cells [8]. However, apoptotic-like cell death is a term that indicates PCD in plants and presents similar features to animal apoptosis [9].

Apart from the mitochondrial roles in eukaryotic cell death, analysis of the plant plasma membrane also reveals acute changes in the morphology of the cells, such as blebbing, cell shrinkage, and cytoplasmic condensation indicating programmed cell death, typical of the concerted dismantling of the cellular structure known as apoptosis [10]. At this juncture, it is worth noting that calcium signaling pathway is inductively related to the architectural integrity of plasma membrane. In other words, the integrity of the cell membrane is affected at the prompt of recognition, and opening of the Ca^{2+} channel is activated, thereby generating more Ca^{2+} in the cytosol [34]. Ca^{2+} influx and efflux depend on the severity of the stress leading to a unique Ca^{2+} signature [35]. More so, ROS produced in response to the stress are activated by the calcium signaling pathway, and alongside NO are required for the activation of plant defense genes [36]. Cytochrome c which chiefly induces PCD genes transcription is released into the cytosol through the permeable mitochondrial pore [37] and ultimately results in apoptosis. Again, during the host-pathogen interaction, JA and other hormones such as salicylic acid and ethylene function along with the signaling molecule in plant defense [38]. JA is particularly important in the activation of defense against necrotrophy [39]. Gene encoding for JA signaling and biosynthesis are expressed upon triggering by the activities of plant necrotrophic pathogen [39]. Localized cell death at the infection site presents cysteine protease activation, the release of cytochrome c, chromatin condensation, loss of membrane integrity, and cytoplasm diminution, all occurring as a result of the activity of several signaling molecules and defense regulation [40, 41]. The release of apoptotic factors ultimately leads to cell death.

Unlike apoptotic pathway, autophagy is an intracellular recycling process involving lysosomes or plant vacuoles that occurs in both plants and animals. PCD can be caused by upregulation of autophagy, which causes enzymatic cell degradation. The mitochondrial morphological transition (MMT) and DNA damage are the first steps in this pathway's induction of PCD. Autophagy is initially induced as a defensive mechanism as a result of this. As autophagy progresses, damaged cell components are engulfed in the vacuole/lysosome or the vacuole membrane is ruptured, resulting in breakdown and PCD [33]. Programmed cell death occurs following significant signalling events of which an important and well-studied one is JA-mediated.

9.3 OXYLIPIN (JASMONATE) BIOSYNTHESIS

There are several studies pointing to the rapid generation of JA in response to stress-associated molecular patterns [42, 43] as recognized by the pattern recognition receptor (PRR) of a stressed plant [44]. This section summarizes recent advances in our understanding of how jasmonate biosynthesis is controlled, as well as its enzymatic activity in the synthesis of oxylipins.

9.3.1 Alpha (A)- Dioxygenases and Their Role in Programmed Cell Death

Dioxygenase (DOX) gene in plants was first discovered to be a homolog of a cyclooxygenase gene involved in the conversion of arachidonic acid to prostaglandins in mammals before Hamberg et al. [45] later observed that the enzyme activities of plant cyclooxygenase homologs created chemically unstable 2(R)-hydroperoxy fatty acids. The proteins were eventually designated α-DOXs [46]. Following that, α-DOX homologs were recovered from various plant species including *Solanum lycopersicum, Oryza sativa, Capsicum annuum, and Nicotiana attenuata*, among others [26]. Pepper α-DOX (Ca-DOX; from *Capsicum annuum*) gene was linked to biotic stress and played a role in developmental processes. Hong et al. [47] recently demonstrated that silencing a Ca-DOX gene slows growth and suppresses basal disease resistance responses in *Capsicum annum*.

The roles of α-DOX in oxilipin biosynthesis are currently identified. α-DOX enzyme catalyzes the oxygenation of fatty acids into the formation of oxylipin [48]. A vital intermediate in the oxylipin pathway of fatty acid oxygenation in plants is the fatty acid hydroperoxide [45]. After several enzymatic catalyzation, a particular hydroperoxide isomer from the derivatives is converted into the oxylipin JA [49]. α-DOX has been previously isolated originally as a pathogen-induced oxygenase from tobacco and was discovered to be responsible for the catalysis of fatty acid oxygenation into 2-hydroperoxides [50]. According to the report, the enzyme is involved in the carbon dioxide liberation during the conversion of palmitic acid to pentadecanal, and the liberation appears to involve the α-carbon oxidation (C-2) of the fatty acid chain, hence the term α-oxidation. Furthermore, the α-oxidation enzyme is thought to work in conjunction with aldehyde dehydrogenase and nicotinamide adenine dinucleotide (NAD+), allowing for stepwise degradation of fatty acids into shorter chain homologous. More importantly, members of this family are thought to play a role in plant defenses against pathogens [26].

The formation of 8(*Z*), 11(*Z*), 14(*Z*)-heptadecantrienal during the incubation of linolenic acid with α-DOX1 from tobacco and other plants is accompanied by oxygen uptake, which is significant to the biosynthesis process. At a varied temperature, the product formation is repressed and 2(*R*)-hydroperoxilinolenic acid appears instead as the major product [26]. Study shows that the α-DOX1 enzymes possesses very minute peroxidase activity as observed in tobacco and Arabidopsis α-DOXs as well as the related α-DOXs from cucumber and pea [26, 51]. Further analysis by SDS-PAGE reveals two different subunits, a 50-kDa enzyme identical to turgor-responsive NAD^+ aldehyde dehydrogenase from pea and another 70-kDa enzyme with similarity to α-DOX from tobacco and Arabidopsis. These enzymes are discovered to be the cause of the uptake of molecular oxygen, and oxygenase activity in the presence of polyunsaturated fatty acids [50], which is a vital process in the oxylipin biosynthesis pathway. Importantly, this pathway is central to plant success because of its involvement in the production of compounds that are utilized in plant defense systems against phytopathogens [52].

The presence of peroxidase activities is observed when 2-hydroperoxypalmitic acid is reduced to 2-hydroxypalmitic acid after incubation in the presence of the peroxidase co-substrate guaiacol [45]. The 75-kDa enzyme is generated in tobacco leaves when infected by bacteria and is called pathogen inducible oxygenase, (PIOX) [50]. The proper identity of PIOX has been carried out when tobacco was challenged with the harpin HrpN protein from Erwinia. The HrpN was specifically used because of its capacity to induce hypersensitive response (HR)-like necrosis in the leaves of several plants [53], and elicitation of HR defenses in response to infection [54]. PIOX expression is induced in Arabidopsis challenged with pathogens, salicylic acid ROS promoting chemical [48]. The demonstration of PIOX as an α-DOX enzyme involved in the conversion of linolenic acid to 2-R-hydroperoxide derivative [45], shows the involvement of the enzyme in the synthesis of lipid-derived (oxylipins) signal in infected plants. α-DOX is thus the name given to the PIOX proteins in reflecting its enzymatic activity in the synthesis of oxylipins [48]. García-Marcos et al. [31] demonstrated that silencing α-DOX could reduce the manifestations of PCD associated with viral infection. This is associated with increased expression of oxylipin biosynthesis genes and DOX activity in plant-virus interactions. This implies that oxylipin metabolism is an important component that positively regulates PCD during plant-pathogen interactions.

9.3.2 The Lipoxygenase (LOX) Associated Genes and Their Role in Programmed Cell Death

In oxylipin metabolism, plant LOXs are essential enzymes involved in the production of fatty acid derivatives [55]. The 9- and 13- LOX pathways (LOXs) are popular for their roles in the response of plants to stress. LOX pathways are critical for lipid peroxidation activities during plant defensive responses to pathogen infection [56].

The complex interaction of LOXs with fatty acids results in 9-hydroperoxides, 13-hydroperoxides, and complicated oxylipins arrays are triggered when plants are damaged [57]. 12-oxo-phytodienoic acid (12-OPDA), and its downstream derivatives, known as jasmonates, are formed through the action of 13-LOX on linolenic acid (Figure 9.1). The jasmonates, which act as signals, perform a comparable but distinct role in plant insect and disease resistance control. Through a similar pathway of the 9-LOX activity on linolenic and linoleic acid, the 12-OPDA positional isomers, 10-oxo-11-phytodienoic acid (10-OPDA) and 10-oxo-11-phytoenoic acid (10-OPEA) are both established respectively [57]. It has been shown through various studies of the 9- LOX signaling pathways that their related defense activities are mediated in part by hormonal homeostasis modulation [58], as well as defense response induction through a JA-independent signaling pathway that may be functionally involved in modifications of cell walls [59]. For defense against herbivores attack, the LOX pathway is threaded by the oxylipins including the 10- OPDA, 12- OPDA with the aid of the 13- LOX, and the action of the 9- LOX on the 10- oxo- 11- phytoenoic acid (10- OPEA). Defense against the action of a bacterial pathogen, *Pseudomonas syringae*, has been reported for the 9- LOX pathway. Local defense against the bacteria is found to be activated by 9- LOX oxylipins as observed in a genetic study of *Arabidopsis thaliana* [60], alongside the α-DOX pathways, while the 9-LOX as well activates systemic resistance [59].

Incompatible reactions have been linked to several chloroplastic 13-LOXs [61; 62]. Also, 13-LOX-mediated lipid peroxidation has been connected to defense responses, especially through the formation of jasmonates and oxylipins [61]. Jasmonates, such as JA or 12-OPDA, are a class of lipid-derived signaling molecules that play a variety of activities, from initiating biotic and abiotic stress responses to controlling plant growth and development [63]. They are produced by the octadecanoid branch of the allene oxide synthase branch (AOS) [23]. The production of 13-hydroperoxy derivatives is initiated by the activation of a 13-LOX in chloroplast membranes [64] (Figure 9.1).

Meanwhile, localized formation of 10-OPEA, 10-OPDA, and a variety of other comparable 12- and 14-carbon cyclopente(a)nones, usually referred to as death acids (DAs), causes tissue necrosis in maize infected with the southern leaf blight (*Cochliobolus heterostrophus*) [57]. DAs, which have direct phytoalexin activity against biotic agents, mediate defense gene expression, and can promote cytotoxicity and cell death, are found in greater abundance in infected tissues than jasmonates. The combination of 12-OPDA and 10-OPEA also promotes the transcription of defense genes that encode glutathione S transferases (GST), cytochrome P450s, and pathogenesis-related proteins [57]. GST gene induction or increased GST activity have frequently been found in plants treated with beneficial pathogens and generate a systemic resistance response (ISR) against subsequent pathogen infections. Additionally, numerous GST enzymes have been discovered to have glutathione peroxidase activity, implying that these GSTs can play a role in antioxidative defense [65].

Furthermore, 9-LOX genes have been cloned from a variety of monocot crops, including maize [66], wheat and rice [67]. Six genes that have been linked to LOX [38], and the LOX2 gene, which encodes the 13-LOX, appear to be involved in

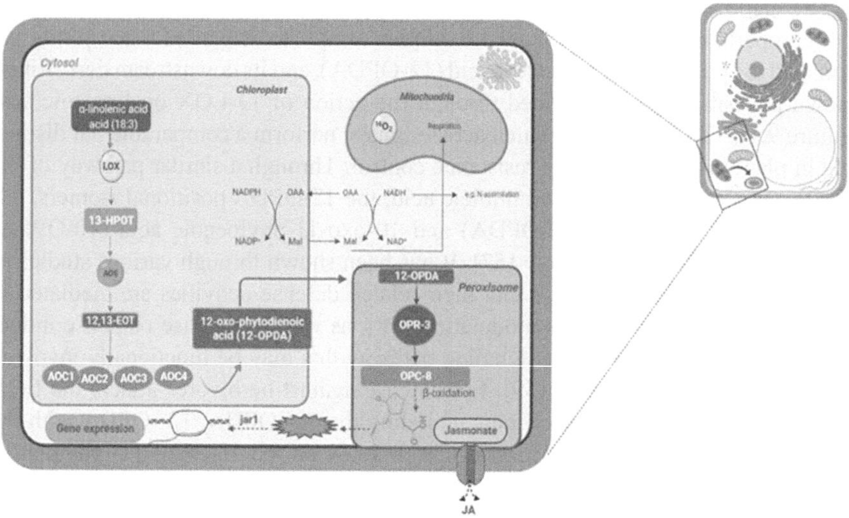

FIGURE 9.1 Induction of defense response mechanism *via* jasmonate synthesis. The octadecanoid pathway is employed in the biosynthesis of jasmonic acid within chloroplasts and peroxisomes. The oxidation of linolenic acid (18:3) initiates this synthesis, which is followed by the generation of cyclopentenone 12-oxo-phytodienoic acid (OPDA), which is catalyzed by allene oxide synthase (AOS) and allene oxide cyclase (AOC). OPDA is then reduced to 3-oxo-2-(2′(Z)-pentenyl)-cyclopentane-1-octanoic acid (OPC-8:0) by OPDA reductase 3 (OPR3). Finally, three cycles of -oxidation are used to shorten OPC:8, resulting in jasmonate (JA). Abbreviations: 13-HPOT, (13S)-hydroperoxy octadecatrienoic acid; JAR1, jasmonoyl amino acid conjugate synthase; JAT1, JA/JA-Ile transporter1.

jasmonate biosynthesis [68]. In maize, the 9-LOX gene ZmLOX3 has multiple activities, one of which is defense against parasitic nematodes [69], and another function is interaction with fungal diseases that affect seed, leaf, and root [69]. Functions of other 9-LOX were elucidated to reveal physiological functions in response to hormonal stress and pathogen infection. Two segmentally-duplicated 9- LOX genes in maize, the ZmLOX4, and ZmLOX5, are induced during infection by the fungal pathogens, *Fusarium verticillioides*, and *Cochliobolus carbonum*, to accomplish an absolute resistance mechanism [70]. In tobacco plants infected with *Phytophthora parasitica* var *nicotianae*, LOX activities and Lox1 mRNA expression increase, but the function of the genes in defenses was not established due to the appearance of disease symptoms [71]. Nonetheless, LOX activities and gene expression occurred faster in an incompatible relationship between the plant and Phytophthora than in a compatible one, demonstrating the role of 9-LOX in plant defense mechanisms against fungal disease [71].

This finding implies that fungal growth occurred as a result of a halt in the synthesis of the LOX pathway with antifungal activity. During the infection of potatoes by P. infestans, two LOX derived compounds with antimicrobial properties, colneleic and colnelenic acids, are synthesized [72], whereas the LOX derivative with antimicrobial properties in the *P. vulgaris-Pseudomonas syringae pv phaseolicola* interaction is (E)-2-hexenal [73]. Another possibility is that some product of LOX metabolism is required to induce HR, a pathogen-induced localized cell death mechanism that stops pathogen spread. This HR is characterized by the loss of membrane integrity and is closely associated with the generation of lipid peroxides and active oxygen species. [74].

Later research implicates 9-LOX and oxidative processes in the HR of tobacco challenged by an avirulent strain of *Pseudomonas syringae* [75]. Cryptogea, a purified protein from *Phytophtora cryptogea*, activates the 9-LOX pathway in tobacco, producing free fatty acid hydroperoxides needed for hypersensitive cell death [76]. The ability of transgenic tobacco plants producing antisense lox to block an incompatible interaction lends credence to the role of LOX in plant disease resistance mechanisms [71]. More importantly, the ability of the LOX pathway to produce hydroperoxides, alkenals, and aldehydes involved in plant cell and pathogen death [52], as well as the activation of the HR, all indicated typical PCD [76].

9.3.3 Monooxygenases that Are Dependent on Cytochrome P450

The role of monooxygenase is the oxidation of fatty acids by a single oxygen atom, which catalyzes in-chain and ω- hydroxylation of saturated and unsaturated C10 to C18 fatty acids. There are differences in the substrate's specificity and the regulation pattern of these oxidases according to evidence from cloning of fatty acids hydroxylases from various plant species [77]. The biological suggestion is that possible harmful effects of free fatty acids accumulation inducible by lipases in their responses to stress are prevented by the enzymes. Members of these groups of enzymes, CYP94A1 and CYP86A8, play roles in the biosynthesis of cutin and in free fatty acids derived signal establishment [78].

A subgroup under the cytochrome p450 group is the CYP74 which includes AOS, HPL, and DES, and EAS. Although reports have indicated certain differences in the function of CYP70 and the cytochrome p450 group [79]. In contrast to these typical p450 enzymes, the CYP74 family uses acyl hydroperoxides as both a substrate and an electron provider, therefore they do not require molecular oxygen or an external electron donor such as the NAD(P)H- dependent cytochrome P450 reductase. However, rather than monoxygenation processes, these enzymes catalyze isomerization reactions. As a result, it has been suggested that these enzymes use a short-circuited catalytic reaction cycle, similar to that of conventional p450 [80].

The function of a cotton P450 gene SILENCE-INDUCED STEM NECROSIS (SSN), named *SSN* (GhCYP82D), has been identified using genetic and metabolic methods in order to determine its role in lesion formation. By influencing a hitherto identified biosynthetic route of oxylipins generated from octadecanoids in cotton, SSN has been found to be crucial for restricting the production of a supposed mobile signal implicated in systemic cell death, and thus thought to be a novel metabolic branch that could modulate the JA signaling pathway [81]. Without a doubt, investigating the roles of the cytochrome p450 subgroup members in oxylipin biosynthesis is critical in order to better understand their enzyme activities in plant defense system.

9.3.4 Allen Oxide Synthase (AOS) Activities in Plant Defense

In the octadecanoic pathway of oxylipin metabolism, JA and similar cyclopenta(e)nones are formed as a result of AOS triggering the 13S- hydroperoxyl-9(Z), 11(E), 15(Z)- octadecatrienoic acid (13-HPOT). [63] (figure 9.1). Both 13S- hydroperoxyl-9(Z), 11(E), 15(Z)- octadecatrienoic acid and 13S- hydroperoxyl-9(Z), 11(E)-octadecadienoic acid were sensitive to AOS. This suggests that AOS plays a role in JA metabolism from 13-HPOT [82]. AOS represents a unique class of cytochrome P450s that is implicated in the rearrangement of fatty acid hydroperoxides. AOS shows a low affinity for carbon monoxide with no need for O_2 or NADPH-dependent cyt P450 reductase in their involvement in the reaction [83].

The AOS as an enzyme is classified as a subfamily of CYP74A within the CYP74 family of the P450s [84]. The 9(S) and the 13(S) produced from the cytosolic 9-LOX and the plastidial 13-LOX respectively are distinct in AOS specificity. The 13-AOS was first cloned in the flaxseed and encodes by a single gene in Arabidopsis while in the tomato it is encoded by two genes [85, 82, 86]. All known 13-AOSs, except the AOS reported in guayule, are consistent with the 13-LOX activities localized in the plastid, where they are found to be associated with the plastid membrane [87]. A large non-polar aspect of 2400 A^2 at the enzyme surface mediates the binding of AOS to the membrane and not the typical transmembrane helices or lipid anchor. AOS has been shown in *Escherichia coli* through the functional expression of the cDNAs to encode the enzymes that metabolize 13- hydroperoxide derivatives of C_{18} fatty acids. Plant resistance is established in Arabidopsis plants expressing the *Castanea crenata* Allen oxide synthase (CcAOS) by a delay in disease growth, according to a study. The plant that expresses CcAOS grows normally and is far more resistant to a pathogen, *Phytophthora cinnamomi* [88].

9.3.5 Allene Oxide Cyclase (AOC) Activities in Plant Defense

In the pathway of oxylipin biosynthesis initiated by LOX, as described earlier, AOC plays a crucial a role in catalyzing the catabolism of (+)-12-oxophytodienoic acid, *cis*(+)-OPDA from α-linolenic acid in a series of reactions [30]. In addition, AOC is an enzyme that catalyzes stereospecific conversion of 12,13(*S*)-epoxy-9(*Z*),11,15(*Z*)-octadecatrienoic acid (12,13-EOT) to *cis*(+)-12-oxophytodienoic acid, during the biosynthesis of JA in plants [89]. Compartmentally, AOC activities are localized to the chloroplast from which the generated *cis*(+)-OPDA moved to the peroxisome where OPDA reductase (OPR) acted on it to reduce it to 3-oxo-2(2'*Z*-pentenyl)-cyclopentane-1-octanoic acid (OPC-8:o) before the final β-oxidation conversion to JA [90] (Figure 9.1).

Deepika and colleagues [91] recently discovered that caAOC1 was localized in other subcellular compartments such as membrane and cytoplasm using in-planta analysis of the chickpea (*Cicer arietinum*) genome [91]. Previously, Schaller and Stintzi [92] demonstrated that in the presence of an AOS, preferential formation of the enantiomer of OPDA occurs, making AOC a key enzyme in establishing the enantiomeric composition of the cyclopentenone ring. When plants are treated with the octadecanoid and jasmonates, products of the AOS branch, there is evidence of a feed-forward regulation in JA biosynthesis, as evidenced by the increase of mRNA coding for AOC and other enzymes [93]. Likewise, transcriptional upregulation of AOC, AOS, and OPR3 accompany endogenous increment of octadecanoids and jasmonates [94].

Several JA biosynthesis-related genes (such as AOC, AOS1, AOS2, and LOX2), as well as signaling genes (such as COI1a and bHLH148) in rice, govern the cellular response to cold stress [95, 96]. Oxylipins are also involved in the activation of singlet oxygen-mediated cell death. Even though, the specific mechanism by which JA signaling promotes cell death is an open question. However, genes implicated in oxylipin biosynthesis, such as AOS, LOX2, and LOX3, show increased expression levels shortly after $^1O_2$ is released, followed by the production of OPDA, dinor-OPDA (dnOPDA), and JA [97]. According to Stintzi et al. [98], a comparison of flu and a flu-opr3 double mutant depleted in JA suggests that JA accelerates PCD produced by ^1O.

9.4 HYDROPEROXIDE LYASE (HPL) ACTIVITIES IN PLANT DEFENSE

The hydroperoxide lyase (HPL) enzyme is an important member of the P450 enzymes involved in the hydroperoxyl acid metabolism to generate jasmonates. The HPL enzyme is implicated in the synthesis of green leaf volatiles (GLVs), which constituted C_6 aldehydes, alcohols and esters that play important roles in the communication between plants stressors [99]. Along with the AOS, the 13-HPL uses (13S)-hydroperoxylinolenic acid (13-HPOT), a product of the regio- and stereospecific 13-LOX, as a substrate in delivering various derivatives. In essence, the function of HPL is cleaving the 13-HPOT to *Z*-3-hexenal and 12- ODA [73; 100].

The unsaturated carbonyl can be isomerized non-enzymatically or enzymatically to produce (E)-2-hexenal and 12-oxo-(E)-10-dodecenoic acid [99]. More so, hexenal is generated from the linoleic acid path as the starting substrate [101]. In effect, the α, β-unsaturated carbonyl group incidentally confers bactericidal properties on the (E)-2-hexenal [102]. Evidence of this can be seen in JA which does not possess the antimicrobial property because it lacks the motif in comparison to the high activity exhibited by 12-oxo-PDA which contains it [101]. Furthermore, the equivalent C6-alcohols are similarly effective antibacterial molecules, and they may work in tandem with their hydrocarbon cousin to create a chemical cocktail for defense [101].

Meanwhile, HPL belongs to the same cytochrome P450 superfamily as AOS, and is allotted CYP74B. O_2 and the reductase activity of NADPH-dependent cytochrome P450 are not required by HPL in its activities, unlike the canonical cytochrome P450s [103, 104], it possesses a moderately conserved amino acid sequence and the catalytic site residues differ from AOS but with similar hydrophobic substrate-binding pocket [105]. Just as for AOS and other CYP74 enzymes, HPL possesses a nine-residue insertion in its proximal Cys loop, which helps to reduce the thiolate's strength and favors the formation of the S-Fe(IV)-OH complex, which in turn easily participates in oxygen rebound [105]. An HPL protein is encoded by the gene At4g15440 which is proposed to be non-chloroplastic in the Subcellular Localization Database for

Arabidopsis protein (SUBA) [106], although expected to contain a 25 amino acid chloroplast transit peptide (cTP) [105].

GmHPL is a hydroperoxide lyase gene identified during the defense response of soybean to bacterial leaf pustule disease. A truncated GmHPL protein in the cultivar showed a significantly reduced GmHPL RNA in the NT302 mutant, possessing an etiolated phenotype with a chlorotic and spontaneous lesion on podding stage leaves [107]. Considerable reduction in photosynthetic pigment content and degradation of the thylakoid membrane in the leaves are observable features of the chlorotic phenotype, thereby linking the oxylipin pathway metabolite with the degraded photosynthetic activities. Previous studies have also shown JA to promote the loss of chlorophyll and suppression of photosynthesis [108]. The OsHPL3 was also identified as an HPL gene and implicated in rice to modulate rice-specific defense responses by impacting levels of JA, GLVs, and other volatiles [109].

9.5 DIVINYL ETHER SYNTHASE (DES) ACTIVITIES IN PLANT DEFENSE

Divinyl ethers are unstable compounds that are infrequently encountered in biological systems [72]. The enzyme DES is known to convert fatty acid hydroperoxides produced by lipoxygenase activity to divinyl ethers [110] while the 9-HPOD and 9-HPOT are metabolic precursors of these compounds [111]. Synthesis of the two divinyl ethers compounds has been reported in potato, garlic, and tomato extract [112–114]. The potato enzyme specifically uses only 9-hydroperoxides and not the 13-hydroperoxides. Thus, divinyl ether oxylipins were considered a unique potato constituent [111].

There is an accumulation of two 18-carbon divinyl ether fatty acids, colneleic acid and colnelenic acid, during the development of late blight caused by *Phytophthora infestans* on potato leaves. DES accumulates faster in the cultivar with increased resistance to late blight than in the susceptible cultivar. *P. infestans* has been reported to be inhibited by both colneleic and colnelenic acid, implying a role for divinyl ethers in plant defense. There is the possibility that the compounds may diffuse and degrade within *P. infestans* as a phytoalexin, to yield cytotoxic carbonyl fragments because phytoalexin has been encountered in potato tubers during late blight infection [115]. Colneleic and Colnelenic acid accumulate lately during the disease development which correlates with the development of HR symptoms, thus, relating the production of divinyl ethers acids in the system to cell death [72].

9.6 OXYLIPINS AND PROGRAMMED CELL DEATH

A form of ROS generated during oxygenated photosynthesis known as singlet oxygen (represented by $^1O_2$) has been shown to aid in the synthesis of JA [116], in a singlet oxygen-dependent signaling pathway that controls growth and cell viability [117]. This singlet oxygen can cause damage to membrane structure [117]. In a study involving a mutant Arabidopsis thaliana (*flu*), cell death has been observed to be triggered in a nonpermissive dark-to-light cycle involving JA [118]. A large number of genes are identified with different responses to singlet oxygen. Some of the genes are downregulated while others are overexpressed. Among the upregulated genes by singlet oxygen are genes encoding enzymes involved in the biosynthesis of ethylene and JA [119]. Study shows that 13-hydro(pero)xy octadecatrienoic acid, an intermediate in the pathway of JA biosynthesis, is induced by singlet oxygen in the mature *flu* plants. During the re-illumination of the flu mutant, various singlet oxygen-mediated stress responses such as the death of cells and seedlings have been characterized [118]. These responses to stress are a result of the activation of genetic stress response program rather than photo-oxidative program [120].

The *flu* plants were later found to generate large amounts of JA and OPDA, where the JA is required for cell death manifestation while the OPDA is an antagonist to the cell death manifestation [120]. The mature *flu* plant stops growing once the singlet oxygen is released within the chloroplast causing the seedlings to blight and die off [121]. This occurs with concomitant induction of spontaneous change in expression of a nuclear gene affecting a part of the total genome. Genes previously identified to be associated with plant resistance to biotic stress are among those affected [122]. One such gene upregulated after the release of singlet oxygen is the *EDS1* [121]. The EDS1 initially suggested to aid plant disease resistance was observed to repress SA accumulation which has a role in facilitating the hypersensitive cell death, and impairing gene-mediated resistance (R) to bacterial and oomycetes [123]. The EDS1 was later found to take part in an EDS1-dependent synthesis of SA proposed to induce an improved light-dependent formation of H_2O_2 thereby stimulating the spread of necrotic lesions during the HR [124].

EDS1 is thus essential for the accumulation of SA mediated by singlet oxygen and the upregulation of other plant defense genes that are necessary for local and systemically acquired defense processes against pathogens [121]. Cell death reactions observed in the mature leaves were suppressed when the *EDS1* gene was inactivated [121]. The release of singlet oxygen triggers the synthesis of oxylipins that are known to be associated with the cytosol [38]. The induction of the free oxylipin following the release of singlet oxygen [118] occurs simultaneously with a swift accumulation of the *ESD1* transcripts [121].

Active oxygen species include singlet oxygen, superoxide radical, and hydrogen peroxide which are produced by plants as a consequence of cellular metabolism. These active oxygen species are generated in excess when plants are exposed to stressors [125]. Although when active oxygen species are not efficiently metabolized, they damage membrane lipid, protein, and other cellular components and ultimate cell death [125], they are however important part of the plant defense signaling pathway [126]. JA is required as a downstream component of AOS for complete induction of defense gene and cell death [127, 128].

Evidence has shown that precise plant responses to pathogen attack may not be activated by JA only but the outcome of adjunct interaction between different signaling pathways [129]. There are reports on different examples of crosstalk between JA and other hormonal pathways, in response to pathogen attacks, such as salicylic acid, auxin, and ethylene [130]. Cooperation between JA and ethylene (ET) signals in activating plant defense is observed during a plant interaction with a necrotrophic pathogen where ERF1 (ethylene-response-factor1) plays a vital role [131]. The

AtMYC2 transcription factor which functions as a member of the MYC-based regulatory system is implicated in JA-induced defense gene activation [132]. Identification of some jasmonate-insensitive (jai) loci especially jai/jin1 with a branch that is negatively regulated by the AtMYC2 transcription factor shows that there is an interplay between AtMYC2 and ERF1 that are selected by plants in response to different stimuli [129]. In Arabidopsis, the MYC2 functions as an activator and a repressor of the unique expression of JA-responsive genes [146]. MYC2-regulated genes identified include the JA-responsive pathogen defense genes, $PDF_{1.2.}$ CHIB/PR3, and HEL/PR4. MYC2/jin1 mutants are observed to be highly resistant to fungal pathogens[133] and *Pseudomonas syringae* [151], indicating that MYC2 is negatively regulating the defense genes [129].

9.7 OXYLIPIN AND CELL DEATH REGULATIONS

In comparison to other kinds PCD, particularly in animals, our understanding of plant PCD regulation is still limited. Despite the importance of PCD in plant development and as a response to biotic and abiotic stressors, the complex molecular processes that control various kinds of plant PCD are still emerging. ROS have been identified as significant modulators of plant PCD throughout the previous decade. Plant mutations and genomic studies related to ROS-mediated PCD have uncovered a diverse set of plant-specific cell death regulators, contributing to the understanding of the complex redox signaling network.

Today, phytotoxic ozone (O_3) has been shown to be an inducer of the accumulation and spread of lesions in plants [134, 135]. More so, wound stress leading to necrosis is also attributed of the ozone by oxidizing and damage of plasma membrane [136]. The ozone is implicated as a component of HRs present in compatible plant-pathogen interactions [137]. Oxidative bursts alongside the accumulation of active oxygen species are activated by ozone, just like in plant response to pathogens [138]. Active oxygen species generation and lipid peroxide production correlate with membrane damage incidents during the hypersensitive reaction [139]. Several works have attributed the regulation of cell death, in response to $O_{3,}$ to ET. Synthesis of ET upon exposure of plants to O_3 occurs due to specific activation of 1-aminocyclopropane-1-carbocyclic acid (ACC) synthase and ACC oxidase genes [140]. ET is thus required for O_3 damage, whereas jasmonic acid has been shown to protect tobacco plants against O_3 [138].

Signaling pathways that are salicylic-, ET-, and JA-dependent are activated by ozone-induced active oxygen species. Despite this, there are still suggestions of antagonistic interactions between SA-, JA-, and ET signaling pathways leading to plant cell death [138]. In a previous work by Overmyer and coworkers [138], while ET biosynthesis promotes cell death, it is shown that JA signaling on the other hand protects the plant from further spread of lesions.

Expression of JA signaling encoding gene is important to plant defense mechanism against plant pathogenic necrotrophs [141]. In a study involving Arabidopsis thaliana, the *Thi2.1* and *pdf1.2* genes were shown to be inducible by necrotrophic fungi [142]. Constitutive expression of the Thi2.1 gene was observed in Arabidopsis *cet* mutant displaying spontaneous leaf necrosis in association with the systemic acquired resistance pathway. These *cet* genes' action lies within the signaling pathway from which the JA-dependent signals leading to cell death branched [143]. Ceramide accumulation in Arabidopsis acd5 mutant incites the activation of the jasmonates pathway and the accumulation hastened alongside cell death upon treatment with methyl jasmonate [144]. This apparent involvement of JA pathway in acd5-mediated cell death was further confirmed when cell death was delayed in the jasmonic resistant1–1 and coronatine insensitive1–2 mutant [144].

During a mixed viral infection of *Nicotiana benthamiana* with potato virus X (PVX) and potato virus Y (PVY), a synergistic relationship leads to necrosis of the emerging leaves and plant death. Oxylipins biosynthesis genes were especially upregulated and were expressed. This cell death caused by the synergism was slowed down upon silencing of α-dioxygenase1, transcription analysis implicated the expression of reactive oxygen species generating enzymes [145]. Oxidative stress parameters implicated in susceptible virus-host interaction include an increase in lipid peroxidation and an imbalance in the antioxidative system of the infected plant [146]. In a detailed characterization of the resistance response of tobacco to tobacco mosaic virus interaction, there is evidence of activation of the oxylipins metabolism in the tobacco defense system [145]. Accumulation of 12-OPDA) and JA occurred after a high generation of soluble phospholipase A_2 (PLA_2) activity. The steady rise in OPDA level in a tobacco HR indicated that OPDA is a primary octadecanoid signal in the HR [147]. In the HR, OPDA has been found in association with the affected tissue while JA leads to defense response [148]. Chloroplast galactolipids are a primary provider of fatty acids in the production of cell death-promoting free fatty acid hydroperoxide during induced HR of tobacco [139].

JA accumulation in tobacco leaves infected with *Pseudomonas syringae* pv. *phaseolicola* during the hypersensitive response, and involves protein loss, malondialdehyde accumulation, and cell death [149]. A hypersensitive reaction is triggered in resistant plants in response to invading avirulent plant viruses. The HR is associated with a reduction in virus replication and programmed cell death, two situations that have been noticed in systemic necrosis caused by viral infection whereby the latter is triggered by an unidentified pathway separate from the former [150]. During suitable plant-virus interaction, oxylipin metabolism is a crucial component that positively modulates the process of PCD but has no identified effect on viral accumulation in plants [151].

HR presents a sort of membrane damage observed to be closely associated with lipid peroxide production [152], initiated by AOS generation in an autoxidation process [153]. An early response in the event of plant-pathogen interaction correlates with the production of AOS through an oxidative burst [154]. A later response in the HR is lipid peroxidation which as well correlates with the initiation of necrosis [76]. This asserts the assumption that AOS production, followed by the peroxidation of lipid, has a role in the onset of membrane damage, thus, programmed cell death.

9.8 CONCLUSION

There is overwhelming evidence from gene expression profiles in different pathosystems that oxylipin biosynthetic genes are a critical component that positively regulates the process of programmed cell death under various biotic and abiotic threats in plants. This process is orchestrated through regulations of various enzymatic activities involving 9-lipoxygenase (LOX), 13-LOX, α-dioxygenase-1 (α-DOX-1), among others. This demonstrates that when susceptible plants are attacked by any pathogen, a group of defense-related genes are expressed, suggesting that even vulnerable plants recognize pathogens and mount defense responses. However, while plant-pathogen interactions may help overcome any biotic or abiotic threat, changes in defense gene expression may not only provide a line of defense against the pathogen, but they may also pose negative consequences on host metabolism, leading to the development of illness symptoms.

REFERENCES

1. M. Deponte, Programmed cell death in protists, *Biochimica et Biophysica Acta (BBA) — Molecular Cell Research*, vol. 1783, no. 7, pp. 1396–1405, Jul. 2008, doi: 10.1016/J.BBAMCR.2008.01.018.
2. W. Bayles, Bacterial programmed cell death: making sense of a paradox, *Nat Rev Microbiol*, vol. 12, no. 1, pp. 63–69, Jan. 2014, doi: 10.1038/NRMICRO3136.
3. N. Dauphinee and A. N. Gunawardena, An overview of programmed cell death research: From canonical to emerging model species, *Plant Programmed Cell Death*, pp. 1–31, Jan. 2015, doi: 10.1007/978–3-319–21033–9_1.
4. G. Kroemer et al., Classification of cell death: recommendations of the Nomenclature Committee on Cell Death 2009, *Cell Death Differ*, vol. 16, no. 1, p. 3, 2009, doi: 10.1038/CDD.2008.150.
5. J. F. R. Kerr, A. H. Wyllie, and A. R. Currie, Apoptosis: A Basic Biological Phenomenon with Wide-ranging Implications in Tissue Kinetics, *British Journal of Cancer*, vol. 26, no. 4, p. 239, 1972, doi: 10.1038/BJC.1972.33.
6. L. Galluzzi et al., Molecular mechanisms of cell death: recommendations of the Nomenclature Committee on Cell Death 2018, *Cell Death Differ*, vol. 25, no. 3, pp. 486–541, Mar. 2018, doi: 10.1038/S41418–017–0012–4.
7. E. Dykhuizen, Means to an End: Apoptosis and Other Cell Death Mechanisms. By Douglas R. Green. Cold Spring Harbor (New York): Cold Spring Harbor Laboratory Press. $79.00 (hardcover); $45.00 (paper). xii + 220 p.; ill.; index. ISBN: 978–0-87969–887–4 (hc); 978–0-87969–888–1 (pb). 2011., *The Quarterly Review of Biology*, vol. 87, no. 1, pp. 68–68, Mar. 2012, doi: 10.1086/663910.
8. V. Locato and L. de Gara, Programmed Cell Death in Plants: An Overview, *Methods in Molecular Biology*, vol. 1743, pp. 1–8, 2018, doi: 10.1007/978–1-4939–7668–3_1.
9. T. J. Reape and P. F. McCabe, Apoptotic-like programmed cell death in plants, *New Phytologist*, vol. 180, no. 1, pp. 13–26, Oct. 2008, doi: 10.1111/J.1469–8137.2008.02549.X.
10. A. Levine, R. I. Pennell, M. E. Alvarez, R. Palmer, and C. Lamb, Calcium-mediated apoptosis in a plant hypersensitive disease resistance response, *Curr Biol*, vol. 6, no. 4, pp. 427–437, 1996, doi: 10.1016/S0960–9822(02)00510–9.
11. Y. Tsujimoto and S. Shimizu, Another way to die: autophagic programmed cell death, *Cell Death Differ*, vol. 12 Suppl 2, pp. 1528–1534, 2005, doi: 10.1038/SJ.CDD.4401777.
12. G. Mariño, M. Niso-Santano, E. H. Baehrecke, and G. Kroemer, Self-consumption: the interplay of autophagy and apoptosis, *Nat Rev Mol Cell Biol*, vol. 15, no. 2, pp. 81–94, Feb. 2014, doi: 10.1038/NRM3735.

13. W. X. Zong and C. B. Thompson, Necrotic death as a cell fate, *Genes & Development*, vol. 20, no. 1, pp. 1–15, Jan. 2006, doi: 10.1101/GAD.1376506.
14. M. Delledonne, Y. Xia, R. A. Dixon, and C. Lamb, Nitric oxide functions as a signal in plant disease resistance, *Nature*, vol. 394, no. 6693, pp. 585–588, Aug. 1998, doi: 10.1038/29087.
15. O. van Aken and B. J. Pogson, Convergence of mitochondrial and chloroplastic ANAC017/PAP-dependent retrograde signalling pathways and suppression of programmed cell death, *Cell Death & Differentiation 2017–24:6*, vol. 24, no. 6, pp. 955–960, May 2017, doi: 10.1038/cdd.2017.68.
16. L. Prasad, S. Katoch, and S. Shahid, Microbial interaction mediated programmed cell death in plants, *3 Biotech 2022–12:2*, vol. 12, no. 2, pp. 1–18, Jan. 2022, doi: 10.1007/S13205–021–03099–7.
17. J. Glazebrook, Contrasting mechanisms of defense against biotrophic and necrotrophic pathogens, *Annu Rev Phytopathol*, vol. 43, pp. 205–227, 2005, doi: 10.1146/ANNUREV.PHYTO.43.040204.135923.
18. Y. Okazaki and K. Saito, Roles of lipids as signaling molecules and mitigators during stress response in plants, *The Plant Journal*, vol. 79, no. 4, pp. 584–596, Aug. 2014, doi: 10.1111/TPJ.12556.
19. N. Fitoussi et al., Oxylipins are implicated as communication signals in tomato–root-knot nematode (Meloidogyne javanica) interaction, *Scientific Reports 2021–11:1*, vol. 11, no. 1, pp. 1–16, Jan. 2021, doi: 10.1038/s41598–020–79432–6.
20. X. Wang, S. Devaiah, W. Zhang, R. W.-P. in lipid research, and undefined 2006, Signaling functions of phosphatidic acid, *Elsevier*, Accessed: Mar. 21, 2022. Online]. Available: www.sciencedirect.com/science/article/pii/S0163782706000142
21. Y. Li-Beisson et al., Acyl-Lipid Metabolism, *The Arabidopsis Book / American Society of Plant Biologists*, vol. 11, p. e0161, Jan. 2013, doi: 10.1199/TAB.0161.
22. A. Grechkin, Recent developments in biochemistry of the plant lipoxygenase pathway, *Progress in Lipid Research*, vol. 37, no. 5, pp. 317–352, Nov. 1998, doi: 10.1016/S0163–7827(98)00014–9.
23. I. Feussner and C. Wasternack, THE LIPOXYGENASE PATHWAY, http://dx.doi.org/10.1146/annurev.arplant.53.100301.135248, vol. 53, pp. 275–297, Nov. 2003, doi: 10.1146/ANNUREV.ARPLANT.53.100301.135248.
24. E. Blée, Phytooxylipins and plant defense reactions, *Progress in Lipid Research*, vol. 37, no. 1, pp. 33–72, May 1998, doi: 10.1016/S0163–7827(98)00004–6.
25. M. J. Mueller, Archetype signals in plants: the phytoprostanes, *Curr Opin Plant Biol*, vol. 7, no. 4, pp. 441–448, Aug. 2004, doi: 10.1016/J.PBI.2004.04.001.
26. M. Hamberg, I. P. de Leon, M. J. Rodriguez, and C. Castresana, Alpha-dioxygenases, *Biochem Biophys Res Commun*, vol. 338, no. 1, pp. 169–174, Dec. 2005, doi: 10.1016/J.BBRC.2005.08.117.
27. A. Andreou and I. Feussner, Lipoxygenases — Structure and reaction mechanism, *Phytochemistry*, vol. 70, no. 13–14, pp. 1504–1510, Sep. 2009, doi: 10.1016/J.PHYTOCHEM.2009.05.008.
28. C. Schneider, D. A. Pratt, N. A. Porter, and A. R. Brash, Control of oxygenation in lipoxygenase and cyclooxygenase catalysis, *Chem Biol*, vol. 14, no. 5, pp. 473–488, May 2007, doi: 10.1016/J.CHEMBIOL.2007.04.007.
29. C. Wasternack, Jasmonates: An Update on Biosynthesis, Signal Transduction and Action in Plant Stress Response, Growth and Development, *Annals of Botany*, vol. 100, no. 4, p. 681, Oct. 2007, doi: 10.1093/AOB/MCM079.
30. A. Mosblech, I. Feussner, and I. Heilmann, Oxylipins: Structurally diverse metabolites from fatty acid oxidation, *Plant Physiology and Biochemistry*, vol. 47, no. 6, pp. 511–517, Jun. 2009, doi: 10.1016/J.PLAPHY.2008.12.011.

31. García-Marcos A, Pacheco R, Manzano A, Aguilar E, Tenllado F. Oxylipin biosynthesis genes positively regulate programmed cell death during compatible infections with the synergistic pair potato virus X-potato virus Y and Tomato spotted wilt virus. *J Virol*. 2013 May;87(10):5769–83. doi: 10.1128/JVI.03573–12. Epub 2013 Mar 13. PMID: 23487466; PMCID: PMC3648178.
32. Devarenne TP, Martin GB. Manipulation of plant programmed cell death pathways during plant-pathogen interactions. *Plant Signal Behav*. 2007 May;2(3):188–9. doi: 10.4161/psb.2.3.4150. PMID: 19704693; PMCID: PMC2634054.
33. Scott I, Logan DC. Mitochondria and cell death pathways in plants: Actions speak louder than words. *Plant Signal Behav*. 2008 Jul;3(7):475–7. doi: 10.4161/psb.3.7.5678. PMID: 19704490; PMCID: PMC2634434.
34. N. Tuteja and S. Mahajan, Calcium signaling network in plants: an overview, *Plant Signal Behav*, vol. 2, no. 2, pp. 79–85, 2007, doi: 10.4161/PSB.2.2.4176.
35. J. Bose, I. I. Pottosin, S. S. Shabala, M. G. Palmgren, and S. Shabala, Calcium efflux systems in stress signaling and adaptation in plants, *Front Plant Sci*, vol. 2, no. DEC, Dec. 2011, doi: 10.3389/FPLS.2011.00085.
36. A. Görlach, K. Bertram, S. Hudecova, and O. Krizanova, Calcium and ROS: A mutual interplay, *Redox Biol*, vol. 6, pp. 260–271, Dec. 2015, doi: 10.1016/J.REDOX.2015.08.010.
37. G. Rantong and A. H. L. A. N. Gunawardena, Programmed cell death: genes involved in signaling, regulation, and execution in plants and animals, https://doi.org/10.1139/cjb-2014-0152, vol. 93, no. 4, pp. 193–210, Dec. 2015, doi: 10.1139/CJB-2014–0152.
38. N. Li, X. Han, D. Feng, D. Yuan, and L. J. Huang, Signaling Crosstalk between Salicylic Acid and Ethylene/Jasmonate in Plant Defense: Do We Understand What They Are Whispering?, *Int J Mol Sci*, vol. 20, no. 3, Feb. 2019, doi: 10.3390/IJMS20030671.
39. L. Zhang, F. Zhang, M. Melotto, J. Yao, and S. Y. He, Jasmonate signaling and manipulation by pathogens and insects, *Journal of Experimental Botany*, vol. 68, no. 6, pp. 1371–1385, Mar. 2017, doi: 10.1093/JXB/ERW478.
40. C. Chibucos et al., Programmed cell death in host-symbiont associations, viewed through the Gene Ontology, *BMC Microbiology*, vol. 9, no. SUPPL. 1, pp. 1–10, Feb. 2009, doi: 10.1186/1471–2180–9-S1-S5/FIGURES/2.
41. Z. Liu and H. M. Lam, Signal Transduction Pathways in Plants for Resistance against Pathogens, *International Journal of Molecular Sciences 2019, Vol. 20, Page 2335*, vol. 20, no. 9, p. 2335, May 2019, doi: 10.3390/IJMS20092335.
42. L. Li, C. Li, G. I. Lee, and G. A. Howe, Distinct roles for jasmonate synthesis and action in the systemic wound response of tomato, *Proc Natl Acad Sci U S A*, vol. 99, no. 9, pp. 6416–6421, Apr. 2002, doi: 10.1073/PNAS.072072599/ASSET/8336DE62–67B9–4D5E-B9F0-AFAA9C15CD51/ASSETS/GRAPHIC/PQ0720725005.JPEG.
43. L. Campos, J. H. Kang, and G. A. Howe, Jasmonate-triggered plant immunity, *J Chem Ecol*, vol. 40, no. 7, pp. 657–675, 2014, doi: 10.1007/S10886–014–0468–3.
44. Y. Yamaguchi, G. Pearce, and C. A. Ryan, The cell surface leucine-rich repeat receptor for AtPep1, an endogenous peptide elicitor in Arabidopsis, is functional in transgenic tobacco cells, *Proc Natl Acad Sci U S A*, vol. 103, no. 26, pp. 10104–10109, Jun. 2006, doi: 10.1073/PNAS.0603729103/ASSET/21265A27–765D-4066-BD4F-E2A4607DDF28/ASSETS/GRAPHIC/ZPQ0250625910005.JPEG.
45. M. Hamberg, A. Sanz, and C. Castresana, α-Oxidation of Fatty Acids in Higher Plants: IDENTIFICATION OF A PATHOGEN-INDUCIBLE OXYGENASE (PIOX) AS AN α-DIOXYGENASE AND BIOSYNTHESIS OF 2-HYDROPEROXYLINOLENIC ACID, *Journal of Biological Chemistry*, vol. 274, no. 35, pp. 24503–24513, Aug. 1999, doi: 10.1074/JBC.274.35.24503.

46. Bannenberg G, Martínez M, Rodríguez MJ, López MA, Ponce de León I, Hamberg M, Castresana C (2009) Functional analysis of α-DOX2, an active α-dioxygenase critical for normal development in tomato plants. *Plant Physiol* 151:1421–1432.
47. Hong CE, Ha YI, Choi H, Moon JY, Lee J, Shin AY, Park CJ, Yoon GM, Kwon SY, Jo IH, Park JM. Silencing of an α-dioxygenase gene, Ca-DOX, retards growth and suppresses basal disease resistance responses in Capsicum annum. *Plant Mol Biol.* 2017 Mar;93(4–5):497–509. doi: 10.1007/s11103–016–0575–3. Epub 2016 Dec 21. PMID: 28004240.
48. P. de León, A. Sanz, M. Hamberg, and C. Castresana, Involvement of the Arabidopsis alpha-DOX1 fatty acid dioxygenase in protection against oxidative stress and cell death, *Plant J*, vol. 29, no. 1, pp. 61–72, 2002, doi: 10.1046/J.1365–313X.2002.01195.X.
49. M. J. Mueller, Enzymes involved in jasmonic acid biosynthesis, *Physiologia Plantarum*, vol. 100, no. 3, pp. 653–663, Jul. 1997, doi: 10.1111/J.1399–3054.1997.TB03072.X.
50. A. Sanz, J. I. Moreno, and C. Castresana, PIOX, a new pathogen-induced oxygenase with homology to animal cyclooxygenase., *The Plant Cell*, vol. 10, no. 9, p. 1523, 1998, doi: 10.1105/TPC.10.9.1523.
51. T. Koeduka, K. Matsui, Y. Akakabe, and T. Kajiwara, Catalytic Properties of Rice α-Oxygenase: A COMPARISON WITH MAMMALIAN PROSTAGLANDIN H SYNTHASES *, *Journal of Biological Chemistry*, vol. 277, no. 25, pp. 22648–22655, Jun. 2002, doi: 10.1074/JBC.M110420200.
52. E. E. Farmer and C. A. Ryan, Interplant communication: Airborne methyl jasmonate induces synthesis of proteinase inhibitors in plant leaves, *Proc Natl Acad Sci U S A*, vol. 87, no. 19, pp. 7713–7716, 1990, doi: 10.1073/PNAS.87.19.7713.
53. Z. M. Wei et al., Harpin, elicitor of the hypersensitive response produced by the plant pathogen Erwinia amylovora, *Science (1979)*, vol. 257, no. 5066, pp. 85–88, 1992, doi: 10.1126/science.1621099.
54. J. Baker, E. W. Orlandi, and N. M. Mock, Harpin, An Elicitor of the Hypersensitive Response in Tobacco Caused by Erwinia amylovora, Elicits Active Oxygen Production in Suspension Cells, *Plant Physiol*, vol. 102, no. 4, pp. 1341–1344, 1993, doi: 10.1104/PP.102.4.1341.
55. S. Hwang and B. K. Hwang, The Pepper 9-Lipoxygenase Gene CaLOX1 Functions in Defense and Cell Death Responses to Microbial Pathogens, *Plant Physiology*, vol. 152, no. 2, p. 948, 2010, doi: 10.1104/PP.109.147827.
56. R. Casey and R. K. Hughes, Recombinant Lipoxygenases and Oxylipin Metabolism in Relation to Food Quality, http://dx.doi.org/10.1081/FBT-200025673, vol. 18, no. 2, pp. 135–170, 2007, doi: 10.1081/FBT-200025673.
57. S. A. Christensen et al., Maize death acids, 9-lipoxygenase-derived cyclopente(a)nones, display activity as cytotoxic phytoalexins and transcriptional mediators, *Proc Natl Acad Sci U S A*, vol. 112, no. 36, pp. 11407–11412, Sep. 2015, doi: 10.1073/PNAS.1511131112.
58. T. Vellosillo, J. Vicente, S. Kulasekaran, M. Hamberg, and C. Castresana, Emerging complexity in reactive oxygen species production and signaling during the response of plants to pathogens, *Plant Physiol*, vol. 154, no. 2, pp. 444–448, 2010, doi: 10.1104/PP.110.161273.
59. J. Vicente, T. Cascón, B. Vicedo, P. García-Agustín, M. Hamberg, and C. Castresana, Role of 9-Lipoxygenase and α-Dioxygenase Oxylipin Pathways as Modulators of Local and Systemic Defense, *Molecular Plant*, vol. 5, no. 4, pp. 914–928, Jul. 2012, doi: 10.1093/MP/SSR105.

60. M. A. Lõpez et al., Antagonistic role of 9-lipoxygenase-derived oxylipins and ethylene in the control of oxidative stress, lipid peroxidation and plant defence, *Plant J*, vol. 67, no. 3, pp. 447–458, Aug. 2011, doi: 10.1111/J.1365–313X.2011.04608.X.
61. H. Porta, R. E. Figueroa-Balderas, and M. Rocha-Sosa, Wounding and pathogen infection induce a chloroplast-targeted lipoxygenase in the common bean (Phaseolus vulgaris L.), *Planta*, vol. 227, no. 2, pp. 363–373, Jan. 2008, doi: 10.1007/S00425–007–0623-Y.
62. Y. L. Peng, Y. Shirano, H. Ohta, T. Hibino, K. Tanaka, and D. Shibata, A novel lipoxygenase from rice. Primary structure and specific expression upon incompatible infection with rice blast fungus., *Journal of Biological Chemistry*, vol. 269, no. 5, pp. 3755–3761, Feb. 1994, doi: 10.1016/S0021–9258(17)41924–7.
63. R. A. Creelman and J. E. Mullet, BIOSYNTHESIS AND ACTION OF JASMONATES IN PLANTS, *Annu Rev Plant Physiol Plant Mol Biol*, vol. 48, pp. 355–381, 1997, doi: 10.1146/ANNUREV.ARPLANT.48.1.355.
64. C. Sanier, M. Sayegh-Alhamdia, A. Jalloul, A. Clerivet, M. Nicole, and P. Marmey, A 13-lipoxygenase is Expressed Early in the Hypersensitive Reaction of Cotton Plants to Xanthomonas campestris pv. malvacearum, *Journal of Phytopathology*, vol. 160, no. 6, pp. 286–293, Jun. 2012, doi: 10.1111/J.1439–0434.2012.01900.X.
65. Gullner G, Komives T, Király L, Schröder P. Glutathione S-Transferase Enzymes in Plant-Pathogen Interactions. *Front Plant Sci.* 2018 Dec 21;9:1836. doi: 10.3389/fpls.2018.01836. PMID: 30622544; PMCID: PMC6308375.
66. R. A. Wilson, H. W. Gardner, and N. P. Keller, Cultivar-Dependent Expression of a Maize Lipoxygenase Responsive to Seed Infesting Fungi, http://dx.doi.org/10.1094/MPMI.2001.14.8.980, vol. 14, no. 8, pp. 980–987, Feb. 2007, doi: 10.1094/MPMI.2001.14.8.980.
67. G. K. Agrawal, S. Tamogami, O. Han, H. Iwahashi, and R. Rakwal, Rice octadecanoid pathway, *Biochemical and Biophysical Research Communications*, vol. 317, no. 1, pp. 1–15, Apr. 2004, doi: 10.1016/J.BBRC.2004.03.020.
68. C. Delker, I. Stenzel, B. Hause, O. Miersch, I. Feussner, and C. Wasternack, Jasmonate biosynthesis in Arabidopsis thaliana — Enzymes, products, regulation, *Plant Biology*, vol. 8, no. 3, pp. 297–306, May 2006, doi: 10.1055/S-2006–923935/ID/78.
69. X. Gao et al., Maize 9-Lipoxygenase ZmLOX3 Controls Development, Root-Specific Expression of Defense Genes, and Resistance to Root-Knot Nematodes, http://dx.doi.org/10.1094/MPMI-21-1-0098, vol. 21, no. 1, pp. 98–109, Dec. 2007, doi: 10.1094/MPMI-21–1-0098.
70. Y. S. Park, S. Kunze, X. Ni, I. Feussner, and M. v. Kolomiets, Comparative molecular and biochemical characterization of segmentally duplicated 9-lipoxygenase genes ZmLOX4 and ZmLOX5 of maize, *Planta*, vol. 231, no. 6, pp. 1425–1437, 2010, doi: 10.1007/S00425–010–1143–8.
71. I. Rancé, J. Fournier, and M. T. Esquerré-Tugayé, The incompatible interaction between Phytophthora parasitica var. nicotianae race 0 and tobacco is suppressed in transgenic plants expressing antisense lipoxygenase sequences, *Proc Natl Acad Sci U S A*, vol. 95, no. 11, p. 6554, May 1998, doi: 10.1073/PNAS.95.11.6554.
72. H. Weber, A. Chételat, D. Caldelari, and E. E. Farmer, Divinyl Ether Fatty Acid Synthesis in Late Blight-Diseased Potato Leaves, *The Plant Cell*, vol. 11, pp. 485–493, 1999, Accessed: Apr. 14, 2022. Online]. Available: www.plantcell.org
73. P. C. Croft, F. Jüttner, and A. J. Slusarenko, Volatile Products of the Lipoxygenase Pathway Evolved from Phaseolus vulgaris (L.) Leaves Inoculated with Pseudomonas syringae pv phaseolicola, *Plant Physiol*, vol. 101, no. 1, pp. 13–24, 1993, doi: 10.1104/PP.101.1.13.

74. H. Porta and M. Rocha-Sosa, Plant Lipoxygenases. Physiological and Molecular Features, *Plant Physiology*, vol. 130, no. 1, pp. 15–21, Sep. 2002, doi: 10.1104/PP.010787.
75. L. Montillet et al., Fatty Acid Hydroperoxides and H2O2 in the Execution of Hypersensitive Cell Death in Tobacco Leaves, *Plant Physiology*, vol. 138, no. 3, p. 1516, 2005, doi: 10.1104/PP.105.059907.
76. C. Rustérucci et al., Involvement of lipoxygenase-dependent production of fatty acid hydroperoxides in the development of the hypersensitive cell death induced by cryptogein on tobacco leaves, *J Biol Chem*, vol. 274, no. 51, pp. 36446–36455, Dec. 1999, doi: 10.1074/JBC.274.51.36446.
77. N. Tijet et al., Functional expression in yeast and characterization of a clofibrate-inducible plant cytochrome P-450 (CYP94A1) involved in cutin monomers synthesis, *Biochem. J*, vol. 332, p. 583, 1998.
78. E. Blée, Impact of phyto-oxylipins in plant defense, *Trends Plant Sci*, vol. 7, no. 7, pp. 315–322, Jul. 2002, doi: 10.1016/S1360–1385(02)02290–2.
79. D. S. Lee, P. Nioche, M. Hamberg, and C. S. Raman, Structural insights into the evolutionary paths of oxylipin biosynthetic enzymes, *Nature*, vol. 455, no. 7211, pp. 363–368, Sep. 2008, doi: 10.1038/NATURE07307.
80. R. Brash, Mechanistic aspects of CYP74 allene oxide synthases and related cytochrome P450 enzymes, *Phytochemistry*, vol. 70, no. 13–14, pp. 1522–1531, Sep. 2009, doi: 10.1016/J.PHYTOCHEM.2009.08.005.
81. L. Sun, L. Zhu, L. Xu, D. Yuan, L. Min, and X. Zhang, Cotton cytochrome P450 CYP82D regulates systemic cell death by modulating the octadecanoid pathway, *Nature Communications*, vol. 5, 2014, doi: 10.1038/NCOMMS6372.
82. G. A. Howe, G. I. Lee, A. Itoh, L. Li, and A. E. DeRocher, Cytochrome P450-dependent metabolism of oxylipins in tomato. Cloning and expression of allene oxide synthase and fatty acid hydroperoxide lyase, *Plant Physiol*, vol. 123, no. 2, pp. 711–724, 2000, doi: 10.1104/PP.123.2.711.
83. W. C. Song and A. R. Brash, Purification of an allene oxide synthase and identification of the enzyme as a cytochrome P-450, *Science (1979)*, vol. 253, no. 5021, pp. 781–784, 1991, doi: 10.1126/SCIENCE.1876834.
84. D. R. Nelson, Cytochrome P450 and the individuality of species, *Arch Biochem Biophys*, vol. 369, no. 1, pp. 1–10, Sep. 1999, doi: 10.1006/ABBI.1999.1352.
85. W. C. Song, C. D. Funk, and A. R. Brash, Molecular cloning of an allene oxide synthase: a cytochrome P450 specialized for the metabolism of fatty acid hydroperoxides., *Proc Natl Acad Sci U S A*, vol. 90, no. 18, p. 8519, Sep. 1993, doi: 10.1073/PNAS.90.18.8519.
86. S. Sivasankar, B. Sheldrick, and S. J. Rothstein, Expression of Allene Oxide Synthase Determines Defense Gene Activation in Tomato, *Plant Physiology*, vol. 122, no. 4, p. 1335, 2000, doi: 10.1104/PP.122.4.1335.
87. T. Farmaki et al., Differential distribution of the lipoxygenase pathway enzymes within potato chloroplasts, *J Exp Bot*, vol. 58, no. 3, pp. 555–568, Feb. 2007, doi: 10.1093/JXB/ERL230.
88. S. Serrazina, H. Machado, R. L. Costa, P. Duque, and R. Malhó, Expression of Castanea crenata Allene Oxide Synthase in Arabidopsis Improves the Defense to Phytophthora cinnamomi, *Frontiers in Plant Science*, vol. 12, p. 149, Feb. 2021, doi: 10.3389/FPLS.2021.628697/BIBTEX.
89. S. Yoeun, K. Cho, and O. Han, Structural evidence for the substrate channeling of rice allene oxide cyclase in biologically analogous nazarov reaction, *Frontiers in Chemistry*, vol. 6, no. OCT, p. 500, Oct. 2018, doi: 10.3389/FCHEM.2018.00500/BIBTEX.

90. F. Schaller, C. Biesgen, C. Müssig, T. Altmann, and E. W. Weiler, 12-Oxophytodienoate reductase 3 (OPR3) is the isoenzyme involved in jasmonate biosynthesis, *Planta 2000–210:6*, vol. 210, no. 6, pp. 979–984, 2000, doi: 10.1007/S004250050706.
91. D. Deepika, Ankit, S. Jonwal, K. V. Mali, A. K. Sinha, and A. Singh, Molecular analysis indicates the involvement of Jasmonic acid biosynthesis pathway in low-potassium (K+) stress response and development in chickpea (Cicer arietinum), *Environmental and Experimental Botany*, vol. 194, p. 104753, Feb. 2022, doi: 10.1016/J.ENVEXPBOT.2021.104753.
92. A. Schaller and A. Stintzi, Enzymes in jasmonate biosynthesis—Structure, function, regulation, *Phytochemistry*, vol. 70, no. 13–14, pp. 1532–1538, Sep. 2009, doi: 10.1016/J.PHYTOCHEM.2009.07.032.
93. Y. Sasaki et al., Monitoring of methyl jasmonate-responsive genes in Arabidopsis by cDNA macroarray: self-activation of jasmonic acid biosynthesis and crosstalk with other phytohormone signaling pathways, *DNA Res*, vol. 8, no. 4, pp. 153–161, 2001, doi: 10.1093/DNARES/8.4.153.
94. I. Stenzel et al., Jasmonate biosynthesis and the allene oxide cyclase family of Arabidopsis thaliana, *Plant Molecular Biology*, vol. 51, pp. 895–911, 2003.
95. Du H, Liu H, Xiong L. Endogenous auxin and jasmonic acid levels are differentially modulated by abiotic stresses in rice. *Front Plant Sci*. 2013 Oct 9;4:397. doi: 10.3389/fpls.2013.00397. PMID: 24130566; PMCID: PMC3793129.
96. Hu Y, Jiang Y, Han X, Wang H, Pan J, Yu D. Jasmonate regulates leaf senescence and tolerance to cold stress: crosstalk with other phytohormones. *J Exp Bot*. 2017 Mar 1;68(6):1361–1369. doi: 10.1093/jxb/erx004. PMID: 28201612.
97. Danon A, Miersch O, Felix G, Camp RG, Apel K. Concurrent activation of cell death-regulating signaling pathways by singlet oxygen in Arabidopsis thaliana. *Plant J*. 2005 Jan;41(1):68–80. doi: 10.1111/j.1365–313X.2004.02276.x. PMID: 15610350.
98. Stintzi A, Weber H, Reymond P, Browse J, Farmer EE. Plant defense in the absence of jasmonic acid: the role of cyclopentenones. *Proc Natl Acad Sci U S A*. 2001 Oct 23;98(22):12837–42. doi: 10.1073/pnas.211311098. Epub 2001 Oct 9. PMID: 11592974; PMCID: PMC60140.
99. K. Matsui, Green leaf volatiles: hydroperoxide lyase pathway of oxylipin metabolism, *Curr Opin Plant Biol*, vol. 9, no. 3, pp. 274–280, Jun. 2006, doi: 10.1016/J.PBI.2006.03.002.
100. N. J. Bate and S. J. Rothstein, C6-volatiles derived from the lipoxygenase pathway induce a subset of defense-related genes, *Plant J*, vol. 16, no. 5, pp. 561–569, 1998, doi: 10.1046/J.1365–313X.1998.00324.X.
101. G. Griffiths, Biosynthesis and analysis of plant oxylipins, *Free Radical Research*, vol. 49, no. 5, pp. 565–582, May 2015, doi: 10.3109/10715762.2014.1000318.
102. E. E. Farmer and C. Davoine, Reactive electrophile species, *Curr Opin Plant Biol*, vol. 10, no. 4, pp. 380–386, Aug. 2007, doi: 10.1016/J.PBI.2007.04.019.
103. W. C. Song and A. R. Brash, Purification of an allene oxide synthase and identification of the enzyme as a cytochrome P-450, *Science*, vol. 253, no. 5021, pp. 781–784, 1991, doi: 10.1126/SCIENCE.1876834.
104. E. Froehlich, A. Itoh, and G. A. Howe, Tomato allene oxide synthase and fatty acid hydroperoxide lyase, two cytochrome P450s involved in oxylipin metabolism, are targeted to different membranes of chloroplast envelope, *Plant Physiol*, vol. 125, no. 1, pp. 306–317, 2001, doi: 10.1104/PP.125.1.306.
105. S. Rustgi et al., ALLENE OXIDE SYNTHASE and HYDROPEROXIDE LYASE, Two Non-Canonical Cytochrome P450s in Arabidopsis thaliana and Their Different

Roles in Plant Defense, *International Journal of Molecular Sciences*, vol. 20, no. 12, p. 3064, Jun. 2019, doi: 10.3390/IJMS20123064.
106. C. M. Hooper, I. R. Castleden, S. K. Tanz, N. Aryamanesh, and A. H. Millar, SUBA4: the interactive data analysis centre for Arabidopsis subcellular protein locations, *Nucleic Acids Res*, vol. 45, no. D1, pp. D1064–D1074, Jan. 2017, doi: 10.1093/NAR/GKW1041.
107. Y. Wang et al., Hydroperoxide lyase modulates defense response and confers lesion-mimic leaf phenotype in soybean (Glycine max (L.) Merr.), *The Plant Journal*, vol. 104, no. 5, pp. 1315–1333, Dec. 2020, doi: 10.1111/TPJ.15002.
108. D. Nabity, J. A. Zavala, and E. H. Delucia, Herbivore induction of jasmonic acid and chemical defences reduce photosynthesis in Nicotiana attenuata, *Journal of Experimental Botany*, vol. 64, no. 2, pp. 685–694, Jan. 2013, doi: 10.1093/JXB/ERS364.
109. X. Tong et al., The rice hydroperoxide lyase OsHPL3 functions in defense responses by modulating the oxylipin pathway, *Plant J*, vol. 71, no. 5, pp. 763–775, Sep. 2012, doi: 10.1111/J.1365–313X.2012.05027.X.
110. N. Grechkin and M. Hamberg, Divinyl ether synthase from garlic (Allium sativum L.) bulbs: sub-cellular localization and substrate regio-and stereospecificity, *FEBS Lett*, vol. 388, no. 2–3, pp. 112–114, Jun. 1996, doi: 10.1016/0014–5793(96)00536–4.
111. H. W. Gardner, Recent investigations into the lipoxygenase pathway of plants, *Biochimica et Biophysica Acta (BBA) — Lipids and Lipid Metabolism*, vol. 1084, no. 3, pp. 221–239, Jul. 1991, doi: 10.1016/0005–2760(91)90063-N.
112. N. Grechkin', A. v Ilyasov', M. Hamberg3, and A. E. Arbuzov, On the mechanism of biosynthesis of divinyl ether oxylipins by enzyme from garlic bulbs, 1997.
113. T. Galliard, D. R. Phillips, and D. J. Frost, Novel divinyl ether fatty acids in extracts of Solanum tuberosum, *Chemistry and Physics of Lipids*, vol. 11, no. 3, pp. 173–180, Oct. 1973, doi: 10.1016/0009–3084(73)90017–0.
114. D. Caldelari and E. E. Farmer, A rapid assay for the coupled cell free generation of oxylipins, *Phytochemistry*, vol. 47, no. 4, pp. 599–604, Feb. 1998, doi: 10.1016/S0031–9422(97)00443–3.
115. K. Abenthum, S. Hildenbrand, and H. Ninnemann, Elicitation and accumulation of phytoalexins in stems, stolons and roots of Erwinia-infected potato plants, *Physiological and Molecular Plant Pathology*, vol. 46, no. 5, pp. 349–359, May 1995, doi: 10.1006/PMPP.1995.1027.
116. P. Mühlenbock et al., Chloroplast signaling and lesion simulating disease1 regulate crosstalk between light acclimation and immunity in Arabidopsis, *Plant Cell*, vol. 20, no. 9, pp. 2339–2356, 2008, doi: 10.1105/TPC.108.059618.
117. C. Reinbothe, A. Springer, I. Samol, and S. Reinbothe, Plant oxylipins: Role of jasmonic acid during programmed cell death, defence and leaf senescence, *FEBS Journal*, vol. 276, no. 17, pp. 4666–4681, 2009, doi: 10.1111/J.1742–4658.2009.07193.X.
118. G. L. Op Den Camp et al., Rapid Induction of Distinct Stress Responses after the Release of Singlet Oxygen in Arabidopsis, *The Plant Cell*, vol. 15, no. 10, p. 2320, 2003, doi: 10.1105/TPC.014662.
119. D. Kendrick and C. Chang, Ethylene signaling: new levels of complexity and regulation, *Curr Opin Plant Biol*, vol. 11, no. 5, p. 479, Oct. 2008, doi: 10.1016/J.PBI.2008.06.011.
120. D. Przybyla, C. Göbel, A. Imboden, M. Hamberg, I. Feussner, and K. Apel, Enzymatic, but not non-enzymatic, 1O2-mediated peroxidation of polyunsaturated fatty acids forms part of the EXECUTER1-dependent stress response program in the flu mutant of Arabidopsis thaliana, *Plant J*, vol. 54, no. 2, pp. 236–248, Apr. 2008, doi: 10.1111/J.1365–313X.2008.03409.X.

121. C. Ochsenbein *et al.*, The role of EDS1 (enhanced disease susceptibility) during singlet oxygen-mediated stress responses of Arabidopsis, *The Plant Journal*, vol. 47, no. 3, pp. 445–456, Aug. 2006, doi: 10.1111/J.1365–313X.2006.02793.X.
122. R. Mittler, S. Vanderauwera, M. Gollery, and F. van Breusegem, Reactive oxygen gene network of plants, *Trends in Plant Science*, vol. 9, no. 10, pp. 490–498, Oct. 2004, doi: 10.1016/J.TPLANTS.2004.08.009.
123. E. Parker, E. B. Holub, L. N. Frost, A. Falk, N. D. Gunn, and M. J. Daniels, Characterization of eds1, a mutation in Arabidopsis suppressing resistance to Peronospora parasitica specified by several different RPP genes., *The Plant Cell*, vol. 8, no. 11, p. 2033, 1996, doi: 10.1105/TPC.8.11.2033.
124. A. Mateo et al., LESION SIMULATING DISEASE 1 Is Required for Acclimation to Conditions That Promote Excess Excitation Energy, *Plant Physiology*, vol. 136, no. 1, pp. 2818–2830, Sep. 2004, doi: 10.1104/PP.104.043646.
125. v. Rao, H. Lee, R. A. Creelman, J. E. Mullet, and K. R. Davis, Jasmonic Acid Signaling Modulates Ozone-Induced Hypersensitive Cell Death, *The Plant Cell*, vol. 12, no. 9, p. 1633, Sep. 2000, doi: 10.2307/3871179.
126. E. Alvarez, R. I. Pennell, P. J. Meijer, A. Ishikawa, R. A. Dixon, and C. Lamb, Reactive oxygen intermediates mediate a systemic signal network in the establishment of plant immunity, *Cell*, vol. 92, no. 6, pp. 773–784, Mar. 1998, doi: 10.1016/S0092–8674(00)81405–1.
127. v. Rao and K. R. Davis, Ozone-induced cell death occurs via two distinct mechanisms in Arabidopsis: the role of salicylic acid, *The Plant Journal*, vol. 17, no. 6, pp. 603–614, Mar. 1999, doi: 10.1046/J.1365–313X.1999.00400.X.
128. J. Glazebrook, Genes controlling expression of defense responses in Arabidopsis, *Curr Opin Plant Biol*, vol. 2, no. 4, pp. 280–286, 1999, doi: 10.1016/S1369–5266(99)80050–8.
129. O. Lorenzo, J. M. Chico, J. J. Sánchez-Serrano, and R. Solano, JASMONATE-INSENSITIVE1 Encodes a MYC Transcription Factor Essential to Discriminate between Different Jasmonate-Regulated Defense Responses in Arabidopsis, *The Plant Cell*, vol. 16, no. 7, pp. 1938–1950, Jul. 2004, doi: 10.1105/TPC.022319.
130. E. Rojo, R. Solano, and J. J. Sánchez-Serrano, Interactions between Signaling Compounds Involved in Plant Defense, *Journal of Plant Growth Regulation*, vol. 22, no. 1, pp. 82–98, Mar. 2003, doi: 10.1007/S00344–003–0027–6.
131. O. Lorenzo, R. Piqueras, J. J. Sánchez-Serrano, and R. Solano, ETHYLENE RESPONSE FACTOR1 integrates signals from ethylene and jasmonate pathways in plant defense, *Plant Cell*, vol. 15, no. 1, pp. 165–178, Jan. 2003, doi: 10.1105/TPC.007468.
132. M. Boter, O. Ruíz-Rivero, A. Abdeen, and S. Prat, Conserved MYC transcription factors play a key role in jasmonate signaling both in tomato and Arabidopsis, *Genes & Development*, vol. 18, no. 13, pp. 1577–1591, Jul. 2004, doi: 10.1101/GAD.297704.
133. J. P. Anderson et al., Antagonistic interaction between abscisic acid and jasmonate-ethylene signaling pathways modulates defense gene expression and disease resistance in Arabidopsis, *Plant Cell*, vol. 16, no. 12, pp. 3460–3479, 2004, doi: 10.1105/TPC.104.025833.
134. N. Laurie-Berry, V. Joardar, I. H. Street, and B. N. Kunkel, The Arabidopsis thaliana JASMONATE INSENSITIVE 1 gene is required for suppression of salicylic acid-dependent defenses during infection by Pseudomonas syringae, *Molecular Plant-Microbe Interactions*, vol. 19, no. 7, pp. 789–800, Jul. 2006, doi: 10.1094/MPMI-19–0789.

135. D. Kley, M. Kleinmann, H. Sanderman, and S. Krupa, Photochemical oxidants: state of the science, *Environmental Pollution*, vol. 100, no. 1–3, pp. 19–42, Jan. 1999, doi: 10.1016/S0269–7491(99)00086-X.
136. R. L. Heath and G. E. Taylor, Physiological Processes and Plant Responses to Ozone Exposure, pp. 317–368, 1997, doi: 10.1007/978–3-642–59233–1_10.
137. J. Kangasjärvi, J. Talvinen, M. Utriainen, and R. Karjalainen, Plant defence systems induced by ozone, *Plant, Cell & Environment*, vol. 17, no. 7, pp. 783–794, 1994, doi: 10.1111/J.1365–3040.1994.TB00173.X.
138. K. Overmyer et al., Ozone-sensitive arabidopsis rcd1 mutant reveals opposite roles for ethylene and jasmonate signaling pathways in regulating superoxide-dependent cell death, *Plant Cell*, vol. 12, no. 10, pp. 1849–1862, 2000, doi: 10.1105/TPC.12.10.1849.
139. C. Rustérucci et al., Involvement of Lipoxygenase-dependent Production of Fatty Acid Hydroperoxides in the Development of the Hypersensitive Cell Death induced by Cryptogein on Tobacco Leaves *, *Journal of Biological Chemistry*, vol. 274, no. 51, pp. 36446–36455, Dec. 1999, doi: 10.1074/JBC.274.51.36446.
140. J. Tuomainen et al., Ozone induction of ethylene emission in tomato plants: regulation by differential accumulation of transcripts for the biosynthetic enzymes, *The Plant Journal*, vol. 12, no. 5, pp. 1151–1162, Nov. 1997, doi: 10.1046/J.1365–313X.1997.12051151.X.
141. L. Zhang, F. Zhang, M. Melotto, J. Yao, and S. Y. He, Jasmonate signaling and manipulation by pathogens and insects, *Journal of Experimental Botany*, vol. 68, no. 6, pp. 1371–1385, Mar. 2017, doi: 10.1093/JXB/ERW478.
142. P. Epple, A. Vignutelli, K. Apel, and H. Bohlmann, Differential induction of the Arabidopsis thaliana Thi2.1 gene by Fusarium oxysporum f. sp. matthiolae, *Mol Plant Microbe Interact*, vol. 11, no. 6, pp. 523–529, 1998, doi: 10.1094/MPMI.1998.11.6.523.
143. M. Nibbe, B. Hilpert, C. Wasternack, O. Miersch, and K. Apel, Cell death and salicylate- and jasmonate-dependent stress responses in Arabidopsis are controlled by single cet genes, *Planta 2002–216:1*, vol. 216, no. 1, pp. 120–128, Nov. 2002, doi: 10.1007/S00425–002–0907–1.
144. L. Q. Huang et al., Jasmonates modulate sphingolipid metabolism and accelerate cell death in the ceramide kinase mutant acd5, *Plant Physiology*, vol. 187, no. 3, pp. 1713–1727, Nov. 2021, doi: 10.1093/PLPHYS/KIAB362.
145. S. Dhondt, P. Geoffroy, B. A. Stelmach, M. Legrand, and T. Heitz, Soluble phospholipase A2 activity is induced before oxylipin accumulation in tobacco mosaic virus-infected tobacco leaves and is contributed by patatin-like enzymes, *The Plant Journal*, vol. 23, no. 4, pp. 431–440, Aug. 2000, doi: 10.1046/J.1365–313X.2000.00802.X.
146. P. Díaz-Vivancos et al., Alteration in the chloroplastic metabolism leads to ROS accumulation in pea plants in response to plum pox virus, *J Exp Bot*, vol. 59, no. 8, pp. 2147–2160, May 2008, doi: 10.1093/JXB/ERN082.
147. B. A. Stelmach, A. Müller, P. Hennig, D. Laudert, L. Andert, and E. W. Weiler, Quantitation of the octadecanoid 12-oxo-phytodienoic acid, a signalling compound in plant mechanotransduction, *Phytochemistry*, vol. 47, no. 4, pp. 539–546, Feb. 1998, doi: 10.1016/S0031–9422(97)00547–5.
148. D. Laudert and E. W. Weiler, Allene oxide synthase: a major control point in Arabidopsis thaliana octadecanoid signalling, *The Plant Journal*, vol. 15, no. 5, pp. 675–684, Sep. 1998, doi: 10.1046/J.1365–313X.1998.00245.X.

149. P. Kenton, L. A. J. Mur, R. Atzorn, C. Wasternack, and J. Draper, (—)-Jasmonic Acid Accumulation in Tobacco Hypersensitive Response Lesions, http://dx.doi.org/10.1094/MPMI.1999.12.1.74, vol. 12, no. 1, pp. 74–78, Feb. 2007, doi: 10.1094/MPMI.1999.12.1.74.
150. K. Komatsu et al., Viral-Induced Systemic Necrosis in Plants Involves Both Programmed Cell Death and the Inhibition of Viral Multiplication, Which Are Regulated by Independent Pathways, http://dx.doi.org/10.1094/MPMI-23-3-0283, vol. 23, no. 3, pp. 283–293, Feb. 2010, doi: 10.1094/MPMI-23–3-0283.
151. A. García-Marcos, R. Pacheco, A. Manzano, E. Aguilar, and F. Tenllado, Oxylipin Biosynthesis Genes Positively Regulate Programmed Cell Death during Compatible Infections with the Synergistic Pair Potato Virus X-Potato Virus Y and Tomato Spotted Wilt Virus, *Journal of Virology*, vol. 87, no. 10, p. 5769, May 2013, doi: 10.1128/JVI.03573–12.
152. R. Mittler, V. Shulaev, M. Seskar, and E. Lam, Inhibition of Programmed Cell Death in Tobacco Plants during a Pathogen-Induced Hypersensitive Response at Low Oxygen Pressure., *The Plant Cell*, vol. 8, no. 11, pp. 1991–2001, Nov. 1996, doi: 10.1105/TPC.8.11.1991.
153. N. A. Porter, S. E. Caldwell, and K. A. Mills, Mechanisms of free radical oxidation of unsaturated lipids, *Lipids*, vol. 30, no. 4, pp. 277–290, Apr. 1995, doi: 10.1007/BF02536034.
154. P. Wojtaszek, Oxidative burst: an early plant response to pathogen infection, *Biochem J*, vol. 322 (Pt 3), no. Pt 3, pp. 681–692, Mar. 1997, doi: 10.1042/BJ3220681.

10 The Roles of Oxylipins in Plant Systemic Resistance

Tamana Khan[1*], *Labiba Riyaz Shah*[1], *Nawreen Mir*[2], *Gazala Gulzar*[2], *Bazilla Mushtaq*[3], *Rizwan Rashid*[1], *and Baseerat Afroza*[1]
[1]Division of Vegetable Science; Faculty of Horticulture, Sher e Kashmir University of Agricultural Sciences and Technology of Kashmir, Shalimar, Jammu and Kashmir, India
[2] Division of Plant Pathology; Faculty of Horticulture, Sher e Kashmir University of Agricultural Sciences and Technology of Kashmir, Shalimar, Jammu and Kashmir, India
[3] Division of Fruit Science; Faculty of Horticulture, Sher e Kashmir University of Agricultural Sciences and Technology of Kashmir, Shalimar, Jammu and Kashmir, India
*Email: Khantamana96@gmail.com

CONTENTS

DOI: 10.1201/9781003316558-10

10.1 INTRODUCTION

Key defense response to pathogen infection by plants is hypersensitive cell death, which is accompanied by lipid peroxidation activities. HR (hypersensitive response) which is the most constructive system of defense in plants has a race-specific characteristic of imparting resistance against pathogens [1]. When a protein governing host resistance in plants is recognized by the avirulence protein derived from the pathogen, the HR gets triggered which leads to the death of a small number of cells around the infection site, an oxidative burst, synthesis of anti-pathogenic chemicals, and lastly, development of resistance in distant plant parts. The HR at large is effective at preventing pathogen spread and colonization of the host plant. Activation of HR in plants may take place non-enzymatically as a result of ROS (reactive oxygen species) or can be catalyzed by enzymes such as dioxygenases, lipoxygenases, or peroxidases. Correlative research indicating an increase in 9-LOX products in hypersensitively responding cells has previously proposed that a specific set of 9-lipoxygenases is responsible for lipid peroxidation [2]. The hypersensitivity response (HR) generated by incompatible plant-bacteria interactions has also been related to the activation of the LOX pathway [3–6].

Pathogen detection activates a variety of inducible systemic defenses along with the HR which is effective locally. Systemic reactions generate an improved defensive capacity against subsequent infection in plant sections far from the location of primary infection. Systemic acquired resistance (SAR) is a biologically induced resistance in systemic tissue, which is effective in a varied number of species in plants. Such resistance developed is highly enduring and functions against a diverse range of infection-causing agents like viruses, fungus, and bacteria [7–9]. In both local and systemic tissues, SAR activates an enormous number of genes related to pathogenesis (PR genes) [10, 11] and is assumed to be the consequence of a coordinated action of products produced by many PR genes. PR genes are used as effective genetic markers for the beginning of SAR in plant defense studies [7].

Oxylipins are diverse compounds derived from lipids which play critical functions in plant defense. Some defensive phytohormones like SA, JA and ethylene, which activate the immunity of the plants via established signaling routes, have been demonstrated [12]. Out of these oxylipins, JA being a crucial hormone for plant pathogen defense, plays an important function in several areas of plant development [13–17]. Although JA's direct role as a SAR signal for long-distance is doubtful [18, 19], it has been demonstrated to play a part in the development of SAR after the biotrophic bacteria causes infection [20]. Other 13-LOX derivatives apart from JA, play a part in plant's defense by acting as signaling molecules that control expression of genes, cell death, or antimicrobial compounds [21, 22, 3, 23, 24]. Recent research has shown that the α-dioxygenase and 9-lipoxygenase pathways are involved in the modulation of defense in plants and growth, in addition to the significance of oxylipins generated through13-LOX pathway. Research on α-DOX revealed that it has an antibacterial defense function in plants like tobacco and Arabidopsis, and it probably adjusts the oxidative stress and cell death [25–27], and has also an anti-herbivory function in *N. attenuata* [25, 26]. The function of the 9-lipoxygenase pathway in tobacco and Arabidopsis defense has been discovered by several genetic investigations [28–31]. Results indicating that particular derivatives of α-DOX and 9-LOX impart a protective function by lowering symptoms caused by bacterial infection [27, 23] and signaling defense responses through a JA-independent signaling pathway add to the case for their participation in plant defense [29]. It has been discovered that the 9-lipoxygenase and α-dioxygenase oxylipin pathways, as well as particular dioxygenase derivatives, especially 9-lipoxygenase derivative, 9-KOT (9-ketooctadecatrienoic acid), play an active role in local and systemic defense and protect plant tissues against infections caused by bacteria. Furthermore, studies on the impact of 9-KOT in response to infections caused by bacteria revealed that LOX1 and a-DOX1 modulate hormonal responses and hence contribute to plant defense [32].

10.2 THE ROLE OF OXYLIPINS IN ACQUIRED RESISTANCE

10.2.1 Plant Defense to Biotic Stresses

Plants are constantly prone to attacks by pests and pathogens and have inherited a special metabolic diversity that allows them to embark efficient defense measures [33, 34]. Preformed chemical and physical barriers, as well as effective mechanisms including antibacterial compound secretion, cell wall fortification *via* callose and lignin synthesis, and the stimulation of pathways for defense signaling, are a few defense strategies. When pathogen-derived molecules are recognized, defense signaling pathways are activated, which result in PTI (pathogen associated molecular pattern (PAMP)-triggered immunity) or ETI (effector-triggered immunity). PTI is triggered when the plant's PRRs (pattern recognition receptors) detect conserved microbial factors termed as PAMPs [35]. When a pathogen's strain-specific avirulent (AVR) protein interacts with the resistance (R) protein of plants directly or indirectly, ETI is triggered [36]. ETI results in fast production of ROS (reactive oxygen species) and a hypersensitivity reaction (HR), both of which result in the death of cells at the infection's localized area. Hypersensitivity reaction is a type of programmed, sudden cell death that causes the formation of necrotic lesions due to the expiration of plant cells on and around the contact site of the pathogen. It becomes a nearly observable indication of pathogen-induced host defensive responses and is believed to restrict the pathogen to dead cells, thereby preventing disease dispersal.

On top of local resistance, pathogen identification in systemic tissues frequently causes the production of defense responses. The AVR-R interaction, for example, frequently induces systemic acquired resistance (SAR), which provides immunity against secondary infections by linked and unlinked pathogens [9, 37]. When nonpathogenic rhizobacteria colonize plant roots, another kind of secondary immunity called ISR (induced systemic resistance) is generated [38]. The phytohormones such as auxin, abscisic acid (ABA), SA, JA, and ethylene (ET) are important mediators of signaling pathways for defense in plants [39]. These plant hormones not only trigger defense responses on their own, but they also work together or against each other to coordinate downstream signaling.

Complexly inter-related networks of signaling including various plant hormones facilitate the fine-tuning of pathways for signal transduction, with many identified elements in some plants, such as *Arabidopsis thaliana* [40–43]. Various elements of primary metabolism play a role in controlling plant defense signaling which is clear by the growing evidence [44]. For instance, Glycerol-3-phosphate (G3P), a glycerol-derived molecule, is vital in imparting resistance against the anthracnose fungus *Colletotrichum higginsianum* [45]. In Arabidopsis and rice, respectively, vitamin B1 and sucrose enhance pathogen resistance [46, 47]. Recent studies suggest that fatty acids (FAs), carbohydrates, lipids, and lipases all play essential roles in the defense mechanisms of plants and are engaged in crosstalk with plant hormones such as SA, JA, and ABA [42, 47, 48].

10.2.2 Fatty Acids: Regulators of Immunity

In the cells of the plant, FAs and a few species of lipid represent a keystone of cellular metabolism [49]. FAs have a polar carboxyl-containing head group and a hydrophobic carbon chain, rendering them as amphipathic compounds. Various lengths (number of C atoms) and degrees of unsaturation describe hydrophobic hydrocarbon chains. Linoleic acid ($18{:}2^{\Delta 9,12}$), palmitic acid (16:0), stearic acid (18:0), oleic acid ($18{:}1^{\Delta 9}$), and linolenic acid ($18{:}3^{\Delta 9,12,15}$) are some of the most frequent FAs [50, 51]. Fatty acids and species of lipid have been described as molecules with biological roles in phyto-immunity, such as membrane and cuticle production. In response to damage to the infected plant's cellular membranes and attack by a pathogen, PUFAs (polyunsaturated fatty acids) are released by lipase activity, raising the quantities of accessible free fatty acids (FFAs) [52–54]. The plant-derived FFAs like C18:0, C18:1, C18:2, and C18:3 have been shown to contribute in the defense against a variety of diseases and opportunistic microbes [55, 56]. These FAs either act directly as FAs or indirectly as oxylipins on the pathogen [55]. A free carboxylic acid moiety and the number of double bonds are those structural characteristics that are important for antibacterial activity [49, 51, 55]. Furthermore, FAs with cis-double bonds have been shown to have more antimicrobial activity than their trans counterparts [57].

It has been suggested that the amphipathic character of PUFAs produced from plant membranes allows lipids to associate with the cellular membranes of bacteria. The penetration or destruction of membranous structures has a number of negative consequences for the viability of bacterial cells. When long- or medium-chain unsaturated FAs enter the cellular membrane of bacteria, they cause a rise in overall membrane fluidity, which leads to membrane instability, cytosolic leakage, and cellular lysis [54]. On account of straight interaction with carriers of protein electron, these FAs bring about additional destruction of the lipid bilayer, affecting the transport of electrons and oxidative phosphorylation, which results in cessation of ATP generation [58]. FA can uncouple oxidative phosphorylation in two ways: by disrupting the proton gradient and blocking ADP conversion to ATP, or by directly binding to ATP synthase and inhibiting its activity, thus limiting the ability to produce ATP [59]. Furthermore, FAs which are linked to transportation proteins frequently block nutrient absorption. FAs also serve as significant inhibitors of enzymes in the membrane and cytoplasm, contributing to their antimicrobial properties [51, 60].

FAs are particularly efficient in the case of gram-positive bacteria, owing to their less-complicated cell walls and higher porosity, which allows antimicrobial chemicals to enter the cell more easily [61]. Saturated fatty acids have also been extensively researched in terms of hydrocarbon chain length and antibacterial action [62]. Saturated FAs with hydrocarbon chains ranging from 6–18 carbon atoms have the highest powerful activity against gram-positive bacteria, short chain FAs with 6 or fewer carbon atoms have been reported to influence gram-negative bacteria [63]. This is mainly because the layer of lipopolysaccharide prevents the buildup of long and medium-chain fatty acids on the cell wall, preventing these chemicals from acting as antimicrobials [64].

10.2.3 The Role of Oxylipins in Plant Defense

Lipoxygenase (LOX) activity allows polyunsaturated fatty acids (PUFAs) to produce secondary phytochemicals [65]. Lipoxygenase enzymes are a non-heme iron protein family found throughout plants which start off the hydro-peroxidation of PUFAs with cis, cis-1,4-pentadiene moieties, resulting in the formation of a novel class of species of lipid that are known as oxygenated lipids or oxylipins [55]. These series of oxygenated by-products generated from precursors of PUFA possess a variety of lengths of carbons i.e., C16 to C22 and unsaturation patterns (ω3, ω6, and ω9) through dioxygen-dependent oxidation [66]. Auto-oxidation can also produce oxylipins, in which free radicals and reactive oxygen species trigger non-enzymatic pathways, resulting in the simultaneous synthesis of a variety of oxidized lipids, such as phytoprostanes and hydroxy-FAs [67]. Hydroperoxide aldehydes, alcohol-, oxo-, and fatty aldehydes, cyclized OPDA, hydroxides and epoxides, divinyl ethers, keto-fatty acids (α- and γ-ketols), JA precursors and JA derivatives are among the oxylipin sub-classes [56, 68, 69]. The majority of oxylipin's biological actions are mediated through either jasmonate (JA) perception or signaling networks of RES; reactive electrophilic species [70].

After wounding or pathogen infection, flowering plants produce a variety of oxylipins [71]. Antimicrobial activities [23, 24], cell death regulation [3], callose deposition [29, 31] and stimulation of defense genes [14] have all been attributed to these oxylipins. *Physcomitrella patens* releases a range of oxylipins in response to injury, such as volatiles generated from (3Z)-nonenal (C9) and 12-HPETE e.g., octenols (C8) [72]. C8 volatiles can boost disease resistance by inducing the production of the genes involved in defense of flowering plants [73]. Furthermore, C8 volatiles are biologically active metabolites in case of pests [74] and C9 volatiles show antimicrobial properties against few fungal pathogens such as *Botrytis cinerea* and *Fusarium oxysporum* [75].

Oxygenated lipids are the ions favorably associated with biotic stress, as examined in several metabolomics investigations (Table 10.1) [76, 77]. *Sorghum bicolor* has been shown not only to detect LP (lipopolysaccharides) from *Burkholderia andropogonis*, but also to produce numerous metabolites in the extra-cellular environment also, such as trihydroxyoctadecadienoic acid and trihydroxy-octadecenoic acid, as a plant defense technique [78]. After infection with *Fusarium pseudograminearum*, the seedlings of sorghum primed with *Paenibacillus alvei* show an increase in the rate of metabolic reprogramming [79]. Some oxylipin metabolites whose production is enhanced after pathogen infection in the root, leaf, and stem tissues, are epoxy-hydroxyoctadecanoic

TABLE 10.1
Oxylipins as Potent Biomarkers Against Biotic Stress (Pathogen Attack/Elicitor Induction) in Various Plant Species

Empirical formula	Oxylipin	Plant	Biotic stress	Reference
$C_{13}H_{25}NO_3$	Amino-oxo-tridecanoic acid	*Solanum lycopersicum*	*Ralstonia solanacearum*	76
$C_{16}H_{30}O_2$	Palmitoleic acid	*Arabidopsis thaliana*	LP	80
$C_{16}H_{32}O_3$	Hydroxypalmitate	*Sorghum bicolor*	LP	78
$C_{18}H_{30}O_3$	Hydroxyoctadecatrienoic acid	*S. lycopersicum* *Sorghum bicolor* *Solanum lycopersicum*	*Phytophthoracapsici* *C. sublineolum* *Meloidogyn ejavanica*	92 93 81
$C_{18}H_{32}O_3$	Hydroxy linoleic acid	*Sorghum bicolor*	LP	78
$C_{18}H_{30}O_3$	Hydroxylinolenic acid	*Arabidopsis thaliana*	LP	80
$C_{18}H_{30}O_4$	13S-Hydroperoxy-9Z, 11E, 15Z octadecatrienoic acid	*A. thaliana* *S. bicolor*	LP LP	80 78
$C_{18}H_{32}O_4$	12-oxo-9-hydroxy-10E,15Z-octadecadienoic acid	*Zea mays*	*Trichoderma virens*	77
$C_{18}H_{32}O_5$	Trihydroxyoctade cadienoic acid	*Sorghum bicolor* *S. lycopersicum*	LP *R. solanacearum* *Phytophthora capsici*	78 76 92
$C_{18}H_{34}O_5$	Trihydroxy-octadecenoic acid	*S. bicolor* *S. lycopersicum*	LP *R. solanacearum* *P. capsici*	78 76 92

LP = Lipopolysaccharides

acid and hydroperoxy-epoxy-octadecenoic acid [78]. Differential defense associated perturbations as well as the release of a few oxylipin molecules like hydroperoxyl octadecatrienoic acid and OPDA and some glycoglycerolipid arabidopsides have been observed in *Arabidopsis thaliana* when inoculated with purified LPs from *B. cepacia*, *Xanthomonas campestris* and *Pseudomonas syringae* [80]. Using comprehensive lipid profiling, a plant and nematode interaction investigation on *Solanum lycopersicum* roots identified oxylipins as modulators of plant signaling and essential molecules attenuating nematode parasitism [81]. Multiple enzymes found in solanaceous plants convert eicosapolyenoic FAs like arachidonic acid into physiologically operative oxylipin species [82].

Oomycetes MAMPs are also free fatty acid derivatives that can activate responses for host defense. Increased production of lipoxygenase (9-LOX), α-dioxygenase (α-DOX) and 9-divinyl ether synthase (9-DES) enzymes in tomato roots inoculated with *Phytophthora capsici* implicates oxylipin production in the host for defense against soil-borne diseases [83]. The presence of trihydroxy-octacdecanoic acid, hydroxyocta-decanedioic acid and amino-oxo-tridecanoicacidas as possible markers of tomato bacterial wilt was detected in metabolomics analysis when infected with *Ralstonia solanacearum*[76]. The in vitro actions of oxylipins in the case of necrotrophic, biotrophic, and hemi-biotrophic pathogens, have been the focus of research into their possible antimicrobial properties.

Oxylipins produced from the pathways of α-DOX and 9-LOX have a high antibacterial effect [84]. 9-Keto-10(E),12(Z),15(Z)-octadecatrienoic acid (9- KOT), the main lipoxygenase product from linoleic acid, is extremely potent against *P. syringae* pv. *tomato* (Pst) DC3000 [32]. In consequence, over 50 oxylipins have been tested in vitro against 13 agronomically important pathogens (fungus, oomycetes and bacteria), along with their stability showing that one or more oxylipins suppress the pathogen development [85, 23]. The oxylipins are even more effective at inhibiting the fungal spore germination, with (u-5-Z)-etherolenic acid, colnelenic acid and colneleic acid, showing particularly high efficacy [85, 23, 86]. It is commonly acknowledged that divinyl-, hydroxy- and keto- fatty acids (FAs) and HPOs have potent antimicrobial properties directly, but others, such as jasmonic acid and certain volatile aldehydes, appear to play primarily a role in signaling.

Phyto-oxylipin pathways produce a wide variety of structurally varied metabolites with important functions. Phyto-oxylipins, particularly JA, play a key role in the growth and the development of plants (e.g., pollen, flower, and seed development), as well as responses to numerous stresses [87, 88]. JA is also a pivotal part of plant defenses against herbivores and certain diseases, primarily necrotrophic, via its precursor OPDA (12-oxo-phytodienoic acid) and its derivatives [89–91]. As a result, this might be expanded to all phyto-oxylipins involved in early defense responses to insect or disease attacks. Hitherto, oxylipins function as defense agents by contributing to the improvement of plant tolerance and resistance mechanisms against various biotic stresses. Their role as precursors of phyto-hormone to signaling pathways as well as active metabolites that restrict plant infection, is significant and ponderable.

10.3 THE ROLE OF OXYLIPINS IN INDUCED RESISTANCE

10.3.1 Plant Defense Mechanisms

Plants reside in a fixed habitat throughout their life span owing to their sessile nature and are thus subject to a number of stresses. Plants, over the millions of years of evolutionary progress, have developed a myriad of defense strategies yielding safety against a number of abiotic and biotic stresses. Plants have evolved a variety of physical barriers as defense weapons over time, including cuticle, hairy proturberances, laminar modifications, and sticky hairs, as well as hazardous chemicals or enzymes that are constitutively expressed. Aside from these morphological modifications, inducible systems are also established in plants [91]. The defense plan activated for a particular threat is not just localized and short lived but often is systemic and embedded in plant systems to be used again during the next encounter with the same excitant, in what is called as systemic acquired resistance (SAR). Apart from this type of defense strategy, plants also exhibit a unique type of resistance, termed induced systemic resistance (ISR), whereby a plant infected by a non-pathogenic strain of a micro-organism develops resistance against the pathogenic ones when attacked [38]. This type of resistance is also activated by compounds that are produced in uninfected tissues upon first infection—a phenomenon referred to as priming.

Unlike SAR, ISR does not entail the accumulation of pathogenesis-related proteins or salicylic acid [94]; rather, the two most precisely described forms of induced resistance rely on jasmonate and ethylene-regulated pathways [95, 96]. These molecular analyses, on the other hand, are based on a small number of ISR systems. Other ISR examples are related to PGPR strains producing siderophores or salicylic acid, and hence have more in common with SAR [97]. In plants that acquire pervasive resistance, SAR is contemplated through the salicylic acid signaling pathway, being controlled by the NONEX-PRESSER OF PR GNENS 1 (NPR1), that is a redox-regulated protein [98]. ISR, on the other hand, is affected by the jasmonic acid/ethylene-signaling pathways, and NPR1 plays a key role in the execution of this protective retaliation [99].

10.3.2 Oxylipins as Plant Defenders

A plant is able to defend itself against the attacking pathogen by the various classes of compounds that are either preformed or are generated de novo during the pathogen invasion. Those compounds can have both local and systemic effect and may also be involved in signal transduction. Different classes of compounds like carbohydrates, phenols, and lipids fall under this category. Fatty acids (FAs), along with other lipid species, are essential components of plant cell metabolism. These FFAs can act directly or indirectly as oxylipins on the pathogen [94]. Compounds generated from the conversion of multiple unsaturated bonds containing fatty acids, commonly known as oxylipins, play a critical role in incited reaction systems in plants and animals [91]. Oxylipins in plants are produced in response to a variety of stresses, and while they are acknowledged for activating stress-induced signaling mechanisms and reactions, their non-signaling functions are not well studied [57]. Oxylipins are lipophilic signaling molecules produced from polyunsaturated fatty acids after they have been oxidized. Eukaryotic plants, which include algae, mosses, and angiosperms, have been revealed to contain around 500 distinct oxylipin molecules [100].

The enzymatic or chemical production of fatty acid hydroperoxides is the primary mode of fatty acid oxidation. A variety of further processes convert fatty acid hydroperoxides further, resulting in the production of numerous different types of oxylipins, several of which have been linked to plant signaling associating them with plant resistance. The inclusion of a hydrogenated peroxyl moiety to the lipid molecule, as well as the existence of double bonds, is ascribed to the increased antibacterial activity usually associated with oxylipins. The oxylipins, due to their unique character of interacting with both hydrophobic and hydrophilic substances, are responsible for distortion and fracture of plasma membrane [70].

10.3.3 Antipathic Activity of Oxylipins

Several oxylipin compounds' antipathic properties against various pathogens as bacteria and fungi, including the lower fungi that belong to oomycetes class of Kingdom Chromista, have been studied by various workers (Table 10.2) [85, 84].

TABLE 10.2
Compendium of Most Effective Antimicrobial Free POs as Identified Under In-Vitro Analysis

	Pathogen		
Pos	**Fungi**	**Oomycetes**	**Bacteria**
ω-5(Z)-Etherolenic acid	*Alternaria brassicae, Leptosphaeria maculans, Cladosporium herbarum*	*Phytophthora infestans*	*Pseudomonas syringae*
Epoxy-9-octadecenoic acid	*Alternaria brassicae, Cladosporium herbarum, Rhizopus* sp., *Sclerotinia sclerotiorum*	*Phytophthora parasitica*	
Epoxy-12-octadecenoic acid	*Cladosporium herbarum, Leptosphaeria maculans, Rhizopus* sp.	*Phytophthora parasitica*	*Pseudomonas syringae*
Hydroperoxy--octadecatrienoic acid (13-HPOT)	*Alternaria brassicae, Botrytis cinerea, Cladosporium herbarum, Leptosphaeria maculans, Fusarium oxysporum*	*Phytophthora parasitica*	
Hydroperoxy-octadecatrienoic acid (9-HPOT)	*Botrytis cinerea, Cladosporium herbarum, Fusarium oxysporum, Rhizopus* sp.	*Phytophthora parasitica*	-
Colneleic acid	*Cladosporium herbarum, Fusarium oxysporum,*	-	-
Anacardic acid	*Fusarium oxysporum*	*Phytophthora infestans*	*Xanthomonascampestris*
Oxophytodienoic acid (OPDA)	*Alternaria brassicae, Botrytis cinerea, Cladosporium herbarum, Fusarium oxysporum*	*Phytophthora infestans*	*Pseudomonas syringae*
2(E)-Nonenal	-	-	*Pseudomonas syringae*
2(E)-Hexenal	*Alternaria brassicae, Botrytis cinerea, Cladosporiumherbarum, Fusarium oxysporum, Rhizopus* sp.	*Phytophthorain festans, Phytophthora parasitica*	*Pseudomonas syringae, Xanthomonas campestris*
3(Z)-Hexenal	-	-	*Pseudomonas syringae*

The potential antipathic activity of POs has been studied in vitro for various obligate, perthotrophic, and facultative saprotrophic infections. Plant oxylipins generated from the 9-lipoxygenase and α-Dioxygenase reaction pathways have been shown to have potent antibacterial activity [101]. Keto-octadecatrienoic acid (9- KOT), a lipoxygenase enzyme, the main outcome derived from fatty acid, linoleic acid, is particularly effective for *P. syringae* pv. tomatoDC3000 [102]. As a result, 50 POs were evaluated in vitro for their effect against 13 economically important diseases (bacteria, fungus, and oomycetes). The germination of fungal spores was inhibited more efficiently by (u-5-Z)-etherolenic, colneleic, and colnelenic acids [103]. It is widely believed that fatty acid conjugate compounds like divinyl-, keto-, and hydroxy-FAs have potent and exclusive antipathic properties, but others, such as jasmonic acid and certain aldehydes that are vaporous, are more involved in mechanisms pertaining to signaling. The biocidal effects of POs may be connected to a variety of fatal mechanisms, including increased membrane porosity, membrane disruption, denaturation of vital biological components as proteins and nucleic acids, and oxidative stress. The laboratory tests revealed that 2(E)-hexenal had the maximum efficiency of the POs, with a surfactant-like effect that gravely destroys the cell walls and cell membranes [104]. This type of behavior is common among reactive electrophiles (RES)- α,β-unsaturated carbonyl possessing components, containing molecules that are concentrated in damaged and injured tissues. The chemical structure of the progenitor of oxylipins i.e., PUFAs have a major role to offer in the biological activity of these compounds. This contributor of the biocidal activity of oxylipins, however, remains less explored. The construction (which includes the carbon chain length, and the existence, number of units, location, and navigation of unsaturation) largely determines the antibacterial properties of PUFAs [54]. The antibacterial properties of PUFAs having *cis* double bonds are superior to those possessing *trans* double bonds [54].

The oxylipins were evaluated at concentrations of roughly 100 mM, and observations were recorded after 24 hrs.

10.3.4 Oxylipins as Signaling Molecules

The signaling chemicals belonging to oxylipins have been implicated in a variety of environmental stress conditions. In particular, JA and its precursor, OPDA, as well as other electrophilic species that are reactive, have important parts to play [91]. It starts with the addition of oxygen to polyunsaturated fatty acids by enzymes such as lipoxygenases, to generate hydroperoxides of fatty acids. Such hydroperoxides of fatty acid are transformed to various classes of biologically active chemicals inclusively referred to as oxylipins, which are produced as a result of interaction with various enzymes. Few among these, such as allene oxide synthase, hydroperoxide lyase, and divinyl ether synthase, are especially noteworthy. AOS catalyzes the production of OPDA or dinor-OPDA, that are formed as the earliest intermediaries in the biosynthesis of JA, in conjunction with allene oxide cyclase (AOC). Alternatively, HPL can cleave hydroperoxides into different signaling molecules like volatile aldehydes and oxo-acids. Upon the conclusion of these enzymatic processes, a variety of oxylipins, including jasmonates, aldehydes, ketols, and divinyl ethers—each having a specialized biological function—are produced. In normal physiological conditions, the levels of oxylipins are modest. However, in response to adverse external conditions, including herbivores and pathogens, the rate of rise is quick [105].

The majority of oxylipins' biological actions are mediated by either jasmonate sensing or signaling networks involving reactive electrophilic species [99]. OPDA, JA, JA-Ile, and methyl jasmonate are collectively referred to as jasmonates and are involved in the stress management. JA-dependent reactions are linked to extensive adjustment of gene expression, as well as numerous JA-dependent downstream genes. The generation of mRNA from DNA by JA-responsive genes remains the best-studied jasmonate signaling mechanism. In *Arabidopsis thaliana*, enzymes encoded by JARI bind JA with an amino acid [106]. Jasmonoyl-l-isoleucine, one of the conjugates, plays an irreplaceable part in transcriptional control using jasmonate-ZIM domain repressor proteins [107]. By interacting with its coreceptor, the Skp1-Cullin1-F-box-type (SCF) protein ubiquitin ligase complexSCFCOI1-JAZ, JA-Ile functions as the primary biologically active JA that stimulates primary jasmonic acid dependent signaling [107]. This fundamental JA signaling mediated by JA-Ile plays a crucial function in controlling a variety of processes related to defense against abiotic and biotic vagaries present in the environment, in particular against herbivores and necrotrophic pathogens [108]. Oxylipin signaling also involves signals other than JA-Ile which was proved by using a mutant lacking 12-oxophytodienoatereductase3 (opr3), which is involved in the transformation of *cis*-OPDA to JA [22], that was still able to elicit defense response.

Upon detection of levels of bioavailable JAs, -7-iso-JA-Ile, results in a rapid switch of transcriptional states from repression to activation which is mediated by the interaction of transcriptional factors. MYC (JASMONATE-ZIM) is an activator, while JAZ (JASMONATE-ZIM) is a repressor. *Arabidopsis* MYC3 and MYC4 that are loosely associated with MYC2 and are subclade III members of the basic helix-loop-helix (bHLH) protein family. This group of transcription factors (MYCs) binds to G-box motifs to control the interpretation of a wide range of JA-responsive genes [109]. JAZ proteins play a key function in suppressing MYC transcription factor activity. Higher JA-Ile The MED25 binding site on MYC is unmasked by JAZ degradation, permitting the production of the transcription pre-initiation complex with RNA polymerase II and RNA polymerase III. As a result, core JA signaling is activated [110].

Jasmonic acid is produced in reaction to cell injury (resulting due to abiotic or biotic reasons) and may be carried throughout the body, most likely through the vascular tissues (primarily phloem), to trigger reactions in distant tissues. This occurrence shows that any one type of biotic or abiotic stress results in the development of cross-protection against others. There has been evidence of cross-protection [111, 112]. In fact, even plant tissue invasion by *Pseudomonas fluorescens*, a non-pathogenic bacterium leads to a rise in resistance to pathogens through ISR. The systemic JA signaling after *P. fluorescens* colonization of roots leads to increased MYC2 expression, which was proved by transcriptional profiling and analysis of MYC2- deficient (jai1/jin1) plants. This leads to enhanced expression of genes involved in yielding defense when JA signaling is stimulated by future herbivore or pathogen besiege [113].

10.4 CROSSTALK BETWEEN SALICYLIC ACID AND OXYLIPINS

10.4.1 Overview

Plant defenses against diseases and herbivorous insects constitute a cross-communicating system of signal transduction channels, where salicylic acid and jasmonic acid play crucial tasks. Although oxylipins are thought to work alone, numerous instances were given to show how the crosstalk with various other signaling molecules like ethylene and SA influences the JA-induced responses. Salicylic acid builds up as a result of several plant resistance responses and is a crucial component of plant defense. After the first pathogen attack, SA becomes engaged in signaling pathways that provide systemic-acquired resistance, which protects plants from future infections. Generally, JA signaling provides protection from insect invasion as well as necrotrophic pathogens, whereas SA signaling offers broad-spectrum resistance against the biotrophic pathogens [12].

Recently, it was proposed that oxylipins (JA precursors) have a role in stress responses [22, 68, 114]. While much is already established regarding the functions of jasmonic acid, methyl jasmonate, and JA-Ile, along with their perception and the transduction of signals [14], the function of oxylipins prior to their conversion to jasmonic acid is unclear. Still, some investigations indicate that JA precursors have a role in defensive responses [68, 115]. cis-OPDA, which is the precursor of jasmonic acid, is a recently reported participant in plant defense [15]. Both JA and OPDA function as signaling molecules, activating overlapping but separate sets of genes. While JA-related gene expression is dependent on COI1, cis-OPDA and phytoprostanes trigger gene expression in a way that is independent of COI1 [22, 114, 116]. A transcriptional study of Arabidopsis revealed that cis-OPDA activated more than 150 genes that are not affected by either jasmonic acid or me-JA [114].

10.4.2 Crosstalk

Previous studies hypothesized that plants elicit salicylic acid and jasmonic acid signaling pathways that function in a linear fashion to trigger various plant defensive responses. However, research with Arabidopsis mutants demonstrated that the salicylic acid, jasmonic acid, and ethylene-signaling pathways do not work separately and that there are regulatory elements in plants to limit the amplitude of each of these processes and to govern connections between these varied pathways [117]. SA- and JA-dependent defenses have been found to have both synergistic and antagonistic interactions. The examples below give convincing evidence supporting the concept that crosstalk between JA and SA is critical in fine-tuning complicated defensive responses.

The antagonistic interplay of the SA and JA is well understood [118, 119], however, some studies also report a synergistic interaction between the phytohormones [120]. Early findings from pharmacological investigations indicate that SA inhibits either JA production or JA signaling in flax, tomato, and tobacco [121–123]. As such, SA acts by inhibiting the biosynthesis of JA biosynthesis [124] as well as the JA-dependent induction of proteinase inhibitor genes [121]. SA treatment decreased the expression of basic PR genes induced via methyl-JA in tobacco, whereas MeJA treatment prevented the expression of acidic PR genes induced via SA [123]. NPR1, a key regulator of the SA signaling pathway, has surfaced as a crucial regulator mediating the cross-communication between the salicylic acid and jasmonic acid signals and therefore is expected to help fine-tune the response related to plant defense [119]. Activated by SA, NPR1 monomers enter the nucleus and interact with transcription factors (TGA) to promote the production of a diverse range of proteins [119]. Studies reveal that SA substantially inhibited JA-responsive gene expression in Arabidopsis wild-type plants when treated with SA and MeJA simultaneously, however, SA showed no inhibitory influence on gene expression induced by methyl jasmonate in mutant plants (npr1) [119]. This suggests that SA is essential to activate NPR1 in order to suppress JA signaling. The inhibitory influence of NPR1 on gene expression, responsive to jasmonic acid, is not dependent on its nuclear location, indicating that a cytosolic form of NPR1 protein is engaged in the salicylic acid mediated inhibition of jasmonic acid signaling via an unclear mechanism [125] (Figure 10.1).

Besides NPR1 some more factors have been suggested to be important participants in cross-communication between salicylic acid and jasmonic acid-based defense signaling. SSI1 which was identified during a screen for suppressors of the npr1–5

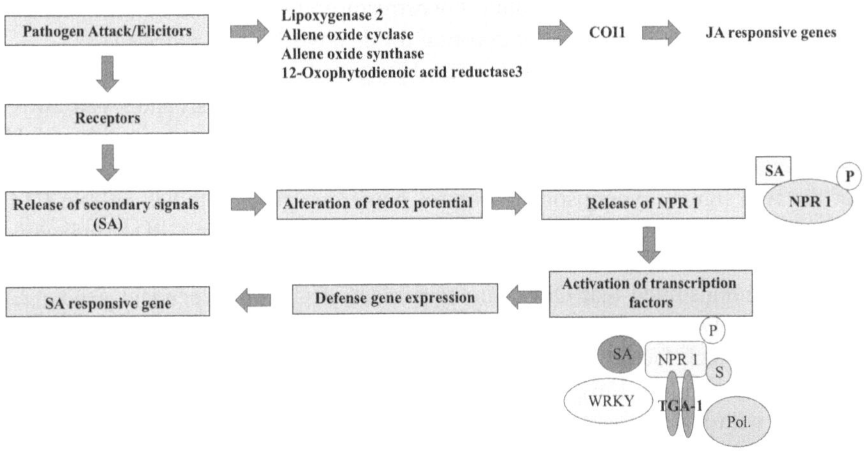

FIGURE 10.1 The diagram illustrated the action of NPR1 in the control of SA-induced inhibition of JA-dependent defense signaling. SA alters the cellular redox potential, facilitating the reduction of intermolecular disulfide bonds at certain cysteine residues in the NPR1 oligomer and the consequent release of NPR1 monomer. The NPR1 monomer relocates to the nucleus and interacts with TGA transcription factors. For interaction with nuclear NPR1 monomer, certain TGA transcription factors (e.g., TGA1) need the SA-induced reduction of intramolecular disulphide bonds, but others (e.g., TGA2) do not. By contrast, cytosolic NPR1 monomer is involved in inhibition of JA signalling. According to the model, NPR1 inhibits JA signaling by suppressing the transcription of JA biosynthetic genes and blocking the SCFCOI1 complex from targeting the repressor (R) of JA-responsive genes for ubiquitin (Ub)-proteasome-mediated destruction. Nuclear NPR1 monomer is indicated by an asterisk [119].

mutation, acts as a switch that controls the expression of salicylic acid and jasmonic acid dependent pathways [126]. Both salicylic acid dependent PR genes and the jasmonic acid dependent PDF1.2 gene are expressed constitutively in mutant ssi1 npr1–5 plants [119]. By and large, SA has the ability to decrease the expression three enzymes engaged in jasmonic acid biosynthesis, out of which two are repressed by NPR1 [119]. Such findings point to SA having an inhibitory effect on both JA biosynthesis and JA activity. In contrast, many lines of evidence suggest that JA suppresses SA signaling. JA reduced the production of SA-induced genes producing acidic PR proteins in tobacco [123]. Furthermore, the discovery of JA signaling mutants such as coi1, mpk4, and ssi2 has indicated that jasmonic acid impedes the activation of salicylic mediated defenses [127–129]. Recent research has found that a mitogen-activated protein (MAP) kinase is involved in fine-tuning the expression of the JA/ethylene and SA signaling pathways [127, 130]. In Arabidopsis, MPK4 may operate as a regulator of the negativecross-communicationn between salicylic acid and jasmonic acid in defense activation by inhibiting SA biosynthesis while stimulating response to JA [131]. However, it is unclear how MPK4 may negatively regulate SA-mediated systemic responses while positively regulating JA-mediated defensive responses. Various other MAPKs may potentially be engaged in crosstalk between the SA and JA in tobacco. MPK4 and WIPK appear to suppress SA production in Arabidopsis and tobacco, although their roles in the defense signaling network may differ significantly. MPK4 has a role in signaling downstream of JA biosynthesis [127]. WIPK activity, on the other hand, may be essential for de novo JA biosynthesis [132].

In addition to antagonistic relationship between the salicylic acid pathway and the jasmonic acid pathway, synergistic interactions between the SA and JA pathways have also been characterized. According to a report [133], exogenous SA and JA co-induced over 50 genes associated with defense in Arabidopsis plants, indicating that the two signals synergistically control numerous genes. Studies on oxo-C14-HSL-induced resistance revealed a buildup of SA and the oxylipin-OPDA, indicating a synergistic cross-communication between oxylipins and SA [133]. Moreover, it has been demonstrated that OPDA induces a set of COI1-independent genes [22, 134] and involve the bZIP transcription factors TGA2, TGA5, and TGA6 [116]. Interestingly, such factors happen to be essential for salicylic acid-dependent gene induction as well [135, 136]. Experiments on tobacco revealed that exogenous JA in combined with SA augmented the accumulation of PR-1b mRNA [137]. According to a recent study, OPDA and SA are engaged in induced stomatal closure [138]. The authors hypothesized that the activation of MPK3 and MPK6 during stomatal defense increased the lipoxygenase, resulting in the peroxidation of polyunsaturated fatty acids into oxylipins and the buildup of salicylic acid. The anion channel, which coordinates the stomatal defensive responses, was controlled downstream of this salicylic acid buildup. The process of priming with oxo-C14-HSL was recently discovered to be dependent on a pathway including oxylipin and SA [133]. Despite the fact that AHLs could not translocate to further tissues, enhanced synthesis of the oxylipin (cis-OPDA) and salicylic acid was detected, showing that systemic signaling is implicated in this event. These findings offer genetic support for both antagonistic and synergistic regulatory mechanisms that govern the interplay of JA and SA-dependent processes.

10.5 CONCLUSION

During plant-pathogen interactions, pathways of lipid metabolism hold great significance, and various modifications in membrane lipids are known to occur in the area of infection. Furthermore, the lipid metabolites released from the membranes act as signaling molecules that activate the mechanisms of defense in plants. The understanding of the key oxylipins' production, biosynthesis pathways, metabolism, and biological activities has undergone significant advances which occur both in regulatory conditions and in response to a variety of stresses. Oxylipin signals are important components of the plant's innate immune system because they play a function in a range of signaling pathways. Salicylic and jasmonic acids are important components of defense signaling in plants, which is a dynamic system of interconnected signals. Antagonism and synergy among the molecules of defense signaling allows the plant to enhance its counter defense against a disease, but it could be a drawback if different pathogens having diverse life cycles and infecting methods are found. A full understanding of the underlying crosstalk mechanism is crucial, in addition to the importance of signal interaction. While oxylipins like OPDA and JA are well known for their production, perception, and physiological roles, the relevance of additional oxylipins involved in various plant functions has been investigated lately. As a result, further research is required to fully comprehend the variation of oxylipins derived from plants, their unique functions in biological processes, and their early signaling mechanisms. The significance of oxylipins in plant defense against pathogen threats was discussed in this chapter, both as precursors of plant hormones to signaling events and as effective metabolites that restrict disease in hosts. These metabolites are the potential biotic stress defense mediators which enhance mechanisms of tolerance and resistance in plants, hence should be investigated further by studying the targeted oxylipin metabolomics and lipidomics in order to obtain a better comprehension of their role during interactions between plant and a pathogen and under conditions of biotic stress.

REFERENCES

1. Nimchuk Z, Eulgem T, Holt Iii BF, Dangl JL. Recognition and response in the plant immune system. Annual Review of Genetics. 2003 Dec;37(1):579–609.
2. Göbel C, Feussner I, Rosahl S. Lipid peroxidation during the hypersensitive response in potato in the absence of 9-lipoxygenases. Journal of Biological Chemistry. 2003 Dec 26;278(52):52834–40.
3. Montillet JL, Chamnongpol S, Rustérucci C, Dat J, Van De Cotte B, Agnel JP, Battesti C, Inzé D, Van Breusegem F, Triantaphylidès C. Fatty acid hydroperoxides and H2O2 in the execution of hypersensitive cell death in tobacco leaves. Plant Physiology. 2005 Jul;138(3):1516–26.
4. Montillet JL, Agnel JP, Ponchet M, Vailleau F, Roby D, Triantaphylidès C. Lipoxygenase-mediated production of fatty acid hydroperoxides is a specific signature of the hypersensitive reaction in plants. Plant Physiology and Biochemistry. 2002 Jun 1;40(6–8):633–9.
5. Göbel C, Feussner I, Hamberg M, Rosahl S. Oxylipin profiling in pathogen-infected potato leaves. Biochimica et Biophysica Acta (BBA)-Molecular and Cell Biology of Lipids. 2002 Sep 5;1584(1):55–64.

6. CACAS JL, Vailleau F, Davoine C, Ennar N, AGNEL JP, Tronchet M, Ponchet M, BLEIN JP, Roby D, Triantaphylidès C, MONTILLET JL. The combined action of 9 lipoxygenase and galactolipase is sufficient to bring about programmed cell death during tobacco hypersensitive response. Plant, Cell & Environment. 2005 Nov;28(11):1367–78.
7. Ryals JA, Neuenschwander UH, Willits MG, Molina A, Steiner HY, Hunt MD. Systemic acquired resistance. The Plant Cell. 1996 Oct;8(10):1809.
8. Sticher L, Mauch-Mani B, Métraux AJ. Systemic acquired resistance. Annual Review of Phytopathology. 1997 Sep;35(1):235–70.
9. Durrant WE, Dong X. Systemic acquired resistance. Annual Review of Phytopathology. 2004 Sep 8;42(1):185–209.
10. Ward, E. R., Uknes, S. J., Williams, S. C., Dincher, S. S., Wiederhold, D. L., Alexander, D. C., Ahl-Goy, P., Métraux, J.-P., and Ryals, J. A. (1991) Coordinate gene activity in response to agents that induce system ic acquired resistance. Plant Cell 3, 1085–109.
11. Maleck, K., Levine, A., Eulgem, T., Morgan, A., Schmid, J., Lawton, K. A., Dangl, J. L., and Dietrich, R. A. (2000) The transcriptome of Arabi dopsis thaliana during systemic acquired resistance. Nature Genetics 26, 403–410.
12. Glazebrook, J. (2005). Contrasting mechanisms of defense against biotrophic and necrotrophic pathogens. Annu. Rev. Phytopathol. 43, 205–227.
13. Staswick, P.E. (2008). JAZing up jasmonate signaling. Trends Plant Sci. 13, 66–71.
14. Browse, J. (2009). Jasmonate passes muster: a receptor and targets for the defense hormone. Annu. Rev. Plant Biol. 60, 183–205.
15. Fonseca, S., Chico, J.M., and Solano, R. (2009). The jasmonate path way: the ligand, the receptor and the core signalling module. Curr. Opin. Plant Biol. 12, 539–547.
16. Koo, A.J., and Howe, G.A. (2009). The wound hormone jasmonate. Phytochemistry. 70, 1571–1580.
17. Wu, J., and Baldwin, I.T. (2010). New insights into plant responses to the attack from insect herbivores. Annu. Rev. Genet. 44, 1–24.
18. Chaturvedi, R., Krothapalli, K., Makandar, R., Nandi, A., Sparks, A.A., Roth, M.R., Welti, R., and Shah, J. (2008). Plastid omega3-fatty acid desaturase-dependent accumulation of a sys temic acquired resistance inducing activity in petiole exudates of Arabidopsis thaliana is independent of jasmonic acid. Plant J. 54, 106–117.
19. Attaran, E., Zeier, T.E., Griebel, T., and Zeier, J. (2009). Methyl salic ylate production and jasmonate signaling are not essential for systemic acquired resistance in Arabidopsis. Plant Cell. 21, 954–971.
20. Truman, W., Bennett, M.H., Kubigsteltig, I., Turnbull, C., and Grant, M. (2007). Arabidopsis systemic immunity uses conserved defense signaling pathways and is mediated by jasmonates. Proc. Natl Acad. Sci. USA. 104, 1075–1080.
21. Vollenweider, S., Weber, H., Stolz, S., Che´telat, A., and Farmer, E.E. (2000). Fatty acid ketodienes and fatty acid ketotrienes: Michael addition acceptors that accumulate in wounded and diseased Arabidopsis leaves. Plant J. 24, 467–476.
22. Stintzi, A., Weber, H., Reymond, P., Browse, J., and Farmer, E.E. (2001). Plant defense in the absence of jasmonic acid: the role of cyclopentenones. Proc. Natl Acad. Sci. USA. 98, 12837–12842.
23. Prost I, Dhondt S, Rothe G, Vicente J, Rodriguez MJ, Kift N, Carbonne F, Griffiths G, Esquerré-Tugayé MT, Rosahl S, Castresana C. Evaluation of the antimicrobial activities of plant oxylipins supports their involvement in defense against pathogens. Plant Physiology. 2005 Dec;139(4):1902–13.

24. Kishimoto, K., Matsui, K., Ozawa, R., and Takabayashi, J. (2008). Direct fungicidal activities of C6-aldehydes are important con stituents for defense responses in Arabidopsis against Botrytis cinerea. Phytochemistry. 69, 2127–2132.
25. Sanz, A., Moreno, J.I., and Castresana, C. (1998). PIOX, a new pathogen-induced oxygenase with homology to animal cycloox ygenase. Plant Cell. 10, 1523–1537.
26. Ponce de León, I., Sanz, A., Hamberg, M., and Castresana, C. (2002). Involvement of the Arabidopsis a-DOX1 fatty acid dioxygenase in protection against oxidative stress and cell death. Plant J. 29, 61–62.
27. Hamberg, M., Sanz, A., Rodríguez, M.J., Calvo, A.P., and Castresana, C. (2003). Activation of the fatty acid a-dioxygenase pathway during bacterial infection of tobacco leaves: formation of oxylipins protecting against cell death. J. Biol. Chem. 278, 51796–51805.
28. Rancé, I., Fournier, J., and Esquerré-Tugayé, M.T. (1998). The incom patible interaction between Phytophthora parasitica var. nico tianae race 0 and tobacco is suppressed in transgenic plants expressing antisense lipoxygenase sequences. Proc. Natl Acad. Sci. USA. 95, 6554–6559.
29. Vellosillo, T., Martínez, M., Lo′ pez, M.A., Vicente, J., Cascón, T., Dolan, L., Hamberg, M., and Castresana, C. (2007). Oxylipins pro duced by the 9-lip- oxygenase pathway in Arabidopsis regulate lateral root development and defense responses through a specific signaling cascade. Plant Cell. 19, 831–846.
30. Hwang, I.S., and Hwang, B.K. (2010). The pepper 9-lipoxygenase gene CaLOX1 functions in defense and cell death responses to microbial pathogens. Plant Physiol. 152, 948–967.
31. López, M.A., Vicente, J., Kulasekaran, S., Vellosillo, T., Martínez, M., Irigoyen, M.L., Cascón, T., Bannenberg, G., Hamberg, M., and Castresana, C. (2011). Antagonistic role of 9-lipoxygenase derived oxylipins and ethylene in the control of oxidative stress, lipid peroxidation and plant defence. Plant J. 67, 447–458.
32. Vicente J, Cascón T, Vicedo B, García-Agustín P, Hamberg M, Castresana C. Role of 9-lipoxygenase and α-dioxygenase oxylipin pathways as modulators of local and systemic defense. Molecular Plant. 2012 Jul 1;5(4):914–28.
33. Zipfel C. Plant pattern-recognition receptors. Trends in immunology. 2014 Jul 1;35(7):345–51.
34. Sanabria NM, Huang JC, Dubery IA. Self/non-self perception in plants in innate immunity and defense. Self/nonself. 2010 Jan 1;1(1):40–54.
35. Ausubel FM. Are innate immune signaling pathways in plants and animals conserved?. Nature Immunology. 2005 Oct;6(10):973–9.
36. Dangl JL, Jones JD. Plant pathogens and integrated defence responses to infection. Nature. 2001 Jun;411(6839):826–33.
37. Vlot AC, Dempsey DM, Klessig DF. Salicylic acid, a multifaceted hormone to combat disease. Annual Review of Phytopathology. 2009 Sep 8;47:177–206.
38. Van Loon LC, Bakker PA, Pieterse CM. Systemic resistance induced by rhizosphere bacteria. Annual Review of Phytopathology. 1998;36:453–83.
39. Spoel SH, Dong X. Making sense of hormone crosstalk during plant immune responses. Cell host & microbe. 2008 Jun 12;3(6):348–51.
40. Glazebrook J. Genes controlling expression of defense responses in Arabidopsis-2001 status. Current Opinion in Plant Biology. 2001 Aug 1;4(4):301–8.
41. Hammond-Kosack KE, Parker JE. Deciphering plant-pathogen communication: fresh perspectives for molecular resistance breeding. Current Opinion in Biotechnology. 2003 Apr 1;14(2):177–93.

42. Kachroo A, Kachroo P. Salicylic acid-, jasmonic acid-and ethylenemediated regulation of plant defense signaling. Genetic engineering. 2007:55–83.
43. Thomma BP, Penninckx IA, Cammue BP, Broekaert WF. The complexity of disease signaling in Arabidopsis. Current Opinion in Immunology. 2001 Feb 1;13(1):63–8.
44. Schaaf J, Walter MH, Hess D. Primary metabolism in plant defense (regulation of a bean malic enzyme gene promoter in transgenic tobacco by developmental and environmental cues). Plant Physiology. 1995 Jul;108(3):949–60.
45. Chanda B, Venugopal SC, Kulshrestha S, Navarre DA, Downie B, Vaillancourt L, Kachroo A, Kachroo P. Glycerol-3-phosphate levels are associated with basal resistance to the hemibiotrophic fungus Colletotrichumhigginsianum in Arabidopsis. Plant Physiology. 2008 Aug;147(4):2017–29.
46. Ahn IP, Kim S, Lee YH. Vitamin B1 functions as an activator of plant disease resistance. Plant Physiology. 2005 Jul;138(3):1505–15.
47. Morkunas I, Marczak L, Stachowiak J, Stobiecki M. Sucrose-induced lupine defense against Fusariumoxysporum: Sucrose-stimulated accumulation of isoflavonoids as a defense response of lupine to Fusariumoxysporum. Plant Physiology and Biochemistry. 2005 Apr 1;43(4):363–73.
48. Scheideler M, Schlaich NL, Fellenberg K, Beissbarth T, Hauser NC, Vingron M, Slusarenko AJ, Hoheisel JD. Monitoring the switch from housekeeping to pathogen defense metabolism in Arabidopsis thaliana using cDNA arrays. Journal of Biological Chemistry. 2002 Mar 22;277(12):10555–61.
49. Reszczynska E, Hanaka A. Lipids composition in plant membranes. Cell Biochemistry and Biophysics. 2020 Dec;78(4):401–14.
50. Casillas-Vargas G, Ocasio-Malave C, Medina S, Morales-Guzman C, Del Valle RG, Carballeira NM, Sanabria-Ríos DJ. Antibacterial fatty acids: An update of possible mechanisms of action and implications in the development of the next-generation of antibacterial agents. Progress in Lipid Research. 2021 Apr 1;82:101093.
51. Schieferle S, Tappe B, Korte P, Mueller MJ, Berger S. Pathogens and elicitors induce local and systemic changes in triacylglycerol metabolism in roots and in leaves of Arabidopsis thaliana. Biology. 2021 Sep;10(9):920.
52. Shah J. Lipids, lipases, and lipid-modifying enzymes in plant disease resistance. Annual Review of Phytopathology. 2005 Sep 1;43:229.
53. Lee HJ, Park OK. Lipases associated with plant defense against pathogens. Plant Science. 2019 Jul 10;279:51–58.
54. Desbois AP, Smith VJ. Antibacterial free fatty acids: activities, mechanisms of action and biotechnological potential. Applied Microbiology and Biotechnology. 2009 Dec 3;85:1629–1642.
55. Kachroo A, Kachroo P. Fatty acid-derived signals in plant defense. Annual Review of Phytopathology. 2009 Jan 1;47(1):153–76.
56. Zheng CJ, Yoo JS, Lee TG, Cho HY, Kim YH, Kim WG. Fatty acid synthesis is a target for antibacterial activity of unsaturated fatty acids. FEBS Letters. 2005 Sep 26;579(23):5157–62.
57. Deboever E, Deleu M, Mongrand S, Lins L, Fauconnier ML. Plant-pathogen interactions: underestimated roles of phyto-oxylipins. Trends in Plant Science. 2020 Jan 1;25:22–34.
58. Stulnig TM, Huber J, Leitinger N, Imre EM, Angelisova P, Nowotny P, Waldhausl W. Polyunsaturated eicosapentaenoic acid displaces proteins from membrane rafts by altering Raft lipid composition. Journal of Biological Chemistry. 2001 Oct;276:37335–37340.

59. Maia MR, Chaudhary LC, Bestwick CS, Richardson AJ, McKain N, Larson TR, Graham IA, Wallace RJ. Toxicity of unsaturated fatty acids to the biohydrogenatingruminal bacterium, Butyrivibriofibrisolvens. BMC Microbiology. 2010 Dec;10(1):1–10.
60. Lim GH, Singhal R, Kachroo A, Kachroo P. Fatty acid-and lipid-mediated signaling in plant defense. Annual Review of Phytopathology. 2017 Aug 4;55(1):505–536.
61. Alves E, Dias M, Lopes D, Almeida A, Domingues MD, Rey F. Antimicrobial lipids from plants and marine organisms: An overview of the current state-of-the-art and future prospects. Antibiotics. 2020 Aug;9(8):441.
62. Yoon BK, Jackman JA, Valle-Gonzalez ER, Cho NJ. Antibacterial free fatty acids and monoglycerides: biological activities, experimental testing, and therapeutic applications. International Journal of Molecular Sciences. 2018 Apr;19(4):1114.
63. McGaw LJ, Jager AK, Van Staden J. Antibacterial effects of fatty acids and related compounds from plants. South African journal of botany. 2002 Dec 1;68(4):417–23.
64. Sheu CW, Freese E. Lipopolysaccharide layer protection of gram-negative bacteria against inhibition by long-chain fatty acids. Journal of Bacteriology. 1973 Sep;115(3):869–75.
65. Pretorius CJ, Zeiss DR, Dubery IA. Mini-Review/Perspective/Commentary: The presence of oxygenated lipids in plant defense in response to biotic stress: a metabolomics appraisal. Plant Signaling & Behavior. 2021 Dec 31:1989215.
66. Wasternack C. Jasmonates: an update on biosynthesis, signal transduction and action in plant stress response, growth and development. Annals of Botany. 2007 Oct 1;100(4):681–97.
67. Mosblech A, Feussner I, Heilmann I. Oxylipins: structurally diverse metabolites from fatty acid oxidation. Plant Physiology and Biochemistry. 2009 Jun 1;47(6):511–7.
68. Blee E. Impact of phyto-oxylipins in plant defense. Trends in Plant Science. 2002 Jul 1;7(7):315–22.
69. Genva M, ObounouAkong F, Andersson MX, Deleu M, Lins L, Fauconnier ML. New insights into the biosynthesis of esterified oxylipins and their involvement in plant defense and developmental mechanisms. Phytochemistry Reviews. 2019 Feb;18(1):343–58.
70. Farmer EE, Mueller MJ. ROS-mediated lipid peroxidation and RES-activated signaling. Annual Review of Plant Biology. 2013 Apr 29;64:429–50.
71. de Leon IP, Hamberg M, Castresana C. Oxylipins in moss development and defense. Frontiers in Plant Science. 2015 Jul 3;6:483.
72. Senger T, Wichard T, Kunze S, Göbel C, Lerchl J, Pohnert G, Feussner I. A multifunctional lipoxygenase with fatty acid hydroperoxide cleaving activity from the moss Physcomitrella patens. Journal of Biological Chemistry. 2005 Mar 4;280(9):7588–96.
73. Kishimoto K, Matsui K, Ozawa R, Takabayashi J. Volatile 1-octen-3-ol induces a defensive response in Arabidopsis thaliana. Journal of General Plant Pathology. 2007 Feb;73(1):35–7.
74. Combet E, Eastwood DC, Burton KS, Henderson J. Eight-carbon volatiles in mushrooms and fungi: properties, analysis, and biosynthesis. Mycoscience. 2006 Dec 1;47(6):317–26.
75. Matsui K, Minami A, Hornung E, Shibata H, Kishimoto K, Ahnert V, Kindl H, Kajiwara T, Feussner I. Biosynthesis of fatty acid derived aldehydes is induced upon mechanical wounding and its products show fungicidal activities in cucumber. Phytochemistry. 2006 Apr 1;67(7):649–57.
76. Zeiss DR, Mhlongo MI, Tugizimana F, Steenkamp PA, Dubery IA. Metabolomic profiling of the host response of tomato (Solanumlycopersicum) following

infection by Ralstoniasolanacearum. International Journal of Molecular Sciences. 2019 Jan;20(16):3945.

77. Wang KD, Gorman Z, Huang PC, Kenerley CM, Kolomiets MV. Trichodermavirens colonization of maize roots triggers rapid accumulation of 12-oxophytodienoate and two α-ketols in leaves as priming agents of induced systemic resistance. Plant Signaling & Behavior. 2020 Sep 1;15(9):1792187.
78. Mareya CR, Tugizimana F, Di Lorenzo F, Silipo A, Piater LA, Molinaro A, Dubery IA. Adaptive defence-related changes in the metabolome of Sorghum bicolor cells in response to lipopolysaccharides of the pathogen Burkholderiaandropogonis. Scientific Reports. 2020 May 6;10(1):1–7.
79. Carlson R, Tugizimana F, Steenkamp PA, Dubery IA, Labuschagne N. Differential metabolic reprogramming in Paenibacillusalvei-primed Sorghum bicolor seedlings in response to Fusariumpseudograminearum infection. Metabolites. 2019 Jul;9(7):150.
80. Tinte MM, Steenkamp PA, Piater LA, Dubery IA. Lipopolysaccharide perception in Arabidopsis thaliana: Diverse LPS chemotypes from Burkholderiacepacia, Pseudomonas syringae and Xanthomonascampestris trigger differential defence-related perturbations in the metabolome. Plant Physiology and Biochemistry. 2020 Nov 1;156:267–77.
81. Fitoussi N, Borrego E, Kolomiets MV, Qing X, Bucki P, Sela N, Belausov E, Braun Miyara S. Oxylipins are implicated as communication signals in tomato-root-knot nematode (Meloidogynejavanica) interaction. Scientific Reports. 2021 Jan 11;11(1):1–6.
82. Dye SM, Yang J, Bostock RM. Eicosapolyenoic fatty acids alter oxylipin gene expression and fatty acid hydroperoxide profiles in tomato and pepper roots. Physiological and Molecular Plant Pathology. 2020 Jan 1;109:101444.
83. Viswanath KK, Varakumar P, Pamuru RR, Basha SJ, Mehta S, Rao AD. Plant lipoxygenases and their role in plant physiology. Journal of Plant Biology. 2020 Apr;63(2):83–95.
84. Schuck S, Kallenbach M, Baldwin IT, Bonaventure G. The Nicotianaattenuata GLA 1 lipase controls the accumulation of Phytophthoraparasitica-induced oxylipins and defensive secondary metabolites. Plant, Cell & Environment. 2014 Jul;37(7):1703–15.
85. Graner G, Hamberg M, Meijer J. Screening of oxylipins for control of oilseed rape (Brassica napus) fungal pathogens. Phytochemistry. 2003 May 1;63(1):89–95.
86. Nakamura S, Hatanaka A. Green-leaf-derived C6-aroma compounds with potent antibacterial action that act on both gram-negative and gram-positive bacteria. Journal of Agricultural and Food Chemistry. 2002 Dec 18;50(26):7639–44.
87. Wasternack C, Feussner I. The oxylipin pathways: biochemistry and function. Annual Review of Plant Biology. 2018 Apr 29;69:363–86.
88. Battilani P, Lanubile A, Scala V, Reverberi M, Gregori R, Falavigna C, Dallasta C, Park YS, Bennett J, Borrego EJ, Kolomiets MV. Oxylipins from both pathogen and host antagonize jasmonic acid-mediated defence via the 9-lipoxygenase pathway in Fusariumverticillioides infection of maize. Molecular Plant Pathology. 2018 Sep;19(9):2162–76.
89. Heitz T, Smirnova E, Widemann E, Aubert Y, Pinot F, Menard R. The rise and fall of jasmonate biological activities. In *Lipids in Plant and Algae Development* 2016 (pp. 405–426). Springer, Cham.
90. Fonseca S, Chini A, Hamberg M, Adie B, Porzel A, Kramell R, Miersch O, Wasternack C, Solano R. (+)-7-iso-Jasmonoyl-L-isoleucine is the endogenous bioactive jasmonate. Nature Chemical Biology. 2009 May;5(5):344–50.

91. Bottcher C, Pollmann S. Plant oxylipins: Plant responses to 12-oxo-phytodienoic acid are governed by its specific structural and functional properties. The FEBS Journal. 2009 Sep;276(17):4693–704.
92. Mhlongo MI, Piater LA, Steenkamp PA, Labuschagne N, Dubery IA. Concurrent metabolic profiling and quantification of aromatic amino acids and phytohormones in Solanumlycopersicum plants responding to Phytophthoracapsici. Metabolites. 2020 Nov;10(11):466.
93. Tugizimana F, Steenkamp PA, Piater LA, Labuschagne N, Dubery IA. Unravelling the metabolic reconfiguration of the post-challenge primed state in Sorghum bicolor responding to Colletotrichumsublineolum infection. Metabolites. 2019 Oct;9(10):194.
94. Vallad G, Robert, MG. Systemic Acquired Resistance and Induced Systemic Resistance in Conventional Agriculture Article. Crop Sci. 2004;44:1920–34.
95. Knoester M, Pieterse CM, Bol JF VLLS. Systemic resistance in Arabidopsis induced by rhizobacteria requires ethylene-dependent signaling at the site of application. Mol Plant-Microbe Interact. 1999;12(8):720–7.
96. Yan Z, Reddy MS, Ryu CM, McInroy JA, Wilson M KJ. induced systemic protection against tomato late blight elicited by plant growth-promoting rhizobacteriae. Phytopathology. 2002;92(12):1329–33.
97. De Meyer G HM. Salicylic acid produced by the rhizobacterium Pseudomonas aeruginosa 7NSK2 induces resistance to leaf infection by Botrytis cinerea on bean. Phytopathology. 87(6):588–93.
98. Cao, H., Glazebrook, J., Clarke, J. D., Volko, S., Dong X. The Arabidopsis NPR1 gene that controls systemic acquired resistance encodes a novel protein containing ankyrin repeats. Cell. 1997;88:57–63.
99. Pieterse CM, Van Wees SC, Van Pelt JA, Knoester M, Laan R, Gerrits H, Weisbeek PJ VLL. A novel signaling pathway controlling induced systemic resistance in Arabidopsis. Plant Cell. 10(9):1571–80.
100. Li M, Yu G, Cao C, Liu, P. Metabolism, signaling, and transport of jasmonates. Plant Communications. 2021;2: 100231.
101. Lupette J, Jaussaud A, Vigor C, Oger C, Galano JM, Reversat G, Vercauteren J, Jouhet J, Durand T, Marechal E. Non-enzymatic synthesis of bioactive isoprostanoids in the diatom Phaeodactylum following oxidative stress. Plant Physiol. 2018;178, 1344–1357.
102. Griffiths G. Biosynthesis and analysis of plant oxylipins. Free Radical Research. 2015 May 4;49(5):565–82.
103. Vellosillo T, Aguilera V, Marcos R, Bartsch M, Vicente J, Cascón T, Hamberg M, Castresana C. Defense activated by 9-lipoxygenase-derived oxylipins requires specific mitochondrial proteins. Plant Physiology. 2013 Feb;161(2):617–27.
104. Ma W, Zhao L, Xie Y. Inhibitory effect of (E)-2-hexenal as a potential natural fumigant on Aspergillus flavus in stored peanut seeds. Industrial Crops and Products. 2017 Nov 15;107:206
105. Santino A, Bonsegna S, De Domenico S, Poltronieri P. Plant oxylipins and their contribution to plant defence. Plant Biology. 2006;1.
106. Staswick PE, Tiryaki I. The oxylipin signal jasmonic acid is activated by an enzyme that conjugates it to isoleucine in Arabidopsis. The Plant Cell. 2004 Aug;16(8):2117–27.
107. Chini A, Fonseca SG, Fernandez G, Adie B, Chico JM, Lorenzo O, García-Casado G, López-Vidriero I, Lozano FM, Ponce MR, Micol JL. The JAZ family of repressors is the missing link in jasmonatesignalling. Nature. 2007 Aug;448(7154):666–71.

108. Wang KD, Borrego EJ, Kenerley CM, Kolomiets MV. Oxylipins other than jasmonic acid are xylem-resident signals regulating systemic resistance induced by Trichoderma virens in maize. The Plant Cell. 2020 Jan;32(1):166–85.
109. Fernández-Calvo P, Chini A, Fernández-Barbero G, Chico JM, Gimenez-Ibanez S, Geerinck J, Eeckhout D, Schweizer F, Godoy M, Franco-Zorrilla JM, Pauwels L. The Arabidopsis bHLHtranscription factors MYC3 and MYC4 are targets of JAZ repressors and act additively with MYC2 in the activation of jasmonate responses. The Plant Cell. 2011 Feb;23(2):701–15.
110. Chen R, Jiang H, Li L, Zhai Q, Qi L, Zhou W, Liu X, Li H, Zheng W, Sun J, Li C. The Arabidopsis mediator subunit MED25 differentially regulates jasmonate and abscisic acid signaling through interacting with the MYC2 and ABI5 transcription factors. The Plant Cell. 2012 Jul;24(7):2898–916.
111. Chassot C, Buchala A, Schoonbeek H-J, M′etraux J-P, LamotteO.Wounding of Arabidopsis leaves causes a powerful but transient protection against Botrytis infection. Plant J. 2008;55:555–67.
112. Conconi A, Smerdon MJ, Howe GA, Ryan CA. The octadecanoidsignalling pathway in plants mediates a response to UV radiation. Nature 1996;383:826–29.
113. Pozo MJ, Van Der Ent S, Van Loon LC, Pieterse CMJ. Transcription factor MYC2 is involved in priming for enhanced defense during rhizobacteria-induced systemic resistance in Arabidopsis thaliana. New Phytol. 2008; 180:511–232008.
114. Taki N, Sasaki-Sekimoto Y, Obayashi T, Kikuta A, Kobayashi K, Ainai T, Yagi K, Sakurai N, Suzuki H, Masuda T, Takamiya KI. 12-oxo-phytodienoic acid triggers expression of a distinct set of genes and plays a role in wound-induced gene expression in Arabidopsis. Plant physiology. 2005 Nov;139(3):1268–83.
115. Dave A, Graham IA. Oxylipin signaling: a distinct role for the jasmonic acid precursor cis-(+)-12-oxo-phytodienoic acid (cis-OPDA). Frontiers in Plant Science. 2012 Mar 8;3:42.7.
116. Stotz HU, Mueller S, Zoeller M, Mueller MJ, Berger S. TGA transcription factors and jasmonate-independent COI1 signalling regulate specific plant responses to reactive oxylipins. Journal of Experimental Botany. 2013 Feb 1;64(4):963–75.
117. Genoud T, Métraux JP. Crosstalk in plant cell signaling: structure and function of the genetic network. Trends in Plant Science. 1999 Dec 1;4(12):503–7.
118. Rojo E, Solano R, Sánchez-Serrano JJ. Interactions between signaling compounds involved in plant defense. Journal of Plant Growth Regulation. 2003 Mar;22(1):82–98.
119. Beckers GJ, Spoel SH. Fine-tuning plant defence signalling: salicylate versus jasmonate. Plant Biology. 2006 Jan;8(01):1–0.
120. Van Wees SC, De Swart EA, Van Pelt JA, Van Loon LC, Pieterse CM. Enhancement of induced disease resistance by simultaneous activation of salicylate-and jasmonate-dependent defense pathways in Arabidopsis thaliana. Proceedings of the National Academy of Sciences. 2000 Jul 18;97(15):8711–6.
121. Doares SH, Narváez-Vásquez J, Conconi A, Ryan CA. Salicylic acid inhibits synthesis of proteinase inhibitors in tomato leaves induced by systemin and jasmonic acid. Plant Physiology. 1995 Aug;108(4):1741–6.
122. Harms K, Ramirez I, Peña-Cortés H. Inhibition of wound-induced accumulation of allene oxide synthase transcripts in flax leaves by aspirin and salicylic acid. Plant Physiology. 1998 Nov 1;118(3):1057–65.
123. Niki T, Mitsuhara I, Seo S, Ohtsubo N, Ohashi Y. Antagonistic effect of salicylic acid and jasmonic acid on the expression of pathogenesis-related (PR) protein genes in wounded mature tobacco leaves. Plant and Cell Physiology. 1998 May 1;39(5):500–7.

124. Pena-Cortés H, Albrecht T, Prat S, Weiler EW, Willmitzer L. Aspirin prevents wound-induced gene expression in tomato leaves by blocking jasmonic acid biosynthesis. Planta. 1993 Jul;191(1):123–8.
125. Spoel SH, Koornneef A, Claessens SM, Korzelius JP, Van Pelt JA, Mueller MJ, Buchala AJ, Métraux JP, Brown R, Kazan K, Van Loon LC. NPR1 modulates cross-talk between salicylate-and jasmonate-dependent defense pathways through a novel function in the cytosol. The Plant Cell. 2003 Mar;15(3):760–70.
126. Shah J, Kachroo P, Klessig DF. The Arabidopsis ssi1 mutation restores pathogenesis-related gene expression in npr1 plants and renders defensin gene expression salicylic acid dependent. The Plant Cell. 1999 Feb;11(2):191–206.
127. Petersen M, Brodersen P, Naested H, Andreasson E, Lindhart U, Johansen B, Nielsen HB, Lacy M, Austin MJ, Parker JE, Sharma SB. Arabidopsis map kinase 4 negatively regulates systemic acquired resistance. Cell. 2000 Dec 22;103(7):1111–20.
128. Kachroo P, Shanklin J, Shah J, Whittle EJ, Klessig DF. A fatty acid desaturase modulates the activation of defense signaling pathways in plants. Proceedings of the National Academy of Sciences. 2001 Jul 31;98(16):9448–53.
129. Kloek AP, Verbsky ML, Sharma SB, Schoelz JE, Vogel J, Klessig DF, Kunkel BN. Resistance to Pseudomonas syringae conferred by an Arabidopsis thaliana coronatine-insensitive (coi1) mutation occurs through two distinct mechanisms. The Plant Journal. 2001 Jun;26(5):509–22.
130. Seo S, Okamoto M, Seto H, Ishizuka K, Sano H, Ohashi Y. Tobacco MAP kinase: a possible mediator in wound signal transduction pathways. Science. 1995 Dec 22;270(5244):1988–92.
131. Creelman RA, Mulpuri R. The oxylipin pathway in Arabidopsis. The Arabidopsis book/American Society of Plant Biologists. 2002;1.
132. Seo S, Sano H, Ohashi Y. Jasmonate-based wound signal transduction requires activation of WIPK, a tobacco mitogen-activated protein kinase. The Plant Cell. 1999 Feb;11(2):289–98.
133. Schenk PM, Kazan K, Wilson I, Anderson JP, Richmond T, Somerville SC, Manners JM. Coordinated plant defense responses in Arabidopsis revealed by microarray analysis. Proc. Natl Acad. Sci. USA. 2000; 97: 11655–11660.
134. Mueller S, Hilbert B, Dueckershoff K, Roitsch T, Krischke M, Mueller MJ, Berger S. General detoxification and stress responses are mediated by oxidized lipids through TGA transcription factors in Arabidopsis. The Plant Cell. 2008 Mar;20(3):768–85.
135. Zhang Y, Fan W, Kinkema M, Li X, Dong X. Interaction of NPR1 with basic leucine zipper protein transcription factors that bind sequences required for salicylic acid induction of the PR-1 gene. Proceedings of the National Academy of Sciences. 1999 May 25;96(11):6523–8.
136. Zhang Y, Tessaro MJ, Lassner M, Li X. Knockout analysis of Arabidopsis transcription factors TGA2, TGA5, and TGA6 reveals their redundant and essential roles in systemic acquired resistance. The Plant Cell. 2003 Nov;15(11):2647–53.
137. Xu YI, Chang PF, Liu D, Narasimhan ML, Raghothama KG, Hasegawa PM, Bressan RA. Plant defense genes are synergistically induced by ethylene and methyl jasmonate. The Plant Cell. 1994 Aug;6(8):1077–85.
138. Montillet JL, Leonhardt N, Mondy S, Tranchimand S, Rumeau D, Boudsocq M, Garcia AV, Douki T, Bigeard J, Lauriere C, Chevalier A. An abscisic acid-independent oxylipin pathway controls stomatal closure and immune defense in Arabidopsis. PLoS Biology. 2013 Mar 19;11(3):e1001513.

11 The Role of Oxylipins in Plant Reproduction, Fruit Maturity, and Development

Ikra Manzoor[1], Momin Showkat Bhat[2], Neha Sharma[3], and Bismat un Nisa[4]*
[1]Division of Fruit Science, Faculty of Horticulture, SKUAST-Kashmir, India
[2]Division of Floriculture and Landscape Architecture, Faculty of Horticulture, SKUAST-Kashmir, India
[3]Division of Vegetable Science, IARI, Pusa, New Delhi, India
[4]Division of Entomology, Faculty of Horticulture, SKUAST-Kashmir, India
*Correspondence: manzoorikra@gmail.com

CONTENTS

11.1 INTRODUCTION

In the lifecycle of a plant, reproduction constitutes a prime place as it ensures a species survival. For switching to an adult stage, a plant needs to undergo juvenility to come into flowering. During this stage, there is dominance of floral physiology over the leafing stage in the apical meristematic part of plant [1]. There are three stages of fruit development. The ovary develops in stage 1 accompanied by division of cells representing fruit set. In stage 2, there is peak period of cell division. Stage 3 involves cell expansion during which fruit size increases. After full expansion of fruit cells with the maturation of the fruits, there is ripening of fruits [2–3]. Phytohormones are vital players in plants for certain physiological and developmental aspects viz., fertility, tolerance to stress, formation of organs of storage,

DOI: 10.1201/9781003316558-11

elongation in roots, determination of sex, ripening in fruits and aging, defense to oxidation, and inter-relation to other hormones [4–11]. An array of physiological functions in plants is influenced by oxylipins viz., transduction of signals, response to various stresses, development and aging [12–14]. The hormone jasmonic acid (JA), an oxylipin, is produced by oxygenation of substrate fatty acids, resulting in hydroperoxides which are further metabolized by secondary enzymes. The source of JA in plants is linolenic acid. There is a study regarding interaction between membrane receptor and elicitors, resulting in formation of 13-hydroperoxylinolenic acid which is actually a release product of linolenic acid through phospholipase or lipase with addition of oxygen via lipoxygenase (LOX) [15]. The first isolation of JA was from the fungus culture *Lasiodiplodia theobromae* [16]. Another oxylipin i.e., 9,10-ketol-octadecadienoic acid (KODA) in apple fruits, effects synthesis of ethylene via two genes viz., *MdACS1* and *MdACO1*, differing with time and concentration of JA [17]. In this chapter, an overview has been presented regarding the role of oxylipins during plant reproduction, fruit maturity, and development.

11.2 JASMONATES REGULATE REPRODUCTIVE DEVELOPMENT

The primary elicitors of differentiation in the cells of meristematic tissues in apex for switching to the phase of reproduction are internal and external influences including period of day length, cold temperature to floral buds i.e., vernalization, and the role of plant growth substances [18]. JA synthesis reaction is catalyzed by a series of enzymes in a developing stamen, as reported by Turner et al. [19]. JA-related compounds are widely distributed among higher plants and are potent inducers of expression of several genes. The proteins implicated in JA signaling are COI1 (CORONATINE INSENSITIVE 1), which has been discovered for *Arabidopsis thaliana*, and JAZ, (JASMONATE ZIM-DOMAIN), which is induced by Jasmonic acid for regulating expression of genes in negative aspect. COI1 is the mutant most strongly influenced by JA signaling [20]. Additionally, a receptor ligand of jasmonic acid is (+)-7-iso-jasmonoyl-L-isoleucine (JA-Ile) [21]. The main function of JA and jasmonates molecules in plants has been defined as signaling molecules that respond to different developmental events such flowering, fruit ripening, and senescence [15]. It has been noted in plant breeding that the synthesis and accumulation of JA is an essential step in the development of flowers. The discovery of a mutant of COI1, which is non-sensitive for jasmonic acids, showing male sterility, provided the first clues about the function of JA in flower development [22]. The analysis of a mutant of *Arabidopsis* which lacks the precursor of jasmonic acid i.e., linolenic acid, demonstrated the crucial role that JA plays in male fertility [23]. Later, it was discovered that mutations that interfere with additional paths for signaling of jasmonic acid biosynthesis result in male sterility further. Numerous studies have shown that *Arabidopsis* plants with mutations suffer protracted male sterility. Defect in dehiscence of anthers, maturation of pollen grains, and anthesis were present in *defective in anther dehiscence1* (*dad1*) mutants. The exogenous administration of jasmonic acid (JA) was successful in preventing these deficits [24–25]. Because of abnormalities in anther and pollen production, the *aos* mutants exhibited severe male sterility, which could be fully cured

TABLE 11.1
The Role of Jasmonates for Regulating Plant Reproduction

S. No.	Crop	Role	Reference
1.	Rice	Floret opening & anther dehiscence	[61]
2.	Rice	Spikelet development	[62]
3.	Maize	Jasmonate treatment of growing inflorescences helped mutants' stamen development	[63]
4.	Maize	To express androgeny and suppress gynogeny	[64]
5.	Tomato	*jai1* mutant showed female sterility	[65]
6.	*Arabidopsis*	*arf6&arf8* double-null mutants hinders flower formation via producing sterile bud closure having curtailed filaments, un-dehisced anthers, and infertile closed buds with long petals	[28]

by exogenous administration of methyl jasmonate [26]. According to reports, the *opr3* mutant plants were also sterile, but exogenous JA rather than OPDA can make them fertile [27]. The expression of *ARF6* and *ARF8* in the filaments induces dehiscence of anthers and controls stamen and gynoecium maturation of androecium and stigma via stimulating synthesis of jasmonic acid, according to the feeding studies and measurements of jasmonic acid [28]. Recent studies on a variety of plant species found that JA signaling is essential for floral development and fertility, but there are noticeable differences. In flowers of various species, including *Pinus mugo*, *Petunia hybrida*, *Vicia faba*, *Phaseolus vulgaris*, etc., various types of jasmonates viz., *JA-Ile*, been reported to be present in abundance [29]. Jasmonates regulating plant reproduction has been mentioned in (Table 11.1).

11.3 THE ROLE OF 9,10-KETOL-OCTADECADIENOIC ACID (KODA) AND JASMONATES IN REGULATING MATURATION OF FRUITS

9-hydroxy-10-oxo-12 (Z), 15(Z)-octadecadienoic acid is the source of KODA with generation from linolenic acid and 9-lipoxygenase (9-LOX) [30]. Duckweed (*Lemna paucicostata*) is the main source from which 9,10-ketol-octadecadienoic acid (KODA) has been extracted having stress inducing activities [30]. Also, during conditions of dark, the levels of endogenous KODA rises with an association to induction of flowering [31]. Besides, in *Dianthus caryophyllus* L., *Dendranthema grandiflorum* Kitam., and *Eustoma russellianum* Griseb., a rise in KODA levels in immature buds of a flower associates to flower formation [32]. All this evidence shows that KODA is responsible for the induction of flowering in fruit trees but the reports regarding the mechanism of KODA is missing for formation of flower buds [33]. Jasmonic acid and methyljasmonic acid (endogenous) content in grape berries varied among seed and seedless berries, where JA content was higher in seeded berries [34]. Jasmonic acid and methyljasmonic acid rates were at a peak during the initial phases of development of fruits for seeded grapes [34], sweet cherry [35] and strawberry fruit [36]. Increased concentration of JA was observed toward the harvest in apple seeds [35], and grapes [34]. Toward the harvest period, increasing concentrations of JA induce seed dormancy in seeds just like abscisic acid. Injuries due to reduced temperature viz., splitting of fruits and spot formation in fruits of apple, are fewer and closure of stomata in leaves of citrus were observed after application of PDJ [37]. Anthocyanin and ABA concentrations were increased after application of PDJ [35]. In apples, endogenous levels of KODA induce formation of flower buds which seem to be influenced by the amount of fruit [33]. The analog of jasmonic acid i.e., n-propyl dihydro-jasmonates (PDJ) enhanced the color of the skin in grapes [38]. The amount of jasmonates in the seed effects the content of the skin or pulp, since the jasmonic acid and methyljasmonic acid range for the seed has been observed at higher levels compared to skin [34]. Increased total yield per plant and accelerated ripening was observed with application of JA (0.5–1 mM) in strawberry plants [39]. Increased uniform stage of ripening and a ripening delay period was observed for tomato fruits kept for 15–30 days at 5°C, after treatment with MeJA as gas, further reduced chilling injury in tomato fruits [40–41]. Mango injury due to chilling was delayed after dipping in PDJ [42]. MeJA increased the beta-carotene content but reduced the lycopene content of tomato fruit [43–44]. At the pre-climacteric phase, there was over-expression of *ACC synthase* (*ACS*) *1* and *ACC oxidase* (*ACO*) 1 genes in apple and pear on treatment with PDJ. On the contrary, during the climacteric phase, the ACS1 mRNA levels were lower [37], suggesting a role of jasmonates in system 2 ethylene biosynthesis in apples and pears [37] as shown in (Figure 11.1). KODA treatment to shoots has no influence on *MdFT1* gene expression, but 49 DAFB *MdTFL1* expression reduced. Implying use of KODA helps to form flower buds by effecting transcription of *MdTFL1* in apples. In apples, transcriptional initiation of *MdFT1* influences flower regulation, through gene expression of *MdMADS12* [45]. Successful formation of KODA for genetically engineered plants with expression of 9-LOX and AOS has been reported in *Nicotiana benthamiana* [46]. Further applications of KODA and jasmonates are mentioned in (Tables 11.2 and 11.3).

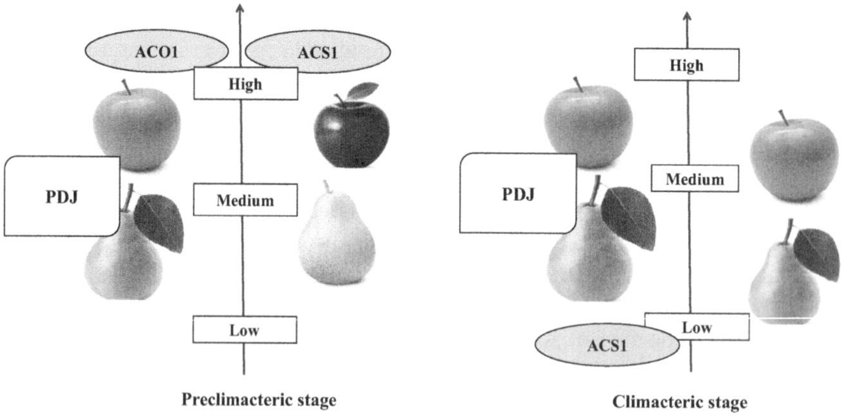

FIGURE 11.1 The role of PDJ in apple and pear at pre-climacteric and climacteric stage.

TABLE 11.2
Applications of KODA in Plants

S. No	Crop	Effect	References
1.	Satsuma Mandarin	Regulate spring shoot occurrence and reduce alternate bearing in satsuma mandarin trees	[66]
2.	Apple	Increase ethylene production in fruit	[17]
3.	Japanese pear	Endo-dormancy stage could effectively promote the breaking of flower buds	[67]
4.	Japanese morning glory	Alpha-ketol linolenic acid levels in short day-induced cotyledons are closely related to flower induction	[31]

TABLE 11.3
Applications of JA in Plants

S. No	Crop	Effect	References
1.	Strawberry	Elevated ripening rates along with yield (26–37%).	[40]
2.	Tomato	Gaseous application of Methyljasmonic acid (0.01 mM) overcomes decay and injury due to chilling for 15–30 days (5°C).	[41–42]
3.	Mango	PDJ dip of mango lowered chilling injury (6°C).	[43]
4.	Raspberry	Methyljasmonic acid promotes SSC with lowering of organic acid loss.	[68]
5.	Garden pea	MeJA (10 μM) reduced photosynthesis.	[69]
6.	Strawberry	Methyljasmonic acid lowers decay of strawberry fruits (5°C or 10°C).	[70]
7.	Zucchini squash	Chilling injury delay for zucchini.	[71–72]
8.	Cucumber	Delayed chilling injury in cucumber fruit.	[71–72]

11.4 THE ROLE OF OXYLIPINS IN FRUIT DEVELOPMENT

Lipoxygenases (LOXs; EC 1.13.11.12) represent dioxygenases (non-heme iron) dioxygenases causing free fatty acids degradation along with those of lipids (esterified) through many links of LOX signaling [47]. LOX depict a primary role in peroxidation of lipids under stress conditions and govern numerous stages of development [48–49]. LOX are lead players in the fruit development and ripening process of avocados, pears and tomatoes and via degradation of membranes and polyunsaturated fatty acids (PUFA) peroxidation which breaks cell and leads to lack of compartments [50–53]. There is loss of firmness in kiwifruit and peaches through increased action of LOX during ripening [54–56]. Also, many oxylipins, controlling quality of fruits, are result of loss of action in LOX enzymes as in tomato, the main flavor compounds are C6 alcohols and aldehydes, and their metabolization takes place via hydroperoxides

(13-HPOs) through the enzyme (13-LOX) [57–58] and in cucumber, (E,Z)-2,6-nonadienal (NDE), an aroma substance generated by 9-LOX activity [59]. In a study conducted by Yang et al. [60] via expression analyses, it was found that there was tissue-specific or preferential accumulation of *LOX* genes in cucumber, with 12 genes expressing in a differential manner during fruit development phase i.e., in exocarp, the endocarp and pulp 5 days after anthesis (DAA) depicting their predominant role in fruit quality via LOX regulatory activities.

11.5 CONCLUSION/FUTURE PERSPECTIVE

The role of oxylipins during flowering and fruiting from the above evidence is quite clear, making the task of biochemists and biotechnologists easy by giving a vast knowledge regarding their signaling pathways. From these studies it is clearly indicated that oxylipins regulate gene expression for proper flowering and fruiting in plants. The major role of oxylipins lies in development of anthers, maturity of pollens, fruit maturation along with development. A mutant showing any variation in the oxylipin biosynthesis pathway will modify their expression and result in male sterility and defected fruit developmental stages with them as exquisite factors responsible for normal flowering and fruiting in plants. A lot of study has been done on the role of oxylipins for regulating the reproductive aspect of a plant in model *Arabidopsis thaliana* (model plant). Research on this aspect should not be confined only to the model plant, so a vast and broader view is quite necessary for control of flowering and fruiting. There should be a proper knowledge to know the physiological role of oxylipins for growth and development in plants which may be done via information on regulation of mutants of oxylipins in varied species of plant kingdom. The receptors of various oxylipins have not yet been reported and tools of molecular biology through which they influence development of male reproduction in plants is still under investigation. So, tackling these issues via molecular approach like genome editing tools will lead to a cognizance regarding the role of oxylipins in order to switch the physiology of plant from vegetative to the reproductive stage.

REFERENCES

1. Koornneef M, Alonso-Blanco C, Blankestijn-de Vries H, Hanhart CJ, Peeters AJ. Genetic interactions among late-flowering mutants of Arabidopsis. Genetics. 1998 Feb;148(2):885–92. Doi: 10.1093/genetics/148.2.885. PMID: 9504934; PMCID: PMC1459831.
2. Gillaspy G, Ben-David H, Gruissem W. Fruits: A developmental perspective. Plant Cell. 1993;5:1439–1451.
3. Ezura H, Hiwasa-Tanase, K. Fruit Development. In E. C. Pua & M. R. Davey (Eds.), Plant Developmental Biology—Biotechnological Perspectives. 2010;1:301–318. Berlin Heidelberg: Springer-Verlag.
4. Browse, J. Jasmonate passes muster: a receptor and targets for the defense hormone. Annual Review of Plant Biology. 2009;60:183–205. Doi: 10.1146/annurev.arplant.043008.092007. PMID: 19025383.

5. Moreno JE, Tao Y, Chory J, Ballare CL. Ecological modulation of plant defense via phytochrome control of jasmonate sensitivity. Proceedings of the National Academy of Sciences of the United States of America. 2009 Mar 24;106(12):4935–40. Doi: 10.1073/pnas.0900701106. Epub 2009 Feb 27. PMID: 19251652; PMCID: PMC2660767.
6. Avanci NC, Luche DD, Goldman GH, Goldman MHS. Jasmonates are phytohormones with multiple functions, including plant defense and reproduction. Genetics and Molecular Research. 2010;9: 484–505. Doi: 10.4238/vol9–1gmr754.
7. Cipollini D. Constitutive expression of methyl jasmonates inducible responses delays reproduction and constrains fitness responses to nutrients in *Arabidopsis thaliana*. Ecology and Evolution. 2010; 24:59–68. Doi: 10.1007/s10682–008–9290–0.
8. Nafie E, Hathout T, Al S, Al M. Jasmonic acid elicits oxidative defense and detoxification systems in *Cucumis melo* L. cells. Brazilian Journal of Plant Physiology. 2011;23: 161–174. Doi: 10.1590/S1677–04202011000200008.
9. Rohwer CL, Erwin JE. Horticultural Applications of Jasmonates: A Review. The Journal of Horticultural Science and Biotechnology. 2008;83:283–304.
10. Ashraf M, Akram NA, Arteca RN, Foolad MR. The physiological, biochemical and molecular roles of brassinosteroids and salicylic acid in plant processes and salt tolerance. Critical Reviews in Plant Sciences. 2010;29:162–190. Doi: 10.1080/07352689.2010.483580.
11. Kumar R, Khurana A, Sharma AK. Role of plant hormones and their interplay in development and ripening of fleshy fruits. Journal of Experimental Botany. 2014;65: 4561–4575. Doi: 10.1093/jxb/eru277.
12. Feussner I, Wasternack C. The lipoxygenase pathway. Annual Review of Plant Biology. 2002;53:275–297.
13. Porta H, Rocha-Sosa M. Plant lipoxygenases. Physiological and molecular features. Plant Physiology. 2002;130:15–21.
14. Liavonchanka A, Feussner I. Lipoxygenases: occurrence, functions and catalysis. Journal of Plant Physiology. 2006;163:348–357.
15. Creelman RA, Mullet JE. Biosynthesis and action of jasmonates in plants. Annual Review of Plant Biology. 1997 Jun;48(1):355–381.
16. Tsukada K, Takahashi K, Nabeta K. Biosynthesis of jasmonic acid in a plant pathogenic fungus, *Lasiodiplodia theobromae*. Phytochemistry. 2010;71:2019–2023. Doi: 10.1016/j.phytochem.2010.09.013.
17. Kondo S, Tomiyama H, Kittikorn M, Okawa K, Ohara H, Yokoyama M, Ifuku O, Saito T, Ban Y, Tatsuki M, Moriguchi T, Murata A, Watanabe N. Ethylene production and 1-aminocyclopropane-1-carboxylate (ACC) synthase and ACC oxidase gene expression in apple fruit are affected by 9,10-ketol-octadecadienoic acid (KODA). Postharvest Biology and Technology. 2012;72:20–26.
18. Campos-Rivero G, Osorio-Montalvo P, Sanchez-Borges R, Us-Camas R, Duarte-Ake F, De-la-Pena C. Plant hormone signalling in flowering: an epigenetic point of view. Journal of Plant Physiology. 2017 Jul 1;214:16–27.
19. Turner JG, Ellis C, Devoto A. The Jasmonate Signal Pathway. The Plant Cell. 2002 Feb; 153–164.
20. Xie DX, Feys BF, James S, Nieto-Rostro M, Turner JG. COI1: an Arabidopsis gene required for jasmonate-regulated defense and fertility. Science. 1998 May 15;280(5366):1091–4.
21. Fonseca S, Chini A, Hamberg M, Adie B, Porzel A, Kramell R, Miersch O, Wasternack C, Solano R. (+)-7-iso-Jasmonoyl-L-isoleucine is the endogenous bioactive jasmonate. Nature Chemical Biology. 2009 May;5(5):344–50.

22. Feys BJ, Benedetti CE, Penfold CN, Turner JG. Arabidopsis mutants selected for resistance to the phytotoxin coronatine are male sterile, insensitive to methyl jasmonate, and resistant to a bacterial pathogen. The Plant Cell. 1994 May;6(5):751–9.
23. McConn M, Browse J. The critical requirement for linolenic acid is pollen development, not photosynthesis, in an Arabidopsis mutant. The Plant Cell. 1996 Mar;8(3):403–16.
24. Ishiguro S, Kawai-Oda A, Ueda J, Nishida I, Okada K. The *DEFECTIVE IN ANTHER DEHISCENCE1* gene encodes a novel phospholipase A1 catalyzing the initial step of jasmonic acid biosynthesis, which synchronizes pollen maturation, anther dehiscence, and flower opening in Arabidopsis. The Plant Cell. 2001 Oct;13(10):2191–209.
25. Sanders PM, Lee PY, Biesgen C, Boone JD, Beals TP, Weiler EW, Goldberg RB. The Arabidopsis DELAYED DEHISCENCE1 gene encodes an enzyme in the jasmonic acid synthesis pathway. The Plant Cell. 2002;12:1041–1062.
26. Park JH, Halitschke R, Kim HB, Baldwin IT, Feldmann KA, Feyereisen R. A knock-out mutation in allene oxide synthase results in male sterility and defective wound signal transduction in *Arabidopsis* due to a block in jasmonic acid biosynthesis. The Plant Journal. 2002 Jul;31(1):1–2.
27. Stintzi A, Browse J. The *Arabidopsis* male-sterile mutant, opr3, lacks the 12-oxophytodienoic acid reductase required for jasmonate synthesis. Proceedings of the National Academy of Sciences. 2000 Sep 12;97(19):10625–30.
28. Nagpal P, Ellis CM, Weber H, Ploense SE, Barkawi LS, Guilfoyle TJ, Hagen G, Alonso JM, Cohen JD, Farmer EE, Ecker JR. Auxin response factors ARF6 and ARF8 promote jasmonic acid production and flower maturation. Development. 2005 Sep;132(18):4107–18.
29. Wasternack C, Forner S, Strnad M, Hause B. Jasmonates in flower and seed development. Biochimie. 2013 Jan 1;95(1):79–85.
30. Yokoyama M, Yamaguchi S, Inomata S, Komatsu K, Yoshida S, Iida T, Yokokawa Y, Yamaguchi M, Kaihara S, Takimoto A. Stress-induced factor involved in flower formation of Lemna is an (α-ketol derivative of linolenic acid. Plant Cell Physiology. 2000;41:110–113.
31. Suzuki M, Yamaguchi S, Iida T, Hashimoto I, Teranishi H, Mizoguchi M, Yano F, Todoroki Y, Watanabe N, Yokoyama M. Endogenous α-ketol linolenic acid levels in short day-induced cotyledons are closely related to flower induction in *Pharbitis nil*. Plant Cell Physiology. 2003;44:35–43.
32. Yokoyama M, Yamaguchi S, Iida T, Suda A, Saeda T, Miwa T, Ujihara K, Nishio J. Transient accumulation of (α-ketol linolenic acid (KODA) in immature flower buds of some ornamental plants. Plant Biotechnology. 2005;22:201–205.
33. Kittikorn M, Shiraishi N, Okawa K, Ohara H, Yokoyama M, Ifuku O, Yoshida S, Kondo S. Effect of fruit load on 9,10-ketol-octadecadienoic acid (KODA), GA and jasmonic acid concentrations in apple buds. Scientia Horticulturae 2010;124:225–230.
34. Kondo S, Fukuda K. Changes of jasmonates in grape berries and their possible roles in fruit development. Scientia Horticulturae. 2001;91: 275–288.
35. Kondo S, Tomiyama A, Seto H. Changes of endogenous jasmonic acid and methyl jasmonate in apples and sweet cherries during fruit development. Journal of the American Society for Horticultural Science. 2000; 125: 282–287.
36. Gansser D, Latza S, Berger RG. Methyl jasmonates in developing strawberry fruit (*Fragaria ananassa* Duch. cv. Kent). Journal of Agricultural and Food Chemistry. 1997;45: 2477–2480.

37. Kondo S. Roles of jasmonates in fruit ripening and environmental stress. Acta Hor ticulturae. 2010;884:711716. https://doi.org/10.17660/Acta Hortic.2010. 884.96
38. Fujisawa H, Seto H, Yoshida S, Kamuro Y. Promoting effects of jasmonic acid analog, n-propyl dihydrojasmonate (PDJ) on plant growth. Procceedings of 23rd Annual Meeting. Plant Growth Regulator. American Society. 1996;111–11.
39. Yilmaz H, Yildiz K, Muradoglu F. Effect of jasmonic acid on yield and quality of two strawberry cultivars. Journal of the American Pomological Society. 2003; 57:32–35.
40. Ding CK, Wang CY, Gross KC, Smith DL. Reduction of chilling injury and transcript accumulation of heat shock proteins in tomato fruit by methyl jasmonate and methyl salicylate. Plant Science. 2001;161: 1153–1159.
41. Ding CK, Wang CY, Gross KC, Smith DL. Jasmonate and salicylate induce the expression of pathogenesis-related-protein genes and increase resistance to chilling injury in tomato fruit. Planta. 2002;214: 895–901.
42. Kondo S, Kittikorn M, Kanlayanarat S. Preharvest antioxidant activities of tropical fruit and the effect of low temperature storage on antioxidants and jasmonates. Postharvest Biology and Technology. 2005;36: 309–318.
43. Saniewski M, Czapski J. The effect of methyl jasmonate on lycopene and β-carotene accumulation in ripening red tomatoes. Experientia. 1983 Dec;39:1373–1374.
44. Saniewski M, Czapski J. stimulation of Ethylene Production and Ethylene –Forming Enzyme Activity in Fruits of the Non- Ripening nor and rin Tomato Mutants by Methyl Jasmonate. Journal of Plant Physiology. 1992 Jan; 139(3): 265–268.
45. Kotoda N, Hayashi H, Suzuki M, Igarashi M, Hatsuyama Y, Kidou S, Igasaki T, Nishiguchi M, Yano K, Shimizu T, Takahashi S, Iwanami H, Moriya S, Abe K. Molecular Characterization of *FLOWERING LOCUS T*-Like Genes of Apple (*Malus × domestica* Borkh.). Plant and Cell Physiology. 2010 April; 51(4):561–575. https://doi.org/10.1093/pcp/pcq021
46. Ihara Y, Wakamatsu T, Yokoyama M, Maezawa D, Ohta H, Shimojima M. Developing a platform for production of the oxylipin KODA in plants. Journal of Experimental Botany. 2022;73(9):3044–3052.
47. Brash AR. Lipoxygenases: occurrence, functions, catalysis, and acquisition of substrate. Journal of Biological Chemistry. 1999;274:23679–23682.
48. Kolomiets MV, Hannapel DJ, Chen H, Tymeson M, Gladon RJ. Lipoxygenase is involved in the control of potato tuber development. Plant Cell. 2001;13:613–626.
49. Porta H, Rueda-Benitez P, Campos F, Colmenero-Flores JM, Colorado JM, Carmona MJ, Covarrubias AA, Rocha-Sosa M. Analysis of lipoxygenase mRNA accumulation in the common bean (*Phaseolus vulgaris* L.) during development and under stress conditions. Plant Cell Physiology. 1999;40:850–858.
50. Thompson JE. The Molecular Basis for Membrane Deterioration During Senescence. In *Senescence and Aging in Plants*; Nooden, L.D., Leopold, A.C., Eds.; Academic Press: San Diego,CA, USA, 1988.
51. Rogiers SY, Kumar GNM, Knowles NR. Maturation and Ripening of Fruit of *Amelanchier alnifolia* Nutt. are Accompanied by Increasing Oxidative Stress. Annals of Botany. 1998;81:203–211.
52. Brennan T, Frenkel C. Involvement of hydrogen peroxide in the regulation of senescence in pear. Plant Physiology. 1977;59:411–416.
53. Brennan T, Rychter A, Frenkel C. Activity of enzymes involved in the turnover of hydrogen peroxide during fruit senescence. Botanical Gazette. 1979;140:384–388.
54. Chen KS, Xu CJ, Lou J, Zhang SL, Ross G. Lipoxygenase in relation to the ripening and softening of Actinidia fruit. Acta Phytophysiologica Sinica 1999;25:138–144.

55. Zhang Y, Chen K, Zhang S, Ferguson I. The role of salicylic acid in postharvest ripening of kiwifruit. Postharvest Biology and Technology. 2003;28:67–74.
56. Wu M, Chen KS, Zhang SL. Involvement of lipoxygenase in the postharvest ripening of peach fruit. Acta Horticulturae Sinica 1999;26:227–231.
57. Baldwin E, Nisperos-Carriedo M, Moshonas M. Quantitative analysis of flavor and other volatiles and for certain constituents of two tomato cultivars during ripening. Journal of the American Society for Horticulture Science.1991;116:265–269.
58. Chen G, Hackett R, Walker D, Taylor A, Lin Z, Grierson D. Identification of a specific isoform of tomato lipoxygenase (TomloxC) involved in the generation of fatty acid-derived flavor compounds. Plant Physiology. 2004;136:2641–2.
59. Buescher R, Buescher R. Production and Stability of (E, Z)-2,6-Nonadienal, the Major Flavor Volatile of Cucumbers. Journal of Food Sciences. 2001;66:357–361.
60. Yang XY, Jiang WJ, Yu HJ. The Expression Prolifing of the Lipo-oxygenase (LOX) Family Genes During Fruit Development, Abiotic Stress and Hormonal Treatments in Cucumber (*Cucumis sativus* L.). International Journal of Molecular Sciences. 2012;13:2482–2500.
61. Xiao Y, Chen Y, Charnikhova T, Mulder PP, Heijmans J, Hoogenboom A, Agalou A, Michel C, Morel JB, Dreni L, Kater MM. OsJAR1 is required for JA-regulated floret opening and anther dehiscence in rice. Plant Molecular Biology. 2014 Sep;86(1):19–33.
62. Cai Q, Yuan Z, Chen M, Yin C, Luo Z, Zhao X, Liang W, Hu J, Zhang D. Jasmonic acid regulates spikelet development in rice. Nature Communications. 2014 Mar 19;5(1):1–3.
63. Acosta IF, Laparra H, Romero SP, Schmelz E, Hamberg M, Mottinger JP, Moreno MA, Dellaporta SL. tasselseed1 is a lipoxygenase affecting jasmonic acid signaling in sex determination of maize. Science. 2009 Jan 9;323(5911):262–5.
64. Yan Y, Christensen S, Isakeit T, Engelberth J, Meeley R, Hayward A, Emery RN, Kolomiets MV. Disruption of OPR7 and OPR8 reveals the versatile functions of jasmonic acid in maize development and defense. The Plant Cell. 2012 Apr;24(4):1420–36.
65. Li L, Zhao Y, McCaig BC, Wingerd BA, Wang J, Whalon ME, Pichersky E, Howe GA. The tomato homolog of CORONATINE-INSENSITIVE1 is required for the maternal control of seed maturation, jasmonate-signaled defense responses, and glandular trichome development. The Plant Cell. 2004 Jan;16(1):126–43.
66. Nakajima N, Ikoma Y, Matsumoto H, Nakamura Y, Yokoyama M, Ifuku O, Yoshida S. Effect of 9,10-α-ketol linolenic acid treatment on flower bearing in Satsuma mandarin. Horticultural Research (Japan). 2011; 10(3):407–411.
67. Sakamoto D, Nakamura Y, Sugiura H, Sugiura T, Asakura T, Yokoyama M, Moriguchi T. Effect of 9-hydroxy-10-oxo-12(Z), 15 (Z)-octadecadienoic acid (KODA) on endodormancy breaking in flower buds of Japanese pear. Hortscience. 2010;45:1470–1474.
68. Wang CY. Maintaining postharvest quality of raspberries with natural volatile compounds. International Journal of Food Science and Technology. 2003;8:869–875.
69. Fedina IS, Tsonev TD. Effect of pretreatment with methyl jasmonate on the response of *Pisum sativum* to salt stress. Journal of Plant Physiology.1997;151: 735–740.
70. Moline HE, Buta JG, Maas JL, Saftner RA. Comparison of three volatile natural products for the reduction of postharvest decay in strawberries. Advances in Strawberry Research.1997;16:13–18.

71. Wang CY, Buta JG. Methyl jasmonate reduces chilling injury in *Cucurbita pepo* through its regulation of abscisic acid and polyamine levels. Environmental and Experimental Botany. 1994;34:427–432.
72. Wang CY, Buta JG. Methyl jasmonate improves quality of stored zucchini squash. Journal of Food Quality. 1997;22:663–670.

12 The Role of Oxylipins (Phyto-Oxylipins) in Moss Development

O.C.U. Adumanya
Department of Biochemistry, the University of Agriculture and Environmental Sciences, Umuagwo, Imo State, Nigeria
Email: oadumanya@gmail.com, adumso@yahoo.com

CONTENTS

12.1 INTRODUCTION

Moss is a non-vascular flowerless plant, bryophyta belonging to a plant sub-kingdom, bryophytes like liverworts and hornworts which exhibit two alternating generation life cycles. The two alternating life cycles are gametophyte and sporophyte generation [1, 2]. Mosses were the first plants to conquest land and have evolved adaptation mechanisms to tolerate extreme conditions such as desiccation and exposure to damaging UV-B radiation, and to resist co-evolving pathogens and herbivores [3]. Mosses use many alternative metabolic pathways, some of which are not present in flowering plants, and probably this has allowed mosses to occupy and function in very different habitats [4]. In addition to polyunsaturated C18 fatty acids, mosses have also large amounts of polyunsaturated C20 fatty acids which are rarely present in flowering plants due to the lack of the corresponding biosynthetic enzymes [5]. It is known that mosses are associated with the production of physiologically important biomolecules called oxylipins or phyto-oxylipins (plant oxylipins). Oxylipins are oxygenated fatty acids derived from polyunsaturated fatty acids that are associated with plant development and defense against stress, pathogen infection, and insects and wounding [6].

Oxylipins are present in most living organisms. In mammals, eicosanoids, notably prostaglandins, leukotrienes, and thromboxanes, are generated mainly by oxygenation

DOI: 10.1201/9781003316558-12

of arachidonic acid (20:4) by lipoxygenases (LOXs) or cyclooxygenases (COXs), and their roles in many physiological processes including the immune response, inflammation, and hemostasis, have been extensively studied [7]. In flowering plants, which lack 20:4, oxylipins are produced mainly from the polyunsaturated C18 fatty acids, linolenic (18:3) and linoleic (18:2) acids by oxygenations catalyzed by LOXs or α-dioxygenases (α-DOXs) [8–10]. DOXs in plants and COXs in mammals are structurally and catalytically related and have similar functions [11, 12]. Non-enzymatic mechanisms in the presence of singlet oxygen or free radical-mediated oxygenation can create oxylipins from polyunsaturated fatty acids [13]. LOX-derived oxylipins are involved in fertilization, seed and root development, germination, fruit development, and senescence, as well as defense responses against microbial diseases, insects, and wounds [14–19]. α-DOXs catalyze the incorporation of molecular oxygen at the α methylene carbon atom of fatty acids. This review aimed at the oxylipins associated in moss development.

12.2 MOSS

Moss is a non-vascular flowerless plant, bryophyta belonging to a plant sub-kingdom, bryophytes like liverworts and hornworts which exhibit two alternating generation life cycles. The two alternating life cycles are gametophyte and sporophyte generation. Mosses contain stems and leaves, but no actual roots. They generate spores and have stems and leaves. Rhizoids, which are tiny hair-like structures, are what they have instead. Their primary purpose is to secure the plant to rock, bark, or soil. Mosses can be found growing in a variety of habitats, from icy snowy mountains to scorching hot deserts. They can live in situations that would otherwise be uninhabitable, such as stony ledges on mountainsides, thanks to their diverse adaptations.

Various moss species have evolved to live in harsh environments. According to studies, they can photosynthesize (convert energy from sunlight into food) in temperatures as low as -15°C and as high as 40°C [20].

Mosses are also important in the formation of new habitats. They are among the first plants to colonize disturbed areas, such as those that have been deforested or have been impacted by forest fires. They assist the growth of new plants by stabilizing the soil top and retaining water [20]. Mosses are essential parts of the vegetation in many parts of the world, and they contribute significantly to biodiversity in wetland, mountain, and tundra habitats. Moss communities provide microhabitats that are essential for a variety of creatures' existence. They provide vital habitat for insects, allowing them to live, lay eggs, and hunt for food. Turtles, for example, can benefit from the mosses' capacity to regulate temperature.

12.3 LIFE CYCLE OF MOSS

Mosses have two generations: an independent gametophyte generation that produces sex organs, sperm, and eggs, and a dependent sporophyte generation that generates spores [21]. The gametophytic (sexual) development of moss plants is made up of stem-like and leaf-like structures. The gametophyte gives rise to the sporophytic (asexual) generation, which usually consists of a raised stalk, or seta, that ends in the sporangium. The sporangium is still reliant on the gametophyte for water and nutrients to varying degrees. Mosses reproduce via branching and fragmenting, as well as by spore production and regeneration from microscopic fragments of photosynthetic tissues. Under favorable conditions, the spore germinates and develops into the protonema, a branching green thread. The gametophyte eventually develops from a tiny bud formed by a protonema cell that splits and differentiates.

12.3.1 Economic Importance of Moss

- Serves as biofuel
- Serves bio-fertilizer
- Buffer system for ecosystem
- Ornaments in landscaping and green roof
- Medicinal uses

As moss grows, it pushes down old mosses (peat) and thereby creates dense mats which can be burnt in a fire or stove for cooking (biofuel). The peat moss can also serve as fertilizer (bio-fertilizer) and growing medium for mushrooms. Moss is becoming useful as an ornament landscape plant to decorate an outdoor space like a grass turf lawn [22]. Its use as base for a green roof to reduce the urban heat effect is gaining attention [23]. Ecologically, mosses break down exposed substrata in the environment, releasing nutrients for use by more complex plants that come after them. They also contribute in soil erosion control by providing surface cover and absorbing water, and they play a significant role in some vegetation types' nutrient and water economies [24, 21]. Dried moss is highly absorbent and can be used as a bandage for wounded soldiers in the field due to its antibacterial qualities [25–27].

12.4 MOSS DEVELOPMENT

Mosses are terrestrial plants that have a very straightforward developmental pattern, with haploid gametophyte and diploid sporophyte generations alternated. Because its genome was sequenced a decade ago, the moss Physcomitrella patens is receiving increased scientific attention among moss species [28]. The gametophyte has two separate developmental stages: juvenile filamentous sprotonema with chloronema and caulonema types of cells, and adult gametophores, which are leafy shoots made of a non-vascular stem with leaves, reproductive organs, and filamentous rhizoids [1]. When a haploid spore germinates or a protoplast divides, chloronema cells form, with perpendicular cross walls and a high concentration of chloroplasts. Chloronemal filaments give rise to caulonemal cells with oblique cross walls and poor chloroplast density. Caulonemal cell branching results in secondary chloronemal or caulonemal filaments and buds, as well as new chloronemal or caulonemal cells [29, 30]. Buds develop into leafy gametophores, which give rise to a diploid sporophyte generation, which creates new haploid spores [30]. Figure 12.1 shows the life cycle of *P. patens* at

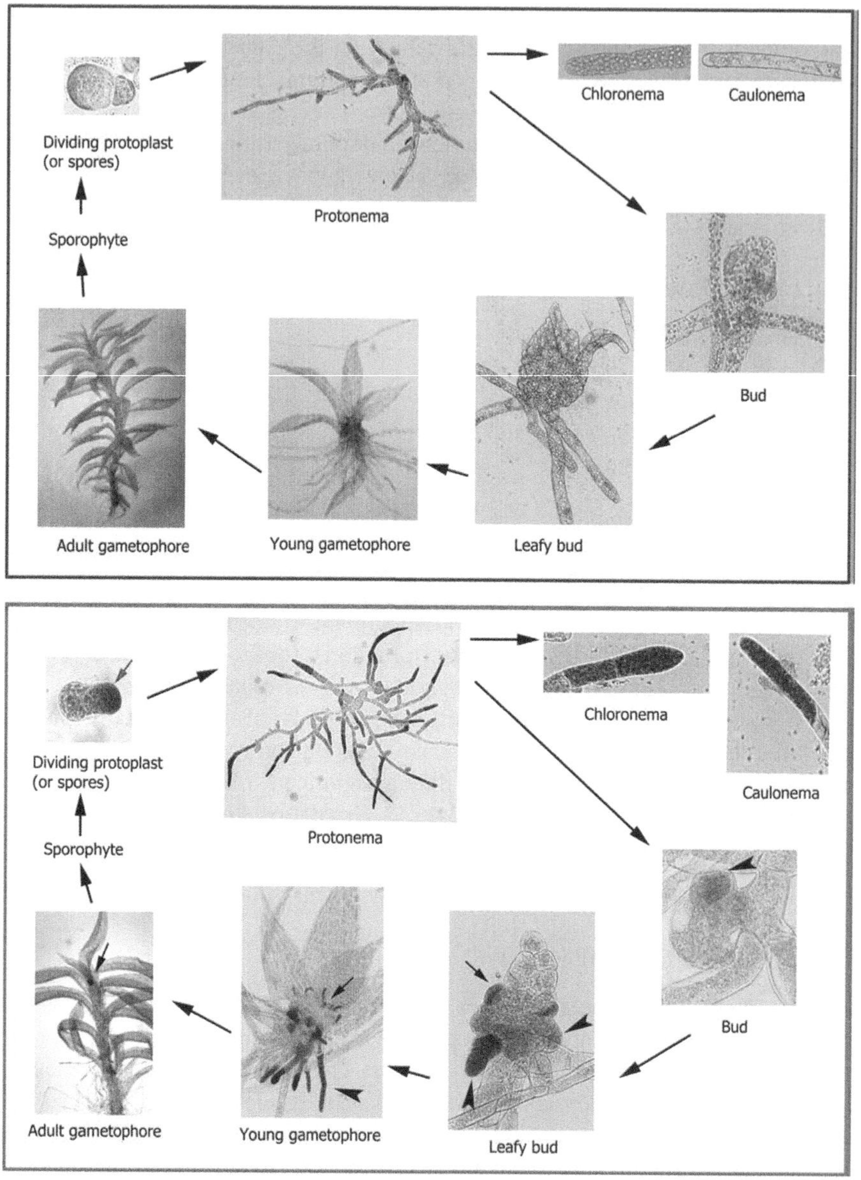

FIGURE 12.1 Physcomitrella patens life cycle.

various stages. Toluidine blue was used to stain the protoplast and protonema for good visibility. Protonema are moss spore-derived thread-like structures. The chloroplasts in the protonema clump together to receive the most amount of available light, and the lens-shaped cells aid in focusing the light.

12.5 MOSS DEVELOPMENT AND POLYUNSATURATED FATTY ACIDS

The fatty acid composition of mosses varies depending on the tissue type. While the content of 16:0 and 20:4 is equal in protonemal filaments and leafy gametophores of different moss species, gametophores and protonemal tissues have more 18:2 and 18:3, respectively [31]. These metabolic changes are linked to variances in the expression levels of genes that code for fatty acid desaturases [31]. The most abundant fatty acids in growing sporophytes of the moss *Mnium cuspidotum* are 16:0 and 20:4, but 18:2 increases after spores have grown and are ready for dispersal, reaching similar levels to 16:0 [32]. The most abundant free hydro (per)oxy fatty acids found in *P. patens* protonemal tissues are 13-hydroperoxylinoleic acid and 12-HPETE [33], which can be processed by the relevant enzymes to produce oxylipins that may play a role in moss development. The specific functions of the C18:2, C18.3, and C20:4 pathways in various tissues and during moss growth are still being discovered.

12.6 OXYLIPINS AND MOSS DEVELOPMENT

Oxylipins are oxygenated fatty acids derived from polyunsaturated fatty acids that are associated with plant development and defense against stress, pathogen infection, and insects and wounding [6]. In moss it is mainly derived enzymatically from arachidonic acid (C20) and C18 fatty acids (linoleic or linolenic acid). This oxygenation is catalyzed mainly by lipoxygenases (LOXs) and alpha-dioxygenase (α-DOXs) or via auto-oxidation (non-enzymatic) resulting in hydroperoxides production, which is further metabolized to oxylipins in moss. Recent findings have associated oxylipins in moss development. Such oxylipins includes oxo-phytodienoic acid (OPDA) like 12-oxo-phytodienoic acid, 11-Oxo-5, 9, 14-prostatrienoic acid derived from C_{20} and C_{18} fatty acids via LOX enzymatic action and heptadecatrienal derived from C_{18} fatty acids via the action of α-DOX. Alteration of these plant oxylipins changes the colonies and protonemal tissues of moss. That is moss colonies are reduced and have less protonemal tissues as the case may be on the alteration of 13-LOX-derived oxylipins, like OPDA. Similarly, alteration of α-DOX- derived aldehyde, heptadecatrienal, lead to reduced protonemal filament growth of moss.

Using a novel moss, *P. patens* Pp-DOX-GUS reporter lines, [34] discovered that Pp-DOX is expressed in the tips of protonemal filaments during development, with maximal expression levels in mitotically active undifferentiated apical chloronemal and caulonemal cells [35]. Pp-DOX-GUS is also abundantly expressed in other mitotically active cells, such as regenerating protoplast apical cells. The role of Pp-DOX-derived oxylipins in undifferentiated apical cells, which are self-renewing stem cells, has to be investigated further. When wild-type tissues are incubated with Pp-DOX-derived oxylipins or when Pp-DOX is overexpressed, *P. patens* develops differently, resulting in smaller moss colonies with fewer protonemal tissues [35]. Heptadecatrienal, a Pp-DOX-derived aldehyde, is responsible for the diminished protonemal filament development (Figure 12.2). *P. patens* development is altered when wild-type tissues are incubated with Pp-DOX-derived oxylipins or when Pp-DOX is overexpressed, resulting in smaller moss colonies with fewer protonemal

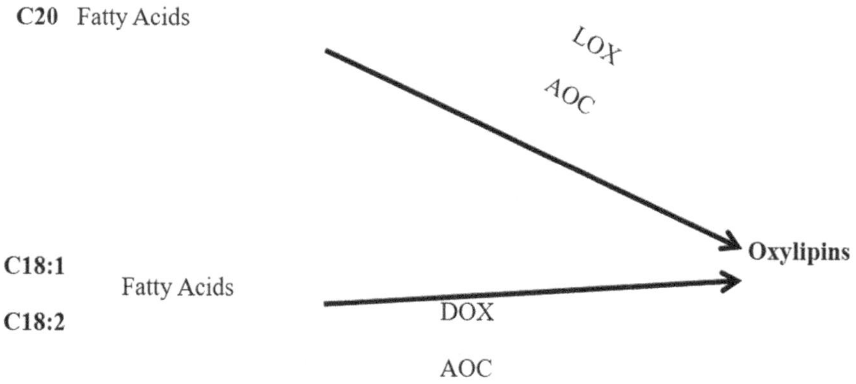

FIGURE 12.2 Schematic biosynthetic pathway of oxylipins in moss.

AOC: Allene oxide cyclase, LOX: Lipoxygenase, DOX: Dioxygenase

tissues [35]. Heptadecatrienal, a Pp-DOX generated aldehyde, is responsible for the reduced protonemal filament development. When moss tissues are grown in the presence of 13-LOX-derived oxylipins, such as OPDA and methyl jasmonate, moss colonies are smaller and have less protonemal tissues [6]. The expression of p-DOX-GUS during *P. patens* development. A red arrow points to the apical cell of a dividing protoplast. An arrowhead indicates GUS-stained cells leading to rhizooids, rhizoid primordial, and rhizoidoids. Therefore oxylipins (plant oxylipins), also called phyto-oxylipins especially 13-LOX-derived like OPDA and α-DOX- derived like heptadecatrienal are associated with moss development and growth.

12.7 CONCLUSION

Oxylipins are polyunsaturated fatty acids that have been linked to plant growth and defense against stress, pathogen invasion, insects, and wounds. It is mostly generated enzymatically from arachidonic acid (C20) and C18 fatty acids in moss (linoleic or linolenic acid). This oxygenation is mostly mediated by lipoxygenases (LOXs) and alpha-dioxygenases (-DOXs), or by auto-oxidation (non-enzymatic), leading in the creation of hydroperoxides, which are then converted to oxylipins in moss. Recent research has linked oxylipins to moss development. Oxylipins (plant oxylipins or phytoxylipins) especially C20 and C18 fatty acids 13-LOX-derived and α-DOX- derived ones are implicated in moss development. The specific functions of the C18:2, C18.3, and C20:4 pathways in various tissues and during moss growth are still being investigated.

REFERENCES

1. Reski, R. (1998). Development, genetics and molecular biology of mosses. *Bot.Acta* 111:1–15.
2. Sabovljevic M, Vujicic M and Sabovljevic A (2014). Plant growth regulators in bryophytes, *Botanica Serbica* 38(1):99–107.

3. Rensing, S.A., Lang, D., Zimmer, A.D., Terry, A., Salamov, A. and Shapiro, H. (2008). The Physcomitrella genome reveals evolutionary insights into the conquest of land by plants. *Science* 319: 64–69.
4. Rensing, S.A., Ick, J., Fawcett, J.A., Lang, D., Zimmer, A. and VandePeer, Y. (2007). An ancient genome duplication contributed to the abundance of Metabolic genes in the moss Physcomitrella patens. *BMC Evol. Biol.* 7:130.
5. Gill, I. and Valivety, R. (1997). Polyunsaturated fatty acids, part1: occurrence, Biological activities and applications. *Trends Biotechnol.* 15:401–409.
6. Ponce de León I, Hamberg M and Castresana C (2015) Oxylipins in moss development and defense. *Front. Plant Sci.* 6:483.
7. Smith, W.L., DeWitt, D.L. and Garavito, R.M. (2000). Cyclooxygenases: structural, cellular, and molecular biology. *Annu. Rev. Biochem.* 69:145–182.
8. Hamberg, M., Ponce de León, I., Sanz, A. and Castresana, C. (2002). Fatty acid alpha-dioxygenases. *Prostaglandins Other Lipid Mediat.* 68–69:363–374.
9. Andreou, A., Brodhun, F., and Feussner, I. (2009). Biosynthesis of oxylipins in non mammals. *Prog. Lipid Res.* 48: 148–170.
10. Mosblech, A., Feussner, I. and Heilmann, I. (2009). Oxylipins structurally diverse metabolites from fatty acid oxidation. *Plant Physiol. Biochem.* 47: 511–517.
11. Sanz, A., Moreno, J.I., and Castresana, C. (1998). PIOX, a new pathogen-induced Oxygenase with homology to animal cyclooxygenase. *Plant Cell* 10:1523–1537.
12. Goulah, C. C., Zhu, G., Koszelak-Rosenblum, M., and Malkowski, M.G. (2013). The crystal structure of α-dioxygenase provides insight into diversity in the cyclooxygenase-peroxidase superfamily. *Biochemistry* 26:1364–1372.
13. Mueller, M.J., and Berger, S. (2009). Reactive electrophilic oxylipins: pattern recognition and signalling. *Phytochemistry* 70: 1511–1521.
14. Howe, G.A. and Schilmiller, A.L. (2002). Oxylipin metabolism in response to stress. *Curr. Opin. Plant Biol.* 5:230–236.
15. Browse, J. (2005). Jasmonate: an oxylipin signal with many roles in plants. *Vitam. Horm.* 72: 431–456.
16. Vellosillo, T., Martínez, M., López, M.A., Vicente, J., Cascón, T., and Dolan, L. (2007). Oxylipins produced by the 9-lipoxygenase pathway in Arabidopsis regulate lateral root development and defense responses through a specific signaling cascade. *Plant Cell* 19:831–846.
17. Kachroo, A., and Kachroo, P. (2009). Fatty acid-derived signals in plant defense. *Annu. Rev. Phytopathol.* 47:153–176.
18. López, M.A., Vicente, J., Kulasekaran, S., Vellosillo, T., Martínez, M., and Irigoyen, M.L. (2011). Antagonistic role of 9-lipoxygenase-derived oxylipins and ethylene in the control of oxidative stress, lipid peroxidation and plant defence. *Plant J.* 67: 447–458.
19. Wasternack, C., and Hause, B. (2013). Jasmonates: biosynthesis, perception, signal transduction and action in plan tstress response, growth and development. An Update to the 2007 review in Annals of Botany. *Ann.Bot.* 111: 1021–1058.
20. Mchale, E (2020). Mosses Growing on Rocks. www.kew.org/read-and-watch/moss www.britannica.com/plant/moss-plant.(2022). "moss"
21. Kimmerer, R W (2003). *Gathering Moss*. Corvallis, Oregon: Oregon State University www. "RoofTopGarden" (2011). www.plant-ark-moss.com what are Mosses?
22. Stalheim, T.; Ballance, S.; Christensen, B. E. and Granum, P. E. (2009). Sphagnan—a pectin-like polymer isolated from Sphagnum moss can inhibit the growth of some typical food spoilage and food poisoning bacteria by lowering the pH. *Journal of Applied Microbiology*. 106 (3): 967–976. www.biologydictionary.net

23. Resemann H.C, Lewandowska M, Go¨mann J and Feussner I (2019) Membrane Lipids, Waxes and Oxylipins in the Moss Model Organism Physcomitrella patens *Plant Cell Physiol.* 60(6): 1166–1175.
24. Cove, D.J., and Knight, C.D. (1993). The moss Physcomitrella patens, a model system with potential for the study of plant reproduction. *Plant Cell.* 5:1483–1488.
25. Cove, D., Bezanilla, M., Harries, P., and Quatrano, R. (2006). Mosses as model systems for the study of metabolism and development. *Annu. Rev. Plant Biol.* 57: 497–520.
26. Beike, A.K., Jaeger, C., Zink, F., Decker, E.L., and Reski, R. (2014). High contents of very long-chain polyunsaturated fatty acids in different moss species. *Plant Cell Rep.* 33: 245–254.
27. Anderson, W.H., Gellerman, J.K., and Schlenk, H. (1972). Arachidonic and eicosapentaenoic acids in developing gametophores and sporophytes of the moss, Mnium cuspidotum. *Lipids* 7: 710–714.
28. Stumpe, M., Göbel, C., Faltin, B., Beike, A.K., Hause, B., and Himmelsbach, K. (2010). The moss Physcomitrella patens contains cyclopentenones but no jasmonates: mutations in allene oxide cyclase lead to reduced fertility and altered sporophyte morphology. *New Phytol.* 188: 740–749.
29. Ponce de León, I., Schmelz, E.A., Gaggero, C., Castro, A., Álvarez, A., and Montesano, M. (2012). *Physcomitrella patens* activates reinforcement of the cell wall, programmed cell death and accumulation of evolutionary conserved defence signals, such as salicylic acid and 12-oxo-phytodienoicacid, but not jasmonic acid, upon Botrytiscinerea infection. *Mol. Plant Pathol.* 13: 9.
30. Machado, L., Castro, A., Hamberg, M., Bannenberg, G., Gaggero, C., and Castresana, C. (2015). The Physcomitrella patens unique alpha-dioxygenase participates in both developmental processes and defense responses. *BMC Plant Biol.* 15: 439.
31. Anderson, W.H., Gellerman, J.K., and Schlenk, H. (1972). Arachidonic and eicosapentaenoic acids in developing gametophores and sporophytes of the moss, Mnium cuspidotum. *Lipids* 7: 710–714.
32. Stumpe, M., Göbel, C., Faltin, B., Beike, A.K., Hause, B., and Himmelsbach, K. (2010). The moss Physcomitrella patens contains cyclopentenones but no jasmonates: mutations in allene oxide cyclase led to reduced fertility and altered sporophyte morphology. *New Phytol.* 188: 740–749.
33. Ponce de León, I., Schmelz, E.A., Gaggero, C., Castro, A., Álvarez, A., and Montesano, M. (2012). Physcomitrella patens activates reinforcement of the cell wall, programmed cell death and accumulation of evolutionary conserved defence signals, such as salicylic acid and 12-oxo-phytodienoicacid, but not jasmonic acid, upon Botrytiscinerea infection. *Mol. Plant Pathol.* 13: 9.
34. Machado, L., Castro, A., Hamberg, M., Bannenberg, G., Gaggero, C., and Castresana, C. (2015). The Physcomitrella patens unique alpha-dioxygenase participates in both developmental processes and defense responses. *BMC Plant Biol.* 15: 439.
35. Machado, L., Castro, A., Hamberg, M., Bannenberg, G., Gaggero, C., Castresana, C., & de León, I.P. (2015). The Physcomitrella patens unique alpha-dioxygenase participates in both developmental processes and defense responses. *BMC Plant Biology*, 15(1): 1–19.

13 The Role of Oxylipins in Leaf Senescence

Ikra Manzoor[1], Bismat un Nisa[2], Momin Showkat Bhat[3], Usma Jan[4], and Yathish VC[5]*

[1]Division of Fruit Science, Faculty of Horticulture, SKUAST-Kashmir, India
[2]Division of Entomology, Faculty of Horticulture, SKUAST-Kashmir, India
[3]Division of Floriculture and Landscape Architecture, Faculty of Horticulture, SKUAST-Kashmir, India
[4]Division of Vegetable Science, Faculty of Horticulture, SKUAST-Kashmir, India
[5]Division of Vegetable Crops, ICAR-IIHR, Bengaluru, India
*Correspondence:manzoorikra@gmail.com

CONTENTS

13.1 INTRODUCTION

In the organic world, senescence is a quite pervasive fact [1, 2] and for plants, leaves exhibits this phenomenon significantly in both annuals as well as deciduous trees. Senescence is identified through malfunctioning of organelles during which substances/nutrients are transferred to other plant parts, ultimately leading to the apoptosis of the organ in which senescence has taken place [3, 4]. Senescence is regulated by various endogenous and exogenous factors which are depicted as degeneration of long chain organic molecules viz., chlorophyll, polypeptides, DNA/RNA and fatty acids, nutrient dissemination and cell structure degradation [5, 1]. In leaves, senescence has been discussed at both morphological and molecular levels. During senescence, due to loss of green pigment (chlorophyll) along with degeneration of chloroplast there is yellowing of leaves. Besides, there is a drastic change in expression of genes during senescence. During this process, some genes viz., *SENESCENCE ASSOCIATED GENE* (*SAG*) and *SENESCENCE* (*SEN*), which are

DOI: 10.1201/9781003316558-13

associated with senescence, get activated. There are various encoded proteins which are responsible for degeneration of macromolecules, withdrawal of toxic compounds and mitigation strategies, or signaling cascade [6]. Despite being damaging in nature, senescence advances in an ordered and balanced way and has great importance in the life cycle of an organism. Senescence restricts yield and there is significant loss in the post-harvest phase in agricultural and horticultural crops, which defines its spectacular nature. Besides, being an approachable process, especially the research on *Arabidopsis*, scientists have decoded certain events viz., regulatory, molecular, and biochemical. Therefore, there is an advanced perception regarding leaf senescence which depicts that plant hormones are the main game changers during the control of stress-induced senescence in plants [7]. Among various plant hormones, oxylipins constitute fatty acids having added oxygen molecules with varied structure in the majority of the life forms on earth [8]. As angiosperms lack arachidonic acid (20:4 = 20 carbon atoms in fatty acid chain with 4 double bonds), polyunsaturated fatty acids (PUFA with 18C) viz., linolenic acid (18:3) and linoleic acid (18:2), are the source of oxylipins via addition of oxygen to them and catalysis through lipoxygenases (LOXs) or α-dioxygenases (α-DOXs) [9–11]. In plants, fatty acids with hydroxyl, oxo, or keto groups, hydroperoxides, ethers having two vinyl groups, aldehydes (volatile), or the plant hormone like jasmonic acid, come under oxylipins [12]. Through the enzymatic approach [13], or through the auto oxidation process [14], hydroperoxide formation is the foremost stride for biosynthesis of oxylipins. As in the former process, hydroperoxides which are reactive in nature belonging to fatty acid group viz., LA (18:2), α -LeA (18:3) or roughanic acid (16:3), get synthesized via lipoxygenases (LOXs, EC 1.13.11.12) [15] or through α-dioxygenase (α-DOX) [16]. Hydroperoxides get subsequently transformed via many optional mechanisms, combining those which begin via allene oxide synthase (AOS, EC 4.2.1.92), divinyl ether synthase (DES), hydroperoxide lyases (HPL), peroxygenases (PXG), or epoxy alcohol synthase (EAS). Phytohormones such as JA, along with oxylipins having a prominent reactive epoxide group, α, β-unsaturated carbonyl, or aldehyde group, are the oxygenated end products, while the latter involving auto oxidation constitute hydroxy fatty acids isomers (positional) and at C-9 of linoleic acid and C-13 of α - linolenic acid, molecular oxygen is added by LOXs, whileas reactive oxygen species (ROS) forms hydroxides at (C-10 and C-12) in LA and in α-LeA at (C-15 and C-16) [17–19]. The racemic mixture of radicals in fatty acids having peroxy group, is yielded through oxidation process in LA and α -LeA, which are vulnerable to free radical attack [14]. Racemic fatty acid hydroperoxides (free or esterified) are synthesized and collected by the kind of radicals which initiate oxidative reaction series. By oxidizing radicals of PUFA i.e., hydroperoxides and peroxy types further where the number of double bonds is more than two hydroperoxides having bicyclic endoperoxy groups like phytoprostane (PPG1), which have short half-lives [14]. Phytoprostanes whose structure matches with isoprostanes found in animals are created by another series of reactions which occur naturally. The quantity of phytoprostanes found in the esterified form of some plant membranes are usually at elevating levels than non-esterified ones [20], and by exposing them to oxidative type of stress viz., metal contamination or peroxide treatment or the attack of pathogens the magnitude of phytoprostanes goes up [20–23]. For lipidation of proteins, lipids (oxidized) under the influence of oxidative stress act as ligands influencing patterns for gene expression, and thus, prove to be arbiters for injury due to oxidants. As per Porter [24], fatty acids with two or three hydroxyl groups, epoxy alcohols, dienes and trienes having a keto group and alkenals are included under the peroxy radical chemistry [24]. By comparison with animals, the majority of oxylipins responsible for lipidation of proteins are included under 4- hydroxy-2-alkenals (4-hydroxy nonenal) group [25] with phytoprostanes and keto fatty acids being mostly present in plants [26]. No doubt phytoprostanes are mainly found in plants [27], but cyclopentenone phytoprostanes when used exogenously are responsible for inducing defense mechanism in plants [22, 23]. In plants, a considerable number of oxylipins are produced via the chemical oxidation (non-enzymatic) mode while a small number of the same is produced through enzymatic pathway i.e., LOX mechanism [28]. In this chapter, an overview has been presented regarding the role of oxylipins during the leaf senescence in plants.

13.2 OXYLIPINS AND GENE REGULATION DURING SENESCENCE

Physiological processes begin with senescence of leaves which is depicted by degradation of chlorophyll pigment, blockage of photosynthesis, denaturation of amino acids and DNA/RNA along with other catabolites, transport of nutrients is affected and the response is the death of cells. At the transcriptional level, all these events are programmatically upregulated or knocked down under the control of genes [29]. Following an ordered and regulative pattern of networks during leaf senescence various transcription factor families viz., *NO APICAL MERISTEM/ ARABIDOPSIS TRANSLATION ACTIVATIONFACTOR/ CUP-SHAPED COTYLEDON (NAC), WRKY, bHLH* (basic helix -loop -helix), *APETALA2/ETHYLENE RESPONSE FACTOR* (*AP2/ERF*), and *MYB* (myeloblastosis) play a vital role [30, 29, 31], but as shown in Figure 13.1, few TFs are involved in leaf senescence as per Miao and Zentgraf [32]. *WRKY53* was found to interact with (*EPITHIOSPECIFYING SENESCENCE REGULATOR* [*ESR/ESP*] (JA-inducible protein) which is associated

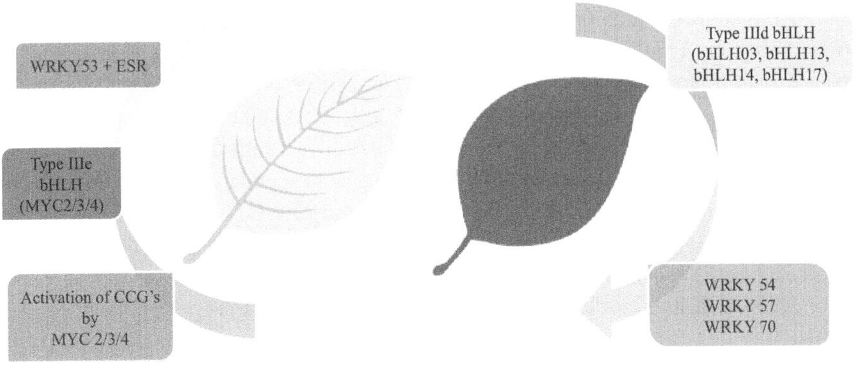

FIGURE 13.1 Transcription factors controlling gene expression (positive and negative) during senescence.

with natural senescence of plants and JA signaling by treating the wild and mutant (*npr1*, *coi1*, and *jar1*) plants with salicylic acid and JA. The studies on expression analyses imply that *WRKY53* shows positive regulation with SA and negative regulation with JA signaling, Besseau et al. [33] confirmed that while studying leaf senescence in *Arabidopsis* it was found that during leaf development, *WRKY54* and *WRKY70* show the same pattern of expression and seem to be negative senescence regulators. Also, *WRKY53* (positive regulator of senescence) interacted independently with *WRKY30* (uncharacterized one), as proved by yeast two-hybrid assaying, and *WRKY57* acts as a negative regulator for leaf senescence in *Arabidopsis* via JA as it attenuates *SEN4* and *SAG12* gene expression [34]. For degradation of chlorophyll, a key enzyme is encoded by pheophorbide (*PAO*) an oxygenase gene whose transcriptional regulation is still unknown. With the help of one-hybrid analysis of yeast, along with in vitro and in vivo studies, it was found that there is association of *Arabidopsis MYC2/3/4* (basic helix-loop-helix proteins) to *PAO* promoter. The upregulation of *MYC*s increase the transcriptional control of *PAO* promoter in the protoplasts of *Arabidopsis*, along with methyl jasmonate treatment which greatly increased the activity of *PAO* in the plants of *Arabidopsis* (wild type) and contrary to the case of its mutants (*myc2 myc3 myc4*). The expression of *NYC1*, which is another gene for catabolism of chlorophyll along with *NYE1/SGR1*, a key regulatory gene for Chl degredation was promoted by *MYC2/3/4* which directly joins to their promoters. The triple mutants, *myc2 myc3 myc4*, depicted the stay-green phenotype whileas overexpression of *MYCs* promoted yellowing of leaves on treatment with MeJA. This study shows that Chl degradation with JA is mediated by *MYC2/3/4* proteins via activation of Chl catabolic genes (*CCG*s) [35]. Downstream from *MYC2/3/4* proteins, *NAC* family proteins (*ANAC092/ANAC019/055/072*) enhance the expression of *CCG*s (*NYE1/SGR1*, *NYE2/SGR2* and *NYC1*) which is a same set of Chl degradation genes while as its triple mutants (*anac019 anac055 anac072*) depicted the stay-green phenotype after treatment with methyl jasmonate. At protein level, *MYC2* and *ANAC019* associate and form a network so they may induce Chl degradation via JA while synergistic regulation with *NYE1* expression [35]. According to Qi et al. [36] the TFs viz., *bHLH03/bHLH13/ bHLH14/bHLH17*, depict a mechanism where the TF type IIIe *bHLH* subgroup (*MYC2*, *MYC3*, and *MYC4*) has JA-induced leaf senescence: antagonistic interactions with type IIId *bHLH* subgroup (*bHLH03*, *bHLH13*, *bHLH14*, and *bHLH17*). The former factors (*MYC2*, *MYC3*, and *MYC4*) act superfluously for activation of leaf senescence via JA induction. Also, for the leaf senescence via JA induction, *MYC2* attaches to and turns on the promoter of *SAG29*, its target gene. Ironically, a regulative feedback mechanism has been evolved by plants for mediating senescence in leaves through JA. The later factors (*bHLH03*, *bHLH13*, *bHLH14*, and *bHLH17*) attach to the *SAG29* promoter so that its expression is reduced for repressing the effect of (*MYC2/MYC3/MYC4*) for leaf senescence through JA. This antagonistic mechanism through activation and repression modulated via JA at optimal ranges for proper plant survival of plants under abnormal environmental conditions. The senescence is also controlled by *TEOSINTEBRANCHED/CYCLOIDEA/PCF* (*TCP*s) which consist of two classes in *Arabidopsis thaliana* viz., (type 1 and type 2) [37, 38]. Type 1 *TCP*s (*TCP20*) is a

TABLE 13.1
Transcription factors (TFs) for positive regulation of leaf senescence

Transcription Factor	Family	References
NtERF3	*AP2/ERF* (*APETALA2/ ETHYLENE RESPONSE FACTOR*)	[41]
AtERF4	*AP2/ERF* (*APETALA2/ ETHYLENE RESPONSE FACTOR*)	[41]
AtERF8	*AP2/ERF* (*APETALA2/ ETHYLENE RESPONSE FACTOR*)	[41]
RAV1	*AP2/ERF* (*APETALA2/ ETHYLENE RESPONSE FACTOR*)	[42]
CIB	*bHLH* (basic helix-loop-helix)	[43]
EIN3	*EIN3* (*ETHYLENE-INSENSITIVE3*)	[44, 45]
NAM-B1	*NAC* (*NO APICAL MERISTEM/ ARABIDOPSIS TRANSLATION ACTIVATIONFACTOR/ CUP-SHAPED COTYLEDON*)	[46]
AtNAP	*NAC* (*NO APICAL MERISTEM/ ARABIDOPSIS TRANSLATION ACTIVATIONFACTOR/ CUP-SHAPED COTYLEDON*)	[47, 48]
ORE1	*NAC* (*NO APICAL MERISTEM/ ARABIDOPSIS TRANSLATION ACTIVATIONFACTOR/ CUP-SHAPED COTYLEDON*)	[49]
OsNAP	*NAC* (*NO APICAL MERISTEM/ ARABIDOPSIS TRANSLATION ACTIVATIONFACTOR/ CUP-SHAPED COTYLEDON*)	[50, 51]
TCP4	*TCP* (*TEOSINTEBRANCHED/ CYCLOIDEA/PCF*)	[52, 41]
TCP5	*TCP* (*TEOSINTEBRANCHED/ CYCLOIDEA/PCF*)	[41]
TCP10	*TCP* (*TEOSINTEBRANCHED/ CYCLOIDEA/PCF*)	[52, 41]

positive regulator, while as type2 *TCP*s (*TB1*) and (*CYC/DICH*) a negative one [39, 40]. Besides this, there are other TFs for leaf senescence which may act either positively or negatively as mentioned in Tables 13.1 and 13.2.

13.3 OXYLIPINS AND CELL DEATH REGULATION

In order to regulate the cell death, oxylipins play a significant role. As discussed earlier by Przybyla et al. [19], it was found that not only do JA control cell death, but some of the substances produced in-between the oxylipin pathway produce JA. Jasmonic acid, 12-oxophytodienoic acid, and its C16 carbon skeleton homologue dinor-oxophytodienoic acid, which depict opposite effects, well-described the control of cell death [19, 60].Wagner et al., and Kim et al. [61–62] explained that two mutants in *Arabidopsis thaliana* viz., *executer* (*exe 1* and *exe 2*) repress the cell death when the singlet oxygen gets accumulated at lower rates with slight cytotoxicity. Genetic studies have shown that in maize (*Zea mays*), JA play a predominant role for surviving

TABLE 13.2
Transcription Factors (TFs) for Negative Regulation of Leaf Senescence

Transcription Factor	Family	References
EDF1	*AP2/ERF* (*APETALA2/ ETHYLENE RESPONSE FACTOR*)	[53]
EDF2	*AP2/ERF* (*APETALA2/ ETHYLENE RESPONSE FACTOR*)	[53]
SUB1A	*AP2/ERF* (*APETALA2/ ETHYLENE RESPONSE FACTOR*)	[54]
CBF2	*AP2/ERF* (*APETALA2/ ETHYLENE RESPONSE FACTOR*)	[55]
VNI2	*NAC* (*NO APICAL MERISTEM/ ARABIDOPSIS TRANSLATION ACTIVATIONFACTOR/ CUP-SHAPED COTYLEDON*)	[56]
MYBR1/MYB44	*MYB* (myeloblastosis)	[57]
TCP19	*TCP* (*TEOSINTEBRANCHED/ CYCLOIDEA/PCF*)	[58]
TCP20	*TCP* (*TEOSINTEBRANCHED/ CYCLOIDEA/PCF*)	[58]
SlZF2	Zn finger	[59]

stress (biotic), regulating senescence, and also controlling cell death with intervention in male sex determination [63–64]. In pepper (*Capsicum annuum*) and *Arabidopsis* through mediation, 9-LOX pathway produced metabolites positively managed cell death reaction to a wide range of pathogens with defense mechansim [65].

As per Ponce de Leon et al. [66], by employing α-DOX *Arabidopsis* plants having transgenic nature, it was found that via α-DOX pathway some of the products generated prevent the hypersensitive reaction leading to extreme cell death in leaf tissues. In infected leaf tissues while detecting 2-hydroxylinolenic acid (2-HOT) as the main product of α-DOX pathway, it was found that this oxylipin has a cell-protecting role. Ironically, by administering (50–100 μM) 2-HOT along with the inoculums of bacteria cell death rates were less [67]. In tobacco and *Arabidopsis*, the genetic research depicted the role of α-DOX-1 and 9-LOX as a defense to fungal and bacterial attack, via controlling cell death and oxidative stress [66–68]. One of the oxylipins from *Physcomitrella patens* (Pp-DOX) in mosses provide cell death protection against *Pectobacterium carotovorum* elicitors which under optimum conditions are produced in filamentous thalloid, in fibrils and in hairs (axillary) acting as a stable defense mechanism protection system [69].

13.4 THE ROLE OF OXYLIPINS DURING LEAF SENESCENCE

The ending of plant growth is characterized by senescence of leaves which might serve as an important physiological aspect during which nutrients from senescent leaves had been redistributed to the new plant parts, enhancing the viability of plants during the coming season [3, 1, 70]. The main feature of leaf senescence involves loss of chlorophyll pigment via degradation, photosynthetic ability gets suppressed and the expression of *SAG12* and *SEN4* is at peak [71–74]. But, early senescence due to abnormal conditions during stress reduces the growth and development phase in crops, which impacts their yield and quality [75–76]. Besides, the senescence of leaves lowers the shelf-life along with the nutritional quality of various leaf type vegetables which is their main post-harvest problem [77–78]. Hence, from the agricultural point of view, the basic understanding of the mechanisms which regulate leaf senescence is of utmost importance to breed higher-yielding varieties of crops having superior nutritional values along with better management for overcoming the post-harvest problems [79]. Senescence of leaves under natural conditions follows a developmental pattern controlled by a myriad of exogenous and endogenous aspects [80]. Oxygenated fatty acid-derivatives (oxylipins) control an array of physiological aspects in plants [81]. Among them, jasmonates (JAs), which are ubiquitous in nature, mediate various physiological processes like the senescence of leaves [82]. Afterward, advances regarding the function of JA to induce senescence were under description [83]. α-linolenic acid (α- LeA) (18:3) is the source of JA and its derivatives in plants and during the biosynthesis, α- LeA produces 12-oxo-phytodienoic acid (12-OPDA) undergoing various reactions which are catalyzed by 13-lipoxygenase (LOX), allene oxide synthase (AOS), and allene oxide cyclise (AOC), respectively. By using OPDA reductase3 (*OPR3*) with three ß-oxidation cycles, 12-OPDA is then changed to JA [84, 30]. The biosynthesis has been already reviewed and it has been found that in chloroplast galactolipids produce α-LeA via phospholipase A1 (*PLA1*) involving hydrolysis with *sn-1* specificity. A (*PLA1*), *DEFECTIVE IN ANTHER DEHISCENCE 1* (*DAD1*), which is a flower specific protein is needed for biosynthesis of Jasmonic acid [85], 13-Lipoxygenase (LOX) produces JA via its AOS branch [86], AOSs is present in gene families in various plants, excluding *Arabidopsis*, in which a the gene with single-copy produced mutants without (JA and OPDA) [87], upregulation of the AOC in *Salvia miltiorrhiza* and in wheat, enhanced JA and its responses in the respective plants [88–89], small gene families include 12-oxo-phytodienoic acid reductase (*OPR*) out of which only *OPR3* in *Arabidopsis* and its homologues biosynthesizes JA. Rice has *OsOPR7* which is the homologue of *AtOPR3* for JA production [90]. The signal of JA is first recognized by *CORONATINE INSENSITIVE1* (*COI1*) receptor F-box protein [91–93] which, along with (*SKP1* and *CULLIN1*), binds *SKP1-Cullin*-F-box complex (*SCFCOI1*), that interacts with *JASMONATE ZIM DOMAIN* (*JAZ*) family proteins in a JA-based pattern [91]. There is ubiquitination of *JAZ* proteins via JA perception and the simultaneous degeneration with the help of *26S*-proteosome. *JAZ* proteins degrade, which switch on many downstream TFs, viz., the IIIe type TF (*bHLH*), *MYC2*, *MYC3*, and *MYC4* [94–96], the IIId type bHLH TFs viz., *bHLH03*, *bHLH13*, *bHLH14*, and *bHLH17* [97, 98, 36] and the *R2R3-MYB* transcription factors, *MYB21* and *MYB24* [99]. A lot of studies have already recognized the regulatory action which control leaf senescence at transcriptional, post-transcriptional, translational, post-translational and chromatin-mediated level [100–102]. It was Ueda and Kato [103] who studied the action of these molecules for enhancement of senescence in the leaves of oat (*Avena sativa*) with MeJa which was extracted from *Artemisia absinthium* [103]. Thereafter, the phenomenon of senescence was seen in other plants also with the use of MeJa exogenously [103–105]. As per molecular studies, MeJa induces senescent leaves due to degredation of chlorophyll and reduction in rubisco along with photosynthesis [104, 106], for years jasmonates have been studied as substances with senescent action on plants, but their activity for senescence under natural conditions has been described crucially in plants [107–111, 81]. The effect of jasmonates in senescence is probably due to up-regulated expression of various enzymes /genes which control biosynthesis of JA viz., AOS and OPDA reductase 3 (*OPR3*), and the enhancement of levels of JA under natural senescence [105, 112]. *Arabidopsis* has reported the endogenous increase of JA level during the senescence of leaves in a dramatic pattern [105]. Nevertheless, application of Jasmonic acid or its derivatives i.e., MeJA promote leaf senescence of various plants like *Arabidopsis* [105, 113–115], wormwood [103], barley [107], maize [116], and rice [117], via upregulation of few *SAG*s. Hisamatsu et al. [118] extracted an oxylipin, namely arabidopside A [*sn*1-*O*-(12-oxophytodienoyl)-*sn*2-*O*-(dinor-oxophytodienoyl)-monogalactosyl diglyceride], using the aerial parts of the ecotype (Col-0) in *Arabidopsis thaliana* L. This oxylipin is rich in OPDA) and (dn-OPDA), acting as source of JA and MeJA [119–120]. It had been defined that in *Arabidopsis thaliana*, the key enzyme *chlorophyllase* for degradation of Chl had been activated by MeJA [121]. Weber [122] reported that arabidopside A has got plant senescence activity, particularly degradation of chlorophyll, as arabidopside A is rich in OPDA and dn-OPDA. The degradation of chlorophyll represents the signature for senescence of leaves under natural and artificial conditions via JA. To overcome damage due to photooxidation, this needs to be controlled and there is the impairment of Chl a / b binding protein system under selective manner, which are the prime light-harvesting complexes bound to PS I and PS II. To regulate the stability of light-harvesting complex, a kind of protein had been discovered [123–124]. In rice, *STAY-GREEN PROTEIN* (*SGR*) had not been found in mature phase of leaves but during the senescence, it was induced in a specific pattern [123]. Under natural, as well as induced environment of senescence, the mutants of rice devoid of *SGR* depict more vitality of chlorophyll. On the contrary, in developing leaves overexpressing of *SGR* promoted degeneration of chlorophyll [123], *SGN1* in *Arabidopsis thaliana* which is a homologue of *SGR* is less in *acd2* which is a mutant that encodes for pheophorbide a oxygenase [125], and red Chl catabolite reductase, encoded by *acd1* [126], describing that senescent chloroplasts depict reverse signaling cascade which regulate stability of light-harvesting complex to release chlorophyll [81]. In tomato plants (*Solanum lycopersicum*) the function of sedoheptulose-1,7-bisphosphatase (SBPase) has been elucidated under MeJA treatment as well as dark-induced senescence of leaves. MeJA repress *SlSBPASE* (*Solyc05g052600*) which is a gene controlling *SBPase* expression in (*Solanum lycopersicum*), along with expression activated in genes associated with senescence. The approach of *CRISPR/Cas9* (clustered regularly interspaced short palindromic repeats (*CRISPR*)/*CRISPR-associated protein 9*)-has modulated the mutation in *SlSBPASE* gene for developing senescent phenotype in tomato plants and also promoting the action of genes associated with senescence, conforming the action of *SBPase* senescence of leaves via JA for plants of tomato [83]. Also, in rice *OsNAP* encoding for *NAC* TF for JA-mediated senescence in leaves has been isolated and screened with the development of the RNAi strains and upregulation of *OsNAP* by analyzing senescence phase in them. Also, the endogenous rates of JA had been estimated gene expression of enzymes encoding biosynthesis of

JA in the transgenic strains of *OsNAP* with some wild-type (non-mutant) plants. These strains show that the *OsNAP* gene produces positive expression in JA biosynthesis for promoting senescence in the leaves of rice plant [50].

Although, it is clear that JA application upgrades the senescence process in plants, but the evident role of JA is still ambiguous. The majority of pathways for JA regulation and transduction in mutant-types is not distinguishable from wild ones for leaf senescence process. Pleiotropic effects like infertility are usually noticed in mutants of JA which show delay of senescence process providing an explanation for already produced senescent phenotypes. In recent times, modifying the biosynthesis of JA has an impact on the overall developmental leaf senescence along with the one induced by stress. To overcome this, genotypes in which LOX2 action has been repressed, were produced and screened to alter levels of JA. It was noticed that in wild-type *Arabidopsis* plants the levels of JA enhanced predominantly under all senescence types, but in plants with LOX2-silencing, the rates of JA had not progressed. Nevertheless, normal initiation and advancement of developmental senescence had been seen in those lines with minimal levels of senescence induced by osmotic stress describing JA not having a prime role to play in those aspects [127].

13.5 CONCLUSION/FUTURE PERSPECTIVE

The evidence of oxylipins having a regulatory function in the senescence of leaves is quite certain. But from the signaling cascade point of view, the information regarding the role of transcription factors is less certain, which could relate the senescence of leaves with other physiological aspects of a plant. The advancement at molecular level to control the action of the oxylipin pathway for senescence reveals only the biosynthetic pathways, with most of the knowledge on the induction of leaf senescence still missing. Also, vast research regarding the function of oxylipins to regulate the phenomenon of senescence is restricted only to *Arabidopsis thaliana* (model plant) which restrains the scope of future research due to lack of information on other plant species. The model plant should be employed for genetic studies at forward and reverse levels, so as to have an idea of the regulatory and biological aspects which control the multiple ways for oxylipin metabolism. Yet, there is a need to study varied plants so as to intensify the knowledge of the metabolism and functioning of oxylipins throughout the plant kingdom. So, the future outlook should unravel the gene expression through a whole-genome approach to screen out the prime steps for biosynthesis and signaling of oxylipins for their upregulation during the senescence phase of a plant. Also, the current tool of biotechnology (clustered regularly interspaced short palindromic repeats (CRISPR)/CRISPR-associated protein 9) may modulate the mutants of certain senescence associated genes for creation of senescent phenotypic expression in various plant species. Above all, an insight into the recognition of genes regulating the oxylipin pathway via bioinformatics will pave the way for understanding the location, control, and the purpose underlying the products of the specified network which may serve as a tool for studying the structural as well as functional aspect to describe the domain of various proteins with catalytic and substrate specificity.

REFERENCES

1. Lim PO, Nam HG. Aging and senescence of the leaf organ. Journal of Plant Biology. 2007;50:291–300.
2. Guo Y. Towards systems biological understanding of leaf senescence. Plant Molecular Biology. 2012;1–10.
3. Hortensteiner S, Feller U. Nitrogen metabolism and remobilization during senescence. Journal of Experimental Botany. 2002;53:927–937.
4. Lim PO, Woo HR, Nam, HG. Molecular genetics of leaf senescence in *Arabidopsis*. Trends in Plant Science. 2003;8:272–278.
5. Lim PO, Kim HJ, Nam HG. Leaf senescence. Annual Review of Plant Biology. 2007;58:115–136.
6. Gepstein S, Sabehi G, Carp MJ, Hajouj T, Nesher MF, Yariv I, Dor C, Bassani M. Large-scale identification of leaf senescence-associated genes. Plant Journal. 2003;36: 629–642.
7. Khan M, Rozhon W, Poppenberger B. The Role of Hormones in the Aging of Plants—A Mini-Review. Gerontology. 2013;60:49–55.
8. Smith WL, DeWitt DL, Garavito RM. Cyclo oxygenases: structural, cellular, and molecular biology. Annual Review of Biochemistry. 2000;69:145–182.
9. Hamberg M, PoncedeLeon I, Sanz A, Castresana C. Fatty acid alpha-dioxygenases. Prostaglandins Other Lipid Mediators. 2002;68–69, 363–374.
10. Andreou A, Brodhun F, Feussner I. Biosynthesis of oxylipins in non-mammals. Progress in Lipid Research. 2009;48:148–170.
11. Mosblech A, Feussner I, Heilmann I. Oxylipins:structurally diverse metabolites from fatty acid oxidation. Plant Physiology and Biochemistry. 2009;47:511–517.
12. Grechkin A. Recent developments in biochemistry of the plant lipoxygenase pathway, Progress in Lipid Research. 1998;37:317–352.
13. Blee E. Phytooxylipins and plant defense reactions. Progress in Lipid Research. 1998;37:33–72.
14. Mueller, MJ. Archetype signals in plants: the phytoprostanes. Current Opinion in Plant Biology. 2004;7:441–448.
15. Feussner I, Wasternack C. The lipoxygenase pathway, Annual Review of Plant Biology. 2002;53:275–297.
16. Hamberg M, PoncedeLeon I, Rodriguez MJ, Castresana C. Alpha-dioxygenases. Biochemical and Biophysical Research Communications. 2005;338:169–174.
17. Mueller MJ, Mene-Saffrane L, Grun C, Karg K, Farmer EE. Oxylipin analysis methods. Plant Journal. 2006;45:472–489.
18. Berger S, Weichert H, Porzel A, Wasternack C, Kuhn H, Feussner I. Enzymatic and non-enzymatic lipid peroxidation in leaf development. Biochimca et Biophysica Acta. 2001;1533:266–276.
19. Przybyla D, Gobel C, Imboden A, Hamberg M, Feussner I, Apel K. Enzymatic, but not non-enzymatic, $^1O_2$-mediated peroxidation of polyunsaturated fatty acids forms part of the EXECUTER1-dependent stress response program in the flu mutant of *Arabidopsis thaliana*. Plant Journal. 2008; 54:236–248.
20. Imbusch R, Mueller MJ. Analysis of oxidative stress and wound-inducible dinor isoprostanes F(1) (phytoprostanes F(1)) in plants. Plant Physiology. 2000;124:1293–1304.
21. Imbusch R, Mueller MJ. Formation of isoprostane F(2)-like compounds (phytoprostanes F(1)) from alpha-linolenic acid in plants. Free Radical Biology and Medicine. 2000;28:720–726.

22. Thoma I, Krischke M, Loeffler C, Mueller MJ. The isoprostanoid pathway in plants. Chemistry and Physics of Lipids. 2004;128:135–148.
23. Thoma I, Loeffler C, Sinha AK, Gupta M, Krischke M, Steffan B, Roitsch T, Mueller MJ. Cyclopentenone isoprostanes induced by reactive oxygen species trigger defense gene activation and phytoalexin accumulation in plants. Plant Journal. 2003;34:363–375.
24. Porter NA. Chemistry of lipid peroxidation. Methods in Enzymology. 1984; 105:273–282.
25. Esterbauer H, Schaur RJ, Zollner H. Chemistry and biochemistry of 4 hydroxynonenal, malonaldehyde and related aldehydes. Free Radical Biology and Medicine. 1991;11:81–128.
26. Farmer EE, Davoine C. Reactive electrophile species. Current Opinion in Plant Biology. 2007;10:380–386.
27. Kohlmann M, Bachmann A, Weichert H, Kolbe A, Balkenhohl T, Wasternack C, Feussner I. Formation of lipoxygenase-pathway-derived aldehydes in barley leaves upon methyl jasmonate treatment. European Journal of Biochemistry. 1999;260:885–895.
28. Blee E. Impact of phytooxylipins in plant defense. Trends in Plant Science. 2002;7:315–322.
29. Koyama T. The roles of ethylene and transcription factors in the regulation of onset of leaf senescence. Frontiers in Plant science. 2014;5:650.
30. Wasternack C, Song S. Jasmonates: biosynthesis, metabolism, and signalling by proteins activating and repressing transcription. Journal of Experimental Botany. 2017;68:1303–1321.
31. Schippers JH. Transcriptional networks in leaf senescence. Current Opinion in Plant Biology. 2015;27:77–83.
32. Miao Y, Zentgraf U. The antagonist function of *Arabidopsis WRKY53* and *ESR/ESP* in leaf senescence is modulated by the jasmonic and salicylic acid equilibrium. The Plant Cell. 2007;19:819–830.
33. Besseau S, Li J, Palva ET. *WRKY54* and *WRKY70* cooperate as negative regulators of leaf senescence in Arabidopsis thaliana. Journal of Experimental Botany. 2012;63:2667–2679.
34. Jiang Y, Liang G, Yang S, Yu D. *Arabidopsis*WRKY57 Functions as a Node of Convergence for Jasmonic Acid– and Auxin-Mediated Signaling in Jasmonic Acid–Induced Leaf Senescence. The Plant Cell. 2014;26:230–245.
35. Zhu X, Chen J, Xie Z, Gao J, Ren G, Gao S, Zhou X, Kuai B. Jasmonic acid promotes degreening via *MYC2/3/4*- and *ANAC019/055/072*-mediated regulation of major chlorophyll catabolic genes. Plant Journal. 2015;84:597–610.
36. Qi T, Wang J, Huang H, Liu B, Gao H, Liu Y, Song S, Xie D. Regulation of Jasmonate-Induced Leaf Senescence by Antagonism between *bHLH* Subgroup IIIe and IIId Factors in *Arabidopsis*. The Plant Cell. 2015;27:1634–1649.
37. Kosugi S, Ohashi Y. *PCF1* and *PCF2* specifically bind to cis elements in the rice proliferating cell nuclear antigen gene. The Plant Cell. 1997; 9:1607–1619.
38. Cubas P, Lauter N, Doebley J, Coen E. The TCP domain: a motif found in proteins regulating plant growth and development. Plant Journal. 1999;18:215–222.
39. Kosugi S, Ohashi Y. DNA binding and dimerization specificity and potential targets for the *TCP* protein family. Plant Journal. 2002;30:337–348.
40. Li C, Potuschak T, Colo n-Carmona A, Gutierreez R, Doermann P. *Arabidopsis TCP29* links regulation of growth and cell division control pathways. Proceedings of National Academy of Sciences of USA. 2005;102:12978–12983.

41. Koyama T, Nii H, Mitsuda N, Ohta M, Kitajima S, Ohme-Takagi M, Sato, F. A regulatory cascade involving class II *ETHYLENE RESPONSE FACTOR* transcriptional repressors operates in the progression of leaf senescence. Plant Physiology. 2013;162(2): 991–1005.
42. Woo HR, Kim JH, Kim J, Kim J, Lee U, Song I, Kim JH, Lee HY, Nam HG, Lim PO. The *RAV1* transcription factor positively regulates leaf senescence in Arabidopsis. Journal of Experimental Botany. 2010; 61: 3947–3957.
43. Meng Y, Li H, Wang Q, Liu B, Lin C. Blue light-dependent interaction between cryptochrome2 and CIB1 regulates transcription and leaf senescence in soybean. Plant Cell. 2013;25:4405–4420.
44. Li Z, Peng J, Wen X, Guo H. Ethylene-insensitive3 is a senescence-associated gene that accelerates age-dependent leaf senescence by directly repressing miR164 transcription in Arabidopsis. Plant Cell. 2013;25:3311–3328.
45. Kim HJ, Hong SH, Kim YW, Lee IH, Jun JH, Phee B, Rupak T, Jeong H, Lee Y, Hong BS, Nam HG, Woo HR, Lim PO. Gene regulatory cascade of senescence-associated *NAC* transcription factors activated by *ETHYLENE-INSENSITIVE2*-mediated leaf senescence signalling in Arabidopsis. Journal of Experimental Botany. 2014;65:4023–4036.
46. Uauy C, Distelfeld A, Fahima T, Blechl A, Dubcovsky J. A *NAC* gene regulating senescence improves grain protein, zinc, and iron content in Wheat. Science. 2006;314: 1298–1301.
47. Guo Y, Gan S. *AtNAP*, a *NAC* family transcription factor, has an important role in leaf senescence. The Plant Journal. 2006;46:601–612.
48. Zhang K, Gan, SS. An abscisic acid-*AtNAP* transcription factor-*SAG113* protein phosphatase 2C regulatory chain for controlling dehydration in senescing *Arabidopsis* leaves. Plant Physiology. 2012;158:961–969.
49. Kim JH, Woo HR, Kim J, Lim PO, Lee IC, Choi SH, Hwang D, Nam HG. Trifurcate feed-forward regulation of age-dependent cell death involving miR164 in Arabidopsis. Science. 2009;323: 1053–1057.
50. Zhou Y, Huang W, Liu L, Chen T, Zhou F, Lin Y. Identification and functional characterization of a rice NAC gene involved in the regulation of leaf senescence. BMC Plant Biology. 2013;13:1.
51. Liang C, Wang Y, Zhu Y, Tang J, Hu B, Liu L, Ou S,Wu H, Sun X, Chu J, Chu C. OsNAP connects abscisic acid and leaf senescence by fine-tuning abscisic acid biosynthesis and directly targeting senescence-associated genes in rice. Proceedings of the National Academy of Sciences of the U.S.A. 2014;111:10013–10018.
52. Schommer C, Palatnik JF, Aggarwal P, Chetelat A, Cubas P, Farmer EE, Nath U, Weigel D. Control of jasmonate biosynthesis and senescence by miR319 targets. PLoS Biology. 2008;6.
53. Chen M, Hsu W, Lee P, Thiruvengadam M, Chen H, Yang C. The MADS box gene, FOREVER YOUNG FLOWER, acts as a repressor controlling floral organ senescence and abscission in Arabidopsis. Plant Journal. 2011;68:168–185.
54. Fukao T, Yeung E, Bailey-serres J. The submergence tolerance gene *SUB1A* delays leaf senescence under prolonged darkness through hormonal regulation in rice. Plant Physiology. 2012;160:1795–1807.
55. Sharabi-Schwager M, Lers A, Samach A, Guy CL, Porat R. Overexpression of the *CBF2* transcriptional activator in *Arabidopsis* delays leaf senescence and extends plant longevity. Journal of Experimental Botany. 2010;61:261–273.
56. Yang SD, Seo PJ, Yoon, HK, Park CM. The *Arabidopsis NAC* transcription factor *VNI2* integrates abscisic acid signals into leaf senescence via the *COR/RD* genes. Plant Cell. 2011;23:2155–2168.

57. Jaradat MR, Feurtado JA, Huang D, Lu Y, Cutler AJ. Multiple roles of the transcription factor *AtMYBR1/AtMYB44* in ABA signaling, stress responses, and leaf senescence. BMC Plant Biology. 2013;13:192.
58. Danisman S, van der Wal F, Dhondt S, Waites R, de Folter S, Bimbo A, van Dijk AD, Muino JM, Cutri L, Dornelas MC, Angenent GC, Immink RG. *Arabidopsis* class I and class II *TCP* transcription factors regulate jasmonic acid metabolism and leaf. Plant Physiology. 2012;159:1511–1523.
59. Hichri I, Muhovski Y, Zi E, Dobrev PI, Franco-zorrilla JM, Solano R, Lopez-Vidriero I, Motyka V, Lutts S. The *Solanum lycopersicum* zinc finger2 cysteine2/histidine2 repressor-like transcription factor regulates development and tolerance to salinity in *Arabidopsis*. Plant Physiology. 2014;64:1967–1990.
60. Ochsenbein C, Przybyla D, Danon A, Landgraf F, Gobel C, Imboden A, Feussner I, Apel K. The role of EDS1 (enhanced disease susceptibility) during singlet oxygen-mediated stress responses of Arabidopsis. Plant Journal. 2006;47: 445–456.
61. Wagner D, Przybyla D, op den Camp R, Kim C, Landgraf F, Lee KP, Wursch M, Laloi C, Nater M, Apel K. The genetic basis of singlet oxygen induced stress responses of *Arabidopsis thaliana*. Science 2004;306:1183–1185.
62. Kim C, Meskauskiene R, Apel K, Laloi C. No single way to understand singlet oxygen signalling in plants. EMBO Rep 2008;9:435–439.
63. Acosta IF, Laparra H, Romero SP, Schmelz E, Hamberg M, Mottinger JP, Moreno MA, Dellaporta SL. Tasselseed1 is a lipoxygenase affecting jasmonic acid signalling in sex determination of maize. Science. 2009;323(5911):262–265.
64. Yan Y, Christensen S, Isakeit T, Engelberth J, Meeley R, Hayward A, Neil Emery RJ, Kolomiets MV. Disruption of *OPR7* and *OPR8* reveals the versatile functions of jasmonic acid in maize development and defense. Plant Cell. 2012;24(4):1420–1436.
65. Hwang IS, Hwang BK. The pepper 9-lipoxygenase gene CaLOX1 functions in defense and cell death responses to microbial pathogens. Plant Physiology. 2010;152(2):948–967.
66. Ponce de Leon I, Sanz A, Hamberg M, Castresana C. Involvement of the *Arabidopsis* 585 -DOX1 fatty acid dioxygenase in protection against oxidative stress and cell death. Plant Journal. 2002;586(29):61–72.
67. Hamberg M, Sanz A, Rodríguez MJ, Calvo AP, Castresana C. 2003. Activation of the fatty acid -dioxygenase pathway during bacterial infection of tobacco leaves. Formation of oxylipins protecting against cell death. Journal of Biological Chemistry. 2003;278:51796–51805.
68. Rance I, Fournier J, Esquerre-Tugaye MT. The incompatible interaction between *Phytophthora parasitica* var.nicotianae race 0 and tobacco is suppressed in transgenic plants expressing antisense lipoxygenase sequences. Proceedings of National Academy Sciences U.S.A. 1998;95:6554–6559.
69. Machado L, Castro A, Hamberg M, Bannenberg G, Gaggero C, Castresana C, de Leon IP. The *Physcomitrella patens* unique alpha-dioxygenase participates in both developmental processes and defense responses. BMC Plant Biology. 2015;15:439.
70. Kim J, Woo, HR Nam HG. Toward systems understanding of leaf senescence: an integrated multi-omics perspective on leaf senescence research. Molecular Plant. 2016;9:813–825.
71. Park JH, Oh SA, Kim YH, Woo HR, Nam HG. Differential expression of senescence-associated mRNAs during leaf senescence induced by different senescence-inducing factors in *Arabidopsis*. Plant Molecular Biology. 1998;37:445–454.

72. Woo HR, Chung KM, Park JH, Oh SA, Ahn T, Hong SH, Jang SK, Nam HG. ORE9, an F-Box protein that regulates leaf senescence in *Arabidopsis*. The Plant Cell. 2001;13:1779–1790.
73. Hortensteiner S. Chlorophyll degradation during senescence. Annual Review of Plant Biology. 2006;57:55–77.
74. Zhao Z, Li Y, Zhao S, Zhang J, Zhang H, Fu B, He F, Zhao M, Liu P. Transcriptome analysis of gene expression patterns potentially associated with premature senescence in *Nicotiana tabacum* L. Molecules 2018;23:2856.
75. Wu XY, Kuai BK, Jia JZ, Jing HC. Regulation of leaf senescence and crop genetic improvement. Journal of Integrative Plant Biology. 2012;54:936–952.
76. Guo Y, Gan SS. Translational researches on leaf senescence for enhancing plant productivity and quality. Journal of Experimental Botany. 2014;65:3901–3913.
77. Al Ubeed HMS, Wills RBH, Bowyer MC, Vuong QV, Golding JB. Interaction of exogenous hydrogen sulphide and ethylene on senescence of green leafy vegetables. Postharvest Biology and Technology. 2017;133:81–87.
78. Fan ZQ, Tan XL, Shan W, Kuang JF, Lu WJ, Chen JY. *BrWRKY65*, a *WRKY* transcription factor, is involved in regulating three leaf senescence-associated genes in Chinese flowering cabbage. International Journal of Molecular Sciences. 2017;18.
79. Tan X, Fan Z, Shan W, Yin X, Kuang J, Lu W, Chen J. Association of *BrERF72* with methyl jasmonate-induced leaf senescence of Chinese flowering cabbage through activating JA biosynthesis-related genes. Horticulture Research. 2018;5:22.
80. Wasternack C, Jasmonates: an update on biosynthesis,signal transduction and action in plant stress response, growth and development. Annals of Botany (Lond). 2007;100:681–697.
81. Reinbothe C, Springer A, Samol I, Reinbothe S. Plant oxylipins: role of jasmonic acid during programmed cell death, defence and leaf senescence. FEBS Journal. 2009;276:4666–4681.
82. Hu Y, Jiang Y, Han X, Wang H, Pan J, Yu D. Jasmonate regulates leaf senescence and tolerance to cold stress: crosstalk with other phytohormones. Journal of Experimental Botany. 2017;68(6):1361–1369.
83. Ding F, Wang M, Zhang S. Sedoheptulose-1,7-Bisphosphatase is Involved in Methyl Jasmonate- and Dark-Induced Leaf Senescence in Tomato Plants. International Journal pf Molecular Sciences. 2018;19:3673.
84. Wasternack C, Hause B. Jasmonates: biosynthesis, perception, signal transduction and action in plant stress response, growth and development. An update to the 2007 review in Annals of Botany. Annals of Botany. 2013;111:1021–1058.
85. Ishiguro S, Kawai-Oda A, Ueda J, Nishida I, Okada K. The defective in anther dehiscence1 gene encodes a novel phospholipase A1 catalyzing the initial step of jasmonic acid biosynthesis, which synchronizes pollen maturation, anther dehiscence, and flower opening in *Arabidopsis*. The Plant Cell. 2001;13:2191–2209.
86. Feussner I, Wasternack C. The lipoxygenase pathway. Annual Review of Plant Physiology and Plant Molecular Biology. 2002;53:275–297.
87. Park JH, Halitschke R, Kim HB, Baldwin IT, Feldmann KA, Feyereisen RA knockout mutation in allene oxide synthase results in male sterility and defective wound signal transduction in *Arabidopsis* due to a block in jasmonic acid biosynthesis. Plant Journal. 2002;31(1):1–12.
88. Gu X, Chen J, Xiao Y, Di P, Xuan H, Zhou X, Zhang L, Chen W. Overexpression of allene oxide cyclase promoted tanshinone/ phenolic acid production in *Salvia miltiorrhiza*. Plant Cell Reports. 2012;31:2247–2259.

89. Zhao Y, Dong W, Zhang N, Ai X, Wang M, Huang Z, Xiao L, Xia G. A wheat allene oxide cyclise gene enhances salinity tolerance via jasmonate signaling. Plant Physiology. 2014;164:1068–1076.
90. Tani T, Sobajima H, Okada K, Chujo T, Arimura S, Tsutsumi N, Nishimura M, Seto H, Nojiri H, Yamane H. Identification of the *OsOPR7* gene encoding 12-oxophytodienoate reductase involved in the biosynthesis of jasmonic acid in rice. Planta. 2008;227(3):517–26.
91. Yan J, Zhang C, Gu M, Bai Z, Zhang W, Qi T, Cheng Z, Peng W, Luo H, Nan F, Wang Z, Xie D. The Arabidopsis *CORONATINE INSENSITIVE1* protein is a jasmonate receptor. The Plant Cell 2009;21:2220–2236.
92. Rowe HC, Walley JW, Corwin J, Chan EKF, Dehesh K, Kliebenstein DJ. Deficiencies in jasmonate-mediated plant defense reveal quantitative variation in *Botrytis cinerea* pathogenesis. PLoS Pathogens. 2010;6.
93. Sheard LB, Tan X, Mao H, Withers J, Ben-Nissan G, Hinds TR, Kobayashi Y, Hsu FF, Sharon M, Browse J, He SY, Rizo J, Howe GA, Zheng N. Jasmonate perception by inositol phosphate-potentiated *COI1- JAZ* co-receptor. Nature. 2010;468(7322):400–405.
94. Cheng Z, Sun L, Qi T, Zhang B, Peng, W, Liu Y, Xie D. The *bHLH* transcription factor *MYC3* interactswith the jasmonate ZIM-domain proteins to mediate jasmonate response in *Arabidopsis*. Molecular Plant. 2011;4:279–288.
95. Fernandez-Calvo P, Chini A, Fernández-Barbero G, Chico JM, Gimenez-Ibanez S, Geerinck J, Eeckhout D, Schweizer F, Godoy M, Franco-Zorrilla JM, Pauwels L, Witters E, Puga MI, Paz-Ares J, Goossens A, Reymond P, De Jaeger G, Solano R. The Arabidopsis *bHLH* transcription factors *MYC3* and *MYC4* are targets of *JAZ* repressors and act additively with MYC2 in the activation of jasmonate responses. The Plant Cell. 2011;23:701–715.
96. Niu Y, Figueroa P, Browse J. Characterization of *JAZ*-interacting *bHLH* transcription factors that regulate jasmonate responses in *Arabidopsis*. Journal of Experimental Botany. 2011;62:2143–2154.
97. Song S, Qi T, Fan M, Zhang X, Gao H, Huang H, Wu D, Guo H, Xie D. The *bHLH* subgroup IIId factors negatively regulate jasmonate-mediated plant defense and development. PLoS Genetics. 2013;9.
98. Fonseca S, Fernandez-Calvo P, Fernandez GM, Diez-Diaz M, Gimenez-Ibanez S, Lopez-Vidriero I, Godoy M, Fernandez-Barbero G, Van Leene J, De Jaeger G, Franco-Zorrilla JM. *bHLH003*, *bHLH013* and *bHLH017* are new targets of *JAZ* repressors negatively regulating JA responses. PLoS ONE. 2014;9.
99. Song S, Qi T, Huang H, Ren Q, Wu D, Chang C, Peng W, Liu Y, Peng J, Xie D. The jasmonate-ZIM domain proteins interact with the *R2R3-MYB* transcription factors *MYB21* and MYB24 to affect jasmonate-regulated stamen development in *Arabidopsis*. The Plant Cell. 2011;23:1000–1013.
100. Jan A, Maruyama K, Todaka D, Kidokoro S, Abo M, Yoshimura E, Shinozaki K, Nakashima K, Yamaguchi-Shinozaki K. *OsTZF1*, a CCCH-tandem zinc finger protein, confers delayed senescence and stress tolerance in rice by regulating stress-related genes. Plant Physiology. 2013;161:1202–1216.
101. Woo HR, Kim HJ, Nam HG, Lim PO. Plant leaf senescence and death — regulation by multiple layers of control and implications for aging in general. Journal of Cell Science. 2013;126:4823–4833.
102. Wang Z, Wang Y, Hong X, Hu D, Liu C, Yang J, Li Y, Huang Y, Feng Y, Gong H, Li Y, Fang G, Tang H, Li Y. Functional inactivation of UDP-N acetylglucosamine

pyrophosphorylase 1 (*UAP1*) induces early leaf senescence and defence responses in rice. Journal of Experimental Botany. 2015;66:973–987.

103. Ueda J, Kato J. Isolation and Identification of a Senescence-promoting Substance from Wormwood (*Artemisia absinthium* L.). Plant Physiology. 1980;66:246–249.
104. Weidhase RA, Kramell HM, Lehmann J, Liebisch HW, Lerbs W, Parthier B. Methyljasmonate-induced changes in the polypeptide pattern of senescing barley leaf segments. Plant Science. 1987a;51:171–186.
105. He Y, Fukushige H, Hildebrand DF, Gan S. Evidence supporting a role of jasmonic acid in Arabidopsis leaf senescence. Plant Physiology. 2002;128:876–884.
106. Weidhase RA, Lehmann J, Kramell HM, Sembdner G, Parthier B. Degradation of ribulose-1,5-bisphosphate carboxylase and chlorophyll in senescing barley leaf segments triggered by jasmonic acid methylester and counteraction by cytokinin. Physiologia Plantarum. 1987b;69: 161–166.
107. Parthier B. Jasmonates: hormonal regulators or stress factors in leaf senescence. Journal of Plant Growth Regulator. 1990;9:57–63.
108. Sembdner G, Parthier. The biochemistry and the physiological and molecular actions of jasmonates. Annual Review of Plant Physiology and Plant Molecular Biology. 1993;44:569–589.
109. Creelman RA, Mullet JE. Biosynthesis and action of jasmonates in plants. Annual Review of Plant Physiology and Plant Molecular Biology. 1997;48:355–381.
110. Wasternack C. Jasmonates: an update on biosynthesis, signal transduction and action in plant stress response, growth and development. Annals of Botany. 2007;100:681–697.
111. Balbi V, Devoto A. Jasmonate signalling network in *Arabidopsis thaliana*: crucial regulatory nodes and new physiological scenarios. New Phytologist. 2008;177: 301–318.
112. Van der Graaff E, Schwacke R, Schneider A, Desimone M, Flugge UI, Kunze R. Transcription analysis of *Arabidopsis* membrane transporters and hormone pathways during developmental and induced leaf senescence. Plant Physiology. 2006;141:776–792.
113. Shan X, Wang J, Chua L, Jiang D, Peng W, Xie, D. The role of *Arabidopsis* Rubisco activase in jasmonate-induced leaf senescence. Plant Physiology. 2011;155:751–764.
114. Jiang Y, Liang G, Yang S, Yu D. *Arabidopsis WRKY57* functions as a node of convergence for jasmonic acid- and auxin-mediated signaling in jasmonic acid-induced leaf senescence. The Plant Cell. 2014;26:230–245.
115. Qi T, Wang J, Huang H, Lui B, Gao H, Lui Y, Song S, Xie D. Regulation of jasmonate-induced leaf senescence by antagonism between *bHLH* subgroup IIIe and IIId factors in *Arabidopsis*. The Plant Cell. 2015;27:1634–1649.
116. Yan Y, Christensen S, Isakeit T, Engelberth, J, Meeley R, Hayward A, Neil Emery RJ, Kolomiets MV. Disruption of *OPR7* and *OPR8* reveals the versatile functions of jasmonic acid in maize development and defense. The Plant Cell. 2012;24(4):1420–1436.
117. Lee SH, Sakuraba Y, Lee T, Kim KW, An G, Lee HY, Paek NC. Mutation of *Oryza sativa* CORONATINE INSENSITIVE 1b (OsCOI1b) delays leaf senescence. Journal of Integrative Plant Biology. 2015;57(6):562–576.
118. Hisamatsua Y, Gotob N, Hasegawaa K, Shigemoria. Senescence-Promoting Effect of Arabidopside A. Z. Naturforsch. 2006;61c.
119. Baertschi SW, Ingram CD, Harris TM, Brash AR. Absolute configuration of *cis*-12-oxophytodienoic acid of flaxseed: implications for the mechanism of biosynthesis from the 13(*S*)-hydroperoxide of linolenic acid. Biochemistry. 1988;27:18–24.

120. Weber H, Vick BA, Farmer EE. Dinoroxo- pytodienoic acid: a new hexadecanoid signal in the jasmonate family. Proceedings of National Academy of Sciences of the USA. 1997;94:10473–10478.
121. Tsuchiya T, Ohta H, Okawa K, Iwamatsu A, Shimada H, Masuda T, Takamiya K. Cloning of chlorophyllase, the key enzyme in chlorophyll degradation: finding of a lipase motif and the induction by methyl jasmonate. Proceedings of National Academy of Sciences of the USA. 1999;96:15362–15367.
122. Weber H. Fatty acid-derived signals in plants. Trends in Plant Science. 2002;7:217–224.
123. Park SY, Yu JW, Park JS, Li J, Yoo SC, Lee SK, Jeong SW, Seo HS, Koh HJ, Park YI, Jeon JS, Paek NC, Lee NY. The senescence-induced stay green protein regulates chlorophyll degradation. The Plant Cell. 2007;19:649–1664.
124. Hortensteiner S. Stay-green regulates chlorophyll and chlorophyll-binding protein degradation during senescence. Trends in Plant Science. 2009;14:155–162.
125. Pruzinska A, Tanner G, Anders I, Roca M, Hortensteiner S. Chlorophyll breakdown: phaeophorbide a oxygenase is a Rieske-type iron-sulfur protein, encoded by the accelerated cell death 1 gene. Proceedings of National Academy of Sciences of the USA. 2003;100:15259–15264.
126. Mach JM, Castillo AR, Hoogstraten R, Greenberg JT. The Arabidopsis accelerated cell death gene ACD2 encodes red chlorophyll catabolite reductase and suppresses the spread of disease symptoms. Proceedings of National Academy of Sciences of the USA. 2001;98:771–776.
127. Seltmann MA, Stingl NE, Lautenschlaeger JK, Krischke M, Mueller MJ, Berger S. Differential impact of lipoxygenase 2 and jasmonates on natural and stress-induced senescence in *Arabidopsis*. Plant Physiology. 2010;152: 1940–1950.

14 Crosstalk Between Oxylipins and Other Metabolites

Abscisic Acid and Salicylic Acid

Mudasir A. Mir[1], Nadia Gul[2], Mohd Ashraf Bhat[1], Zaffar Bashir[3], Firdose A. Malik[4], and Mehrun Nisa[5]*

[1]Division of Plant Biotechnology, Sher-e-Kashmir University of Agricultural Sciences and Technology of Kashmir (SKUAST-K), Shalimar, Srinagar, India

[2]School of Biosciences and Biotechnology, Baba Ghulam Shah Badshah University, Rajouri, India

[3]Department of Microbiology, University of Kashmir, Srinagar, India

[4]College of Temperate Sericulture, Mirgund, Sher-e-Kashmir University of Agricultural Sciences and Technology of Kashmir (SKUAST-K), Srinagar, India

[5]Department of Botany, University of Kashmir, Srinagar, India

Corresponding author:
*Email: drmudasirmir@skuastkashmir.ac.in

CONTENTS

DOI: 10.1201/9781003316558-14

14.1 INTRODUCTION

The name oxylipin was used by Gerwick et al. [1] to designate oxygenated substances generated from fatty acids by a single mono- or dioxygenase enzyme. Additional enzyme families that catalyze the production of oxygenated fatty acid derivatives, such as hydratases, have since been found [2]. As a result, oxylipins may be present in almost every living organism, prokaryotic species like cyanobacteria produce oxylipin molecules from one or two metabolic processes, but eukaryotic plants like algae, mosses, and angiosperms have progressed sophisticated pathways that result in a wide array of over 500 distinct compounds [3]. Oxylipins assist plants in developing and responding to biotic and abiotic environmental cues [4]. The well-studied oxylipin is jasmonic acid (JA) and its precursor 12-oxo-phytodienoic acid (OPDA). The initial stage in the JA signal transduction pathway is the production of JA and JA-isoleucine [5].

Plants have developed a variety of approaches to defend itself against various stressors (Figure 14.1), including the accumulation of significant amounts of salicylic acid-SA [6]. SA is a naturally occurring plant hormone that functions as a signaling molecule, regulates a number of biochemical and physiological processes, and is thus involved in biotic and abiotic stress tolerance [7]. SA and its derivatives (salicylates) are plant-produced signals that activate plant defense genes in response to a stressful situation. An increase in the production of allele-chemicals and defense proteins is triggered when these signals become stronger; SA might be regarded a promising chemical for inducing stress tolerance [8, 9]. Hormones like SA supplemented ABA's activity and SA induces accumulation of ABA [10]. Similarly, many of the secondary messengers elicited by abscisic acid (ABA) can aid in the adaptation of plants to

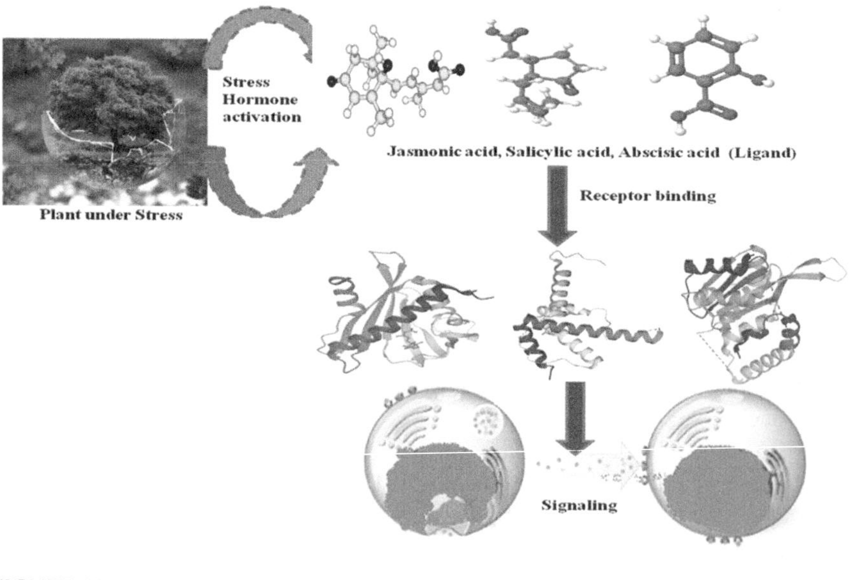

FIGURE 14.1 Stress Signaling in plants.

biotic and abiotic stress like cytosolic free Ca^{2+} and nitric oxide (NO) [11]. Tolerance to stress is promoted by many substances that regulate ABA production and vice versa [12]. The ABA-induced stomatal closure involves signaling pathway. These signaling component' interact with other to synergize the plant tolerance to pathogen invasions. The interactions of ABA with methyl jasmonate (MJ) or salicylic acid (SA) during pathogen resistance and stomatal closure are extensively documented [13].

14.2 THE ROLE OF JAMONATES IN STRESS

Jasmonates serve many purposes in plants during different abiotic and biotic stress [14, 15] and jasmonates are well-studied oxylipins in plants. Oxylipins are used by plants in stressful conditions and to increase systemic immunity. 12 oxo-phytodienoic acid (OPDA) is the main source of JA, during oxidative stress, reactive oxygen species (ROS) are produced and as a defensive response oxylipins are also formed non-enzymatically [16, 17]. Coronatine Insensitive1 (COI1) which is a F-box ubiquitin ligase interacts with transcriptional repressors in response to JA (members of the JAZ family). The repressors of JA including the JIN1-dependent MYC2/JA INSENSITIVE1 (JIN1) are destroyed as a consequence in the downstream [18]. OPDA, on contrary, promotes the expression of a large number of COI1-independent genes [19] which produces more JA. When plants are exposed to diverse abiotic stressors, they develop an osmotic imbalance [20]. The buildup of JA was induced by osmotic stress to counteract the osmotic imbalance [21]. Photosynthesis is inhibited by jasmonates and produce flavonoids buildup which can aid stress adaption [22]. It has been reported that an important artificial JA known as Pro-hydrojasmon improves cold tolerance by inducing anthocyanin and soluble sugars to accumulate, indicating its potential role against cold stress [23]. In the presence of high-intensity light, JA increases the formation of chalcones and flavonoids. JA also stimulates the production of sulfur-derived protective proteins like thionines under such low-light conditions [24]. Further, UVB rays were used to sensitize tobacco plants, increasing their susceptibility to 12OPDA and elicitation of JA production [25]. Hence, new signaling molecules that reconfigure the antioxidant system and restrict the rapid formation of reactive radicals are involved in oxylipin-mediated stress tolerance.

14.3 THE ROLE OF SALICYLIC ACID IN STRESS

Plants have designed a set of ways to protect themselves against various stresses, involving accumulation of large levels of SA [26, 27]. SA is a phenolic molecule that regulates plant growth and development, as well as their reactions to biotic and abiotic stress [28]. It also has a function in the activation of defense-related genes as well as stress tolerance in stressed plants [29]. Recent molecular investigations have shown that SA can control several elements of plant biology at the gene level, allowing plants to better withstand abiotic stress [30]. Several genes encoding chaperones, heat shock proteins (HSPs), antioxidants, and secondary metabolites have been shown to be induced by SA [31]. Furthermore, SA has been shown to have a key role in the regulation of mitogen-activated protein kinase (MAPK), as well as the regulation and activation of non-expressor of pathogenesis-related genes

1 (NPR1) [32]. Through signaling crosstalks with other phytohormones, SA can govern numerous elements of plant responses in both stressful and ideal situations [33]. In *S. lycopersicum*, SA caused the formation of abscisic acid (ABA) in both normal and salinity stressed plants, which aided osmotic adaptation and increased photosynthetic pigments and growth properties [34]. In chilling-exposed Z. mays, ABA treatment generated alterations in the endogenous SA, suggesting that SA-related stress responses may overlap with ABA-induced cold-acclimation [35]. Plant resistance to the biotrophic pathogen *Xanthomonasoryzaepv oryzae* is favorably regulated by JA signaling in rice, probably because both SA and JA activate a similar defense pathway [36–38].

14.4 THE ROLE OF ABSCISIC ACID IN STRESS

Under abiotic stress and pathogen invasion, plants accumulate hormones such as ABA, SA and Methyl Jasmonates [39]. ABA hormone is involved in a variety of abiotic and biotic stress situations, making it an important and versatile molecule. ABA production induces stomatal closure to conserve water under drought, salt, or cold stress, while also upregulating genes to enhance osmotic activities in leaves [40]. In addition to insect herbivores, increased ABA amount in plants facilitate cross-adaptation against diseases and drought [41]. Upon infestation of plants with pathogens, endogenous levels of ABA increased as well [42]. Drought increases ABA in roots as well as in foliar-ABA concentrations, suggesting that drought-induced ABA played a substantial role in modulating leaf water potential [43]. ABA was carried from the roots to the leaves, where it triggered stomatal closure and reduced transpirational water loss [44]. Temperature stress may also produce an increase in ABA levels (low or high) or CLE25, a recently found short peptide [45–47].

14.5 CROSSTALK BETWEEN JASMONATES, ABSCISIC ACID, AND SALICYLIC ACID

JA interacts with various signaling molecules in the stress response, either as a synergist or antagonist. The hormones, elicitors, and metabolites all interact with ABA and work together to increase abiotic stress tolerance [48] (Figure 14.2). The interaction of ABA with SA or MJ during stomatal closure and pathogen resistance is well documented [13]. In Arabidopsis, MJ increased ABA production by increasing the expression of the AtNCED3 gene [49]. ABA was needed during SA-action on stomata [50]. Increased ABA, apart from stomatal closure activates SID2 gene (salicylic acid induction deficient 2) and triggered SA biosynthesis [39]. The synergy of MJ, SA, and ABA during stomatal closure is confirmed by these studies. The formation of JA in soybean leaves before the synthesis of ABA is a quick response to water deficit conditions [51]. Despite the fact that JA and ABA have antagonistic relationships, OPDA functions in tandem with the latter hormone to activate ABA INSENSITIVE 5 (ABI5) translation during seed germination. This causes the polygalacturonase level to rise, allowing the seed to emerge from dormancy [52]. The protection of JA under heat stress is connected to signaling pathways mediated by SA [53]. Plants with a mutant JA dependent signaling system have been shown to react mostly to low light

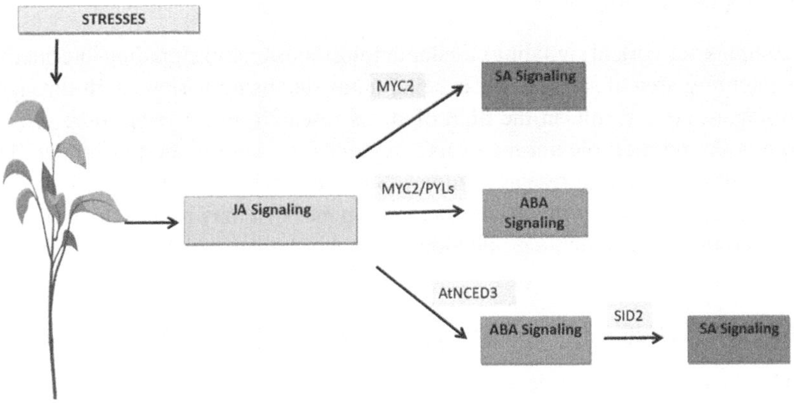

FIGURE 14.2 Oxylipins as central dogma of signaling under stress: Jasmonates as oxylipins have a central role in mediating hormonal signaling under stress conditions. They can directly interact with SA or ABA signaling or can work synergistically to mediate various stress response.

intensity [54]. The binding of the transcription factor MYC2 to the promoters of light-regulated genes is also thought to define crosstalk between the JA, ABA, and light-transduction pathways [55, 56].

ABA's influence on JA signaling may have an indirect effect on SA signaling [57]. Plants generate jasmonate and salicylate, which stimulate plant defense genes in response to herbivore or disease invasion [58]. Although the jasmonate and salicylate pathways are antagonistic, SA inhibits JA signaling through mechanisms involving NPR1, suppressor of salicylic acid insensitivity2 (SSI2), WRKY transcription factors, and MPK4, therefore. there is significant communication between them [59]. SA signaling primarily helps to combat biotrophic diseases and viruses, whereas JA signaling defends against necrotrophic pathogens and insects in pathogen control [60]. Plant responsiveness to herbivorous insect feeding is coordinated by the ABA and JA signaling pathways, which are antagonistic to plant growth and development. JAZs-MYC2 genes affect plant development and defense through interacting with the JA and ABA signaling pathways [61]. Through the JA signaling pathway, ABA receptor PYRABACTIN RESISTANCE1-like proteins (PYLs) govern metabolic reprogramming in *Arabidopsis thaliana* and tobacco [32]. As a result, the crosstalk between the ABA and JA signaling pathways may be used to assess elicitor-induced metabolic and growth reprogramming in plants [62]. Many components, including mitogen-activated protein kinase are involved in crosstalk between the JA and SA signaling pathways (MAPK) [63]. The crosstalk between the JA and SA signaling pathways, which coordinately control plant disease resistance to necrotrophic or hemibiotrophic diseases is mediated by MYC2 and its upstream MPK4 [14]. SA promotes early defense-related gene expression in infected plants, whereas JA causes late defense-related gene expression in infected plants, primarily in necrotrophic or hemibiotrophic pathogens in the necrotrophic stage [64].

14.6 CONCLUSION

The complex network of signaling cascade among thousands of signaling intermediates is an emerging area of science that is being unraveled using various high-throughput technologies. As a result, in the field of stress research, uncovering more crosstalk pathways among multiple hormones like oxylipins in a coordinated fashion will be a major focus of upcoming research studies. Such research will aid in the discovery of crucial genetic regulatory points and candidate genes that may be used to build stress-tolerant crops for sustainable production.

ABBREVIATIONS

OPDA	12-oxo-phytodienoic acid
ROS	reactive oxygen species
COI1	coronatine insensitive
JIN1	JA insensitive
HSPs	heat shock proteins
MAPK	mitogen-activated protein kinase
NPR1	non-expressor of pathogenesis-related genes 1
PYLs	pyrabactin resistance 1-like proteins

REFERENCES

1. Gerwick WH, Moghaddam M, Hamberg M. Oxylipin metabolism in the red alga Gracilariopsis lemaneiformis: mechanism of formation of vicinal dihydroxy fatty acids. Arch Biochem Biophys. 1991;290(2):436–44.
2. Volkov A, Liavonchanka A, Kamneva O, Fiedler T, Goebel C, Kreikemeyer B, et al. Myosin cross-reactive antigen of Streptococcus pyogenes M49 encodes a fatty acid double bond hydratase that plays a role in oleic acid detoxification and bacterial virulence. J Biol Chem. 2010;285(14):10353–61.
3. Andreou A, Brodhun F, Feussner I. Biosynthesis of oxylipins in non-mammals. Prog Lipid Res. 2009;48(3–4):148–70.
4. Pohl CH, Kock JLF. Oxidized fatty acids as inter-kingdom signaling molecules. Molecules. 2014;19(1):1273–85.
5. Thines B, Katsir L, Melotto M, Niu Y, Mandaokar A, Liu G, et al. JAZ repressor proteins are targets of the SCFCOI1 complex during jasmonate signalling. Nature. 2007;448(7154):661–5.
6. Shemi R, Wang R, Gheith E-S, Hussain HA, Hussain S, Irfan M, et al. Effects of salicylic acid, zinc and glycine betaine on morpho-physiological growth and yield of maize under drought stress. Sci Rep. 2021;11(1):1–14.
7. Nazar R, Iqbal N, Syeed S, Khan NA. Salicylic acid alleviates decreases in photosynthesis under salt stress by enhancing nitrogen and sulfur assimilation and antioxidant metabolism differentially in two mungbean cultivars. J Plant Physiol. 2011;168(8):807–15.
8. Tlak Gajger I, Dar SA. Plant allelochemicals as sources of insecticides. Insects. 2021;12(3):189.
9. Wang C-J, Yang W, Wang C, Gu C, Niu D-D, Liu H-X, et al. Induction of drought tolerance in cucumber plants by a consortium of three plant growth-promoting rhizobacterium strains. PLoS One. 2012;7(12):e52565.

10. Wang X, Kong L, Zhi P, Chang C. Update on cuticular wax biosynthesis and its roles in plant disease resistance. Int J Mol Sci. 2020;21(15):5514.
11. Huang H, Ullah F, Zhou D-X, Yi M, Zhao Y. Mechanisms of ROS regulation of plant development and stress responses. Front Plant Sci. 2019;10:800.
12. Adamipour N, Khosh-Khui M, Salehi H, Razi H, Karami A, Moghadam A. Role of genes and metabolites involved in polyamines synthesis pathways and nitric oxide synthase in stomatal closure on Rosa damascena Mill. under drought stress. Plant Physiol Biochem. 2020;148:53–61.
13. Koo YM, Heo AY, Choi HW. Salicylic acid as a safe plant protector and growth regulator. plant Pathol J. 2020;36(1):1.
14. Yang J, Duan G, Li C, Liu L, Han G, Zhang Y, et al. The crosstalks between jasmonic acid and other plant hormone signaling highlight the involvement of jasmonic acid as a core component in plant response to biotic and abiotic stresses. Front Plant Sci. 2019;10:1349.
15. Aslam S, Gul N, Mir MA, Asgher M, Al-Sulami N, Abulfaraj AA, et al. Role of jasmonates, calcium, and glutathione in plants to combat abiotic stresses through precise signaling cascade. Front Plant Sci. 2021;1172.
16. Ghorbel M, Brini F, Sharma A, Landi M. Role of jasmonic acid in plants: The molecular point of view. Plant Cell Rep. 2021;40(8):1471–94.
17. Phua SY, De Smet B, Remacle C, Chan KX, Van Breusegem F. Reactive oxygen species and organellar signaling. J Exp Bot. 2021;72(16):5807–24.
18. Gupta A, Bhardwaj M, Tran L-SP. JASMONATE ZIM-DOMAIN Family Proteins: Important Nodes in Jasmonic Acid-Abscisic Acid Crosstalk for Regulating Plant Response to Drought. Curr Protein Pept Sci. 2021;22(11):759–66.
19. Soriano G, Kneeshaw S, Jimenez-Aleman G, Zamarreño ÁM, Franco-Zorrilla JM, Rey-Stolle MF, et al. An evolutionarily ancient fatty acid desaturase is required for the synthesis of hexadecatrienoic acid, which is the main source of the bioactive jasmonate in Marchantia polymorpha. New Phytol. 2022;233(3):1401–13.
20. Rahman K, Ahmed N, Raihan M, Hossain R, Nowroz F, Jannat F, et al. Jute responses and tolerance to abiotic stress: Mechanisms and approaches. Plants. 2021;10(8):1595.
21. Devireddy AR, Zandalinas SI, Fichman Y, Mittler R. Integration of reactive oxygen species and hormone signaling during abiotic stress. Plant J. 2021;105(2):459–76.
22. Farooq M, Ahmad R, Shahzad M, Sajjad Y, Hassan A, Shah MM, et al. Differential variations in total flavonoid content and antioxidant enzymes activities in pea under different salt and drought stresses. Sci Hortic (Amsterdam). 2021;287:110258.
23. Kondo S. Usage and action mechanism of oxylipins including jasmonic acid on physiological aspects of fruit production. Sci Hortic (Amsterdam). 2022;295:110893.
24. Podolec R, Demarsy E, Ulm R. Perception and signaling of ultraviolet-B radiation in plants. Annu Rev Plant Biol. 2021;72:793–822.
25. Bazinet Q, Tang L, Bede J. Impact of future elevated carbon dioxide on C3 plant resistance to biotic stresses. Mol Plant-Microbe Interact. 2021;(ja).
26. Saleem M, Fariduddin Q, Castroverde CDM. Salicylic acid: A key regulator of redox signalling and plant immunity. Plant Physiol Biochem. 2021;168:381–97.
27. Zulfiqar F, Ashraf M. Bioregulators: unlocking their potential role in regulation of the plant oxidative defense system. Plant Mol Biol. 2021;105(1):11–41.
28. Saleem M, Fariduddin Q, Janda T. Multifaceted role of salicylic acid in combating cold stress in plants: a review. J Plant Growth Regul. 2021;40(2):464–85.
29. Shaukat K, Zahra N, Hafeez MB, Naseer R, Batool A, Batool H, et al. Role of salicylic acid–induced abiotic stress tolerance and underlying mechanisms in plants. In: *Emerging Plant Growth Regulators in Agriculture*. Elsevier; 2022. p. 73–98.

30. Kazerooni EA, Maharachchikumbura SSN, Adhikari A, Al-Sadi AM, Kang S-M, Kim L-R, et al. Rhizospheric Bacillus amyloliquefaciens protects Capsicum annuum cv. Geumsugangsan from multiple abiotic stresses via multifarious plant growth-promoting attributes. Front Plant Sci. 2021;12:821.
31. Ashraf HJ, Aguila LCR, Ahmed S, Haq IU, Ali H, Ilyas M, et al. Comparative transcriptome analysis of Tamarixia radiata (Hymenoptera: Eulophidae) reveals differentially expressed genes upon heat shock. Comp Biochem Physiol Part D Genomics Proteomics. 2022;41:100940.
32. Yang C, Dolatabadian A, Fernando WGD. The wonderful world of intrinsic and intricate immunity responses in plants against pathogens. Can J Plant Pathol. 2022;44(1):1–20.
33. Yusuf M, Khan MTA, Faizan M, Khalil R, Qazi F. Role of Brassinosteroids and Its Cross Talk with Other Phytohormone in Plant Responses to Heavy Metal Stress. In: *Brassinosteroids Signalling*. Springer; 2022. p. 179–201.
34. Mubarik MS, Khan SH, Sajjad M, Raza A, Hafeez MB, Yasmeen T, et al. A manipulative interplay between positive and negative regulators of phytohormones: A way forward for improving drought tolerance in plants. Physiol Plant. 2021;172(2):1269–90.
35. Khan MIR, Fatma M, Per TS, Anjum NA, Khan NA. Salicylic acid-induced abiotic stress tolerance and underlying mechanisms in plants. Front Plant Sci. 2015;6:462.
36. Kanna M, Tamaoki M, Kubo A, Nakajima N, Rakwal R, Agrawal G, et al. Isolation of an Ozone-Sensitive and Jasmonate-Semi-Insensitive Arabidopsis Mutant (oji1). Plant Cell Physiol. 2004;44:1301–10.
37. Yamada S, Kano A, Tamaoki D, Miyamoto A, Shishido H, Miyoshi S, et al. Involvement of OsJAZ8 in jasmonate-induced resistance to bacterial blight in rice. Plant Cell Physiol. 2012;53(12):2060–72.
38. Tamaoki D, Seo S, Yamada S, Kano A, Miyamoto A, Shishido H, et al. Jasmonic acid and salicylic acid activate a common defense system in rice. Plant Signal Behav. 2013;8(6):e24260.
39. Bharath P, Gahir S, Raghavendra AS. Abscisic acid-induced stomatal closure: An important component of plant defense against abiotic and biotic stress. Front Plant Sci. 2021;12:324.
40. Hewage KAH, Yang J, Wang D, Hao G, Yang G, Zhu J. Chemical manipulation of abscisic acid signaling: a new approach to abiotic and biotic stress management in agriculture. Adv Sci. 2020;7(18):2001265.
41. Llorens E, González-Hernández AI, Scalschi L, Fernández-Crespo E, Camañes G, Vicedo B, et al. Priming mediated stress and cross-stress tolerance in plants: Concepts and opportunities. In: *Priming-Mediated Stress and Cross-Stress Tolerance in Crop Plants*. Elsevier; 2020. p. 1–20.
42. Gupta A, Sinha R, Fernandes JL, Abdelrahman M, Burritt DJ, Tran L-SP. Phytohormones regulate convergent and divergent responses between individual and combined drought and pathogen infection. Crit Rev Biotechnol. 2020;40(3):320–40.
43. Hasan MM, Gong L, Nie Z-F, Li F-P, Ahammed GJ, Fang X-W. ABA-induced stomatal movements in vascular plants during dehydration and rehydration. Environ Exp Bot. 2021;186:104436.
44. Haworth M, Marino G, Cosentino SL, Brunetti C, De Carlo A, Avola G, et al. Increased free abscisic acid during drought enhances stomatal sensitivity and modifies stomatal behaviour in fast growing giant reed (Arundo donax L.). Environ Exp Bot. 2018;147:116–24.

45. Takahashi F, Suzuki T, Osakabe Y, Betsuyaku S, Kondo Y, Dohmae N, et al. A small peptide modulates stomatal control via abscisic acid in long-distance signalling. Nature. 2018;556(7700):235–8.
46. Zehra A, Raytekar NA, Meena M, Swapnil P. Efficiency of microbial bio-agents as elicitors in plant defense mechanism under biotic stress: A review. Curr Res Microb Sci. 2021;2:100054.
47. Wang H-Q, Sun L-P, Wang L-X, Fang X-W, Li Z-Q, Zhang F-F, et al. Ethylene mediates salicylic-acid-induced stomatal closure by controlling reactive oxygen species and nitric oxide production in Arabidopsis. Plant Sci. 2020;294:110464.
48. Saijo Y, Loo EP. Plant immunity in signal integration between biotic and abiotic stress responses. New Phytol. 2020;225(1):87–104.
49. Hossain MA, Munemasa S, Uraji M, Nakamura Y, Mori IC, Murata Y. Involvement of endogenous abscisic acid in methyl jasmonate-induced stomatal closure in Arabidopsis. Plant Physiol. 2011;156(1):430–8.
50. Wang P, Zhao Y, Li Z, Hsu C-C, Liu X, Fu L, et al. Reciprocal regulation of the TOR kinase and ABA receptor balances plant growth and stress response. Mol Cell. 2018;69(1):100–12.
51. Youssef MS, Renault S, Hill RD, Stasolla C. The soybean Phytoglobin1 (GmPgb1) is involved in water deficit responses through changes in ABA metabolism. J Plant Physiol. 2021;267:153538.
52. Savchenko T, Kolla VA, Wang C-Q, Nasafi Z, Hicks DR, Phadungchob B, et al. Functional convergence of oxylipin and abscisic acid pathways controls stomatal closure in response to drought. Plant Physiol. 2014;164(3):1151–60.
53. Clarke SM, Cristescu SM, Miersch O, Harren FJM, Wasternack C, Mur LAJ. Jasmonates act with salicylic acid to confer basal thermotolerance in Arabidopsis thaliana. New Phytol. 2009;182(1):175–87.
54. Raza A, Charagh S, Zahid Z, Salman M, Rida M. Jasmonic acid: a key frontier in conferring abiotic stress tolerance in plants. Plant Cell Rep [Internet]. 2020; Available from: https://doi.org/10.1007/s00299-020-02614-z
55. Bhagat PK, Verma D, Sharma D, Sinha AK. HY5 and ABI5 transcription factors physically interact to fine tune light and ABA signaling in Arabidopsis. Plant Mol Biol. 2021;107(1):117–27.
56. Yadav SK, Singla-Pareek SL, Ray M, Reddy MK, Sopory SK. Methylglyoxal levels in plants under salinity stress are dependent on glyoxalase I and glutathione. Biochem Biophys Res Commun. 2005;337(1):61–7.
57. Zamora O, Schulze S, Azoulay-Shemer T, Parik H, Unt J, Brosche M, et al. Jasmonic acid and salicylic acid play minor roles in stomatal regulation by CO2, abscisic acid, darkness, vapor pressure deficit and ozone. Plant J. 2021;108(1):134–50.
58. Kallure GS, Kumari A, Shinde BA, Giri AP. Characterized constituents of insect herbivore oral secretions and their influence on the regulation of plant defenses. Phytochemistry. 2022;193:113008.
59. Wani AB, Chadar H, Wani AH, Singh S, Upadhyay N. Salicylic acid to decrease plant stress. Environ Chem Lett. 2017;15(1):101–23.
60. Yang Y-X, J Ahammed G, Wu C, Fan S, Zhou Y-H. Crosstalk among jasmonate, salicylate and ethylene signaling pathways in plant disease and immune responses. Curr Protein Pept Sci. 2015;16(5):450–61.
61. Zhao B, Liu Q, Wang B, Yuan F. Roles of phytohormones and their signaling pathways in leaf development and stress responses. J Agric Food Chem. 2021;69(12):3566–84.

62. Lackman P, González-Guzmán M, Tilleman S, Carqueijeiro I, Pérez AC, Moses T, et al. Jasmonate signaling involves the abscisic acid receptor PYL4 to regulate metabolic reprogramming in Arabidopsis and tobacco. Proc Natl Acad Sci. 2011;108(14):5891–6.
63. Jagodzik P, Tajdel-Zielinska M, Ciesla A, Marczak M, Ludwikow A. Mitogen-activated protein kinase cascades in plant hormone signaling. Front Plant Sci. 2018;9:1387.
64. Ding L, Xu H, Yi H, Yang L, Kong Z, Zhang L, et al. Resistance to hemi-biotrophic F. graminearum infection is associated with coordinated and ordered expression of diverse defense signaling pathways. PLoS One. 2011;6(4):e19008.

15 Oxylipins in Plant Protection/Disease Management

Barbara Sawicka[1], *Piotr Barbaś*[2], *Dominika Skiba*[1], *Piotr Pszczółkowski*[3], and *Farhood Yeganehpoor*[4]

[1]Department of Plant Production Technology and Commodities Science, University of Life Sciences in Lublin, 20–950 Lublin, Poland; barbara.sawicka@up.lublin.pl; dominika.skiba@up.lublin.pl

[2]Department of Potato Agronomy, Institute of Plant Breeding and Acclimatization—National Research Institute, Jadwisin, 05-140 Serock, Poland; p.barbas@ihar.edu.pl

[3]Experimental Station for Cultivar Assessment of Central Crop Research Centre, Uhnin, 21-211 Dębowa Kłoda, Poland; p.pszczolkowski.inspektor@coboru.gov.pl

[4]Department of Plant Eco-Physiology, University of Tabriz, 51368 Tabriz, Iraq; farhoodyeganeh@yahoo.com

*Correspondence: barbara.sawicka@up.lublin.pl

CONTENTS

DOI: 10.1201/9781003316558-15

15.1 INTRODUCTION

Oxylipins are a group of metabolites produced by the oxidation of polyunsaturated fatty acids that are involved in immunity, vascular function, etc. To date, more than 100 oxylipins have been identified that play overlapping and interrelated roles [1–5]. Oxylipins are also a group of biologically active compounds, the structural diversity of which is generated by the coordinating action of lipases, lipoxygenases, and the group of cytochromes P450 specialized in the metabolism of hydroperoxy-fatty acids. Research to date has focused mainly on the biosynthesis of the plant jasmonic acid (JA) signaling molecule and its role in the regulation of developmental and defense-related processes [5, 6]. Genetic studies indicate that the metabolic precursors of jasmonate are active as signals in themselves, and their synthesis and perception are critical to the induced systemic defense response [7]. More and more evidence indicated that the common biological importance of oxylipins in plants is comparable to the eicosanoid family of lipid mediators in animals [8, 9]. Oxylipins are derived from polyunsaturated fatty acids (PUFAs) via COX (cyclooxygenase) enzymes, LOX (lipoxygenase) enzymes or cytochrome P450 peroxygenase. The bioactive acetylene oxylipins C17 and C18 usually contribute to the anti-inflammatory, cytotoxic, and anti-tumor properties of herbaceous plants. Oxylipins are widely distributed in plants of the *Apiaceae*, *Araliaceae* and *Asteraceae* families and induce cell cycle arrest and/or cancer cell apoptosis in vitro and have a chemopreventive effect on cancer development in vivo. Bioactive acetylene oxylipins C17 and C18 are a group of promising compounds that lead to the development of anti-cancer drugs and pesticides of plant origin [5, 10, 11].

Phytoxylipins are metabolites produced in plants as a result of the oxidative transformation of unsaturated fatty acids through many metabolic pathways. Biochemical analysis and a genetic approach have shown that the oxidized derivatives are actively involved in plant defense mechanisms. During the last decade of the 21st century, interest in this field has focused on the biosynthesis of jasmonic acid (JA) (a branch of the metabolism of C18 polyunsaturated fatty acids) and its relationship with other plant defense signaling pathways. Recently, however, antisense strategies have revealed that oxylipins other than jasmonates are also essential for plant resistance to pathogens [12].

The miRNA with dominance of secondary metabolism is the latest type of research and better information on the peripheral process of metabolism in plants, which will play a key role in achieving new types of results in controlled systems. Research on the production of secondary metabolites by maneuvering the role of miRNAs in various crops, such as medicinal, spice, ornamental, and food plants, may result in improved profitability not only of crops, but also of the food, pharmaceutical, and cosmetic processing industries [11, 12].

There are approximately 67,000 species of weeds, pathogens, and invertebrates in the world that pose the greatest challenge to agriculture. Of these species, 10,000 are arthropods, 30,000 are weeds, about 100,000 are plant pathogenic microorganisms (bacteria, fungi, viruses, viroid's, etc.), and about 1,000 are nematodes. Together, these organisms cause 40% of global food losses [13] despite the use of plant protection products. Weeds are considered the best known and harmful crop reducers [14].

The potential losses caused by weeds (34%) are much higher than those caused by invertebrates (18%) and pathogens (16%) [13]. Losses caused by agricultural pests in developing countries are 40–50% and are much greater, compared with 25–30% of losses in developed countries [13, 14]. It is predicted that these losses will increase even more in the coming future due to the globalization of trade, intensification of agriculture, and climate change [13, 15]. Hence, in order to better manage weeds, diseases, and pests, the aspect of biopesticides has been addressed. As the "European Green Deal" forces producers to change the approach to cultivation, especially plant protection, this chapter emphasizes the importance and advantages of enhancing the natural resistance of plants to pests, with particular emphasis on the importance of oxylipins in plant protection and treatment of plant diseases.

15.2 METHODOLOGY

In order to demonstrate the importance of bioactive compounds of the oxylipin (PO) type in the research and to fully assess the entire context, a quantitative analysis of the literature was carried out, which indicates a great interest in these compounds due to their very favorable properties and protective effects. The search for this group of bioactive compounds and their relationship to plant health was carried out using the Scopus database. The Scopus online database [16] was used to search for bibliometric data using the TITLE-ABS-KEY (Bioactive Compounds and Plant Protection) search. Publications that mentioned these words or their derivatives in the title, abstracts or keywords were identified in the search strategy [17]. The functions of the Scopus internet platform called "Analysis" and "Create a citation report" were used for basic analyses. Complete records and cited references have been exported to VOSviewer for additional processing. Then, the terms used in the titles of papers, abstracts of publications and keywords were analyzed using VOSviewer [17]. As a result of the search, 78 publications from the period from 1990 to 2022 were considered.

15.3 BUILDING THE NATURAL RESISTANCE OF PLANTS

To get to the main topic of the chapter, the process of building plant resistance is briefly presented. Plants have excellent strategies that use many constitutive or induced anatomical, molecular and biochemical defense mechanisms (Figure 15.1).

Induced immune responses, local at first, are triggered in response to a direct, sudden attack by a pathogen, injury or contact with a triggering molecule, or elicitor. They are a signal for the mobilization of the defense system in the entire plant and the appearance of the so-called systemic resistance. There is systemic induced system resistance (ISR), triggered by contact with non-pathogenic organisms or synthetic elicitors, and systemic acquired resistance (SAR), due to earlier contact with the pathogen, but as a result of the appearance of a large number of new data this one undergoes systematic modifications. Plants lack specialized, mobile immune cells and antibodies. This does not mean, however, that they are unable to effectively defend themselves against pathogens [18, 19].

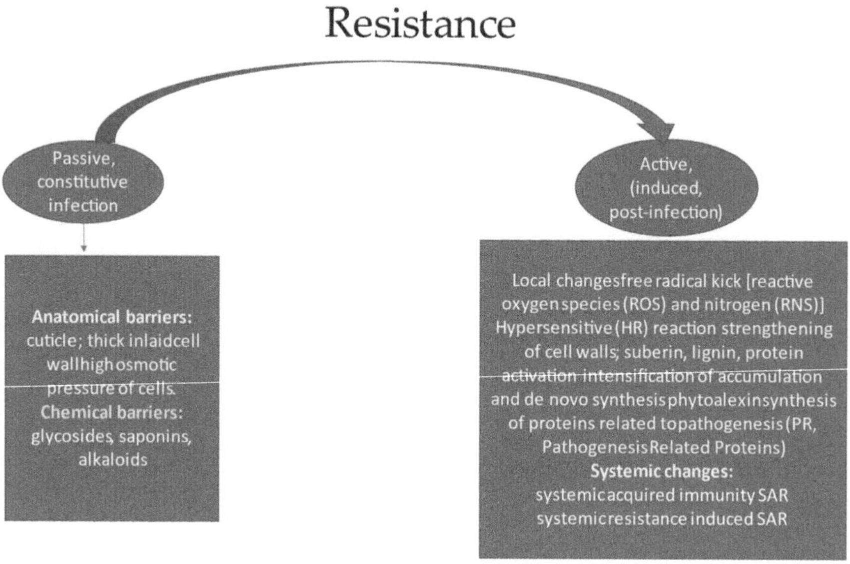

FIGURE 15.1 Types of plant resistance to pathogens.

Almost every plant cell is able to induce an effective defense response thanks to the action of the immune system. One of the models describing the plant immune system is the zigzag model proposed by Jones and Dangl [20], which includes two levels of it. The zigzag model shown in Figure 15.1 illustrates the successive steps in the plant-pathogen interaction. First, it presents pathogen-related molecular patterns (PAMPs). They are recognized by plant transmembrane PRR receptors, which allows for the emergence of molecular pattern induced immunity (PTI) and, finally, for the activation of a defense reaction. In the next phase, the infectious pathogen provides effectors that either interfere with PTI or enhance the nutrition and spread of the pathogen, ultimately leading to the development of sensitivity (ETS). Only in the third phase of this process, effectors can become avirulence factors (avr), when the plant already has the appropriate resistance proteins (R). Recognition of the immune effector by the R protein triggers a specific immune effector-triggered resistance (ETI), which leads to the development of a hypersensitivity reaction (HR). In the next phase, the pathogen may gain a new effector, e.g., in horizontal gene transfer, which may reduce ETI. In response, selection may favor new plant R alleles whose products recognize the new effector, again leading to the activation of the ETI [20, 21].

The effectors of plant (eukaryotic) pathogens are still poorly recognized. Effectors of fungi and oomycetes can act both in the extracellular matrix and inside the host cell. For example, tomato plants RLPs, Cf-2, Cf-4, Cf-5 and Cf-9 respond specifically to extracellular effectors produced by *Cladosporium fulvum* (*C. fulvum*). Other effectors of fungi and oomycetes most likely work inside the host cell. There they are recognized by the NB-LRR proteins. For example, the gene coding for Atr13 of the oomycetes effector of *Hyaloperonospora parasitica* (*H. parasitica*) is characterized by high allelic diversity among *H. parasitica* strains matched by diversity at locus 43 *Arabidopsis* RPP13 NB-LRR. This diversity is also seen within the Atr1 alleles of *H. parasitica* and *Arabidopsis* RPP144. Atr1 and Atr13 transport signal peptides for secretion from *H. parasitica*. They share with each other and with the protein *Phytophthora infestans* Mont. De Barry (*P. infestans*) Avr3a the RxLR motif, which allows the import of *Plasmodium* effectors into the host cells [19, 21].

Pathogens produce small molecule effectors that mimic plant hormones. For example, some strains of *P. syringae* produce coronatin, which mimics jasmonic acid, inhibiting salicylic acid-mediated defense against biotrophic pathogens and inducing stomatal opening, thereby helping pathogenic bacteria gain access to apoplast. PTI involves repression of an auxin response that is mediated in part by micro-RNA that is also induced during a stress response mediated by abscisic acid. Gibberellin, in turn, is produced by the fungal pathogen *Gibberella fujikuroi* (*G. fujikuroi*) leading to the "stupid seedling" syndrome. Cytokinin, which is produced by many pathogens, may promote the growth of pathogens by delaying the aging of infected leaf tissue. The interplay between PTI and normal hormone signaling and pathogen mimics is elucidated [19].

Such conditions arise as a result of the action of biotic factors (pests and pathogens) or abiotic factors, such as: lack or deficiency of water, oxygen, mineral compounds, high air and soil temperature, exposure to ultraviolet rays, deficiency or excess of photosynthetically active light, high concentrations mineral salts in the substrate, excessive concentration of metal ions, the presence of xenobiotics or their residues [18, 19]. The following elements determine plant immunity: 1) genetically determined properties of organism structures, referred to as innate (constitutive) immunity; 2) the ability of plants to regenerate; 3) adaptation abilities of the organism: plant organisms can adapt to life under stressful conditions in order to minimize the effect of stress, ensure the proper course of metabolic processes and produce offspring (adaptation processes, called acclimatization, hardening, and in phytopathology responsible for the acquired induced immunity, reactions to phytopathogens in plants). In nature, there are two types of plant resistance mechanisms: a) mechanisms allowing stress avoidance by preventing its effects, b) tolerance mechanisms enabling plants to survive the negative effects of stress [18, 21, 22]. The first type of mechanisms includes, for example, the creation of a root system or cover tissue with stomatal apparatus in terrestrial plants, morphological adjustments in xerophytic plants, modifications of cell wall structures that limit transpiration, and also hinder the growth of pathogens in the apoplast and are responsible for passive immunity, also called aksenia. Tolerance mechanisms mean, for example, activation of systems counteracting oxidative stress or enabling osmotic adjustments, activation of other, alternative metabolic pathways (allowing for the removal of excess or supplementation of some metabolites), activation of genes responsible for the synthesis of proteins necessary for the survival of stress, and in pathogenesis—the production of cork layer around infected sites, synthesis of phytoalexins (substances produced in response to infections caused by pathogens and inhibiting the development of these pathogens), formation of specific proteins that counteract infection, known as defense mechanisms or active immunity [21, 22, 23].

15.3.1 The Role of Phytohormones in Plant Resistance

Phytohormones are small molecules necessary for the proper growth, development, and reproduction of plants. They usually act as signal particles at low concentrations. Examples of plant phytohormones include: salicylic acid (SA), ethylene (ET), jasmonic acid (JA), auxin, abscisic acid (ABA), brassinosteroids, gibberellic acid and cytokinin [18]. Phytohormones play a very important role in the immune response of plants caused by biotic and abiotic stress factors. As signaling molecules, SA, JA, and ET influence the regulation of processes related to plant resistance. Also, ABA, auxins, as well as brassinosteroids and gibberellins are assigned certain functions in shaping immunity. Pathogenic infections stimulate plants to produce one or more types of hormones depending on the type of pathogen. SA-assisted signaling pathways participate in plant resistance against biotrophic and hemi biotrophic pathogens, while JA and ET dependent pathways participate in resistance against necrotic pathogens [18, 21, 22].

15.3.2 The Role of Jasmonates in Induced Plant Resistance Against Pathogens

Plants can develop local or systemic resistance induced by pathogens. This phenomenon is known as systemic acquired immunity (SAR). Non-pathogenic microorganisms or some elicitors can also induce induced or systemic resistance (ISR). Plant growth regulators such as jasmonates and salicylates play an important role in inducing these types of resistance. JA and MeJA as well as ethylene are components of the signal path that regulates the ISR response in plants, while SA and MeSA are essential for SAR induction [23, 24].

Oxylipins play an important role in plant development and responses to physical damage caused by herbivores and pathogenic microorganisms [8, 23, 24]. The attack of pathogens activates lipases that release unsaturated fatty acids, initiating the synthesis of oxylipins. One of the best known oxylipins is JA, a signaling molecule that supports plant survival in response to the challenges of insects and pathogens [18, 23, 25]. A critical step in the synthesis of oxylipins is the formation of fatty acid hydroperoxides as a catalyzing reaction by the LOX enzymes. *Arabidopsis thaliana* (*A. thalina*), as a reference species, has as many as six LOX genes, four of which encode the 13-LOX enzymes (numbered for the carbon into which oxygen is introduced). 13-LOXs catalyze the first step in the synthesis of oxylipins such as JA. The other genes: LOX, LOX1 and LOX5, encode the 9-LOX enzymes that play a role in plant development and their defense against pathogens [21, 26].

15.3.3 Oxylipin Biosynthesis Activation Specificity

Activation of enzymatic oxylipin biosynthesis after injury, herbivore or attack by pathogens depends on the biochemical activation of lipases that make polyunsaturated fatty acids (PUFA) available to lipoxygenases (LOX) v [26, 27]. The identity and number of lipases involved in this process are controversial and likely vary between plant species. For example, the analysis of transgenic *Nicotiana attenuata* (ir-gla1) plants stably reduced in the expression of the NaGLA1 gene showed that this plastidial glycerolipids is the main supplier of triene fatty acids for JA biosynthesis in leaves and roots after wounding and simulated vegetation, but not during *Phytophthora parasite* infection var. *nicotianae*. NaGLA1 is not necessary to control the development of JA biosynthesis in flowers and the biosynthesis of volatile substances C (6) in the hydroperoxide lyase (HPL) pathway. However, it influences the metabolism of divinyl ethers (DVE) in the early stage of infection with *P. parasitica* var. *nicotianae* and NaDES1 and NaLOX1 mRNA accumulation. Lysolipid profiling by LC-MS / MS has shown that lipase uses different classes of lipids as substrates. The complexity and specificity of the lipase-mediated regulation of oxylipin biosynthesis indicate the existence of pathway and stimulus-specific lipases [9, 28, 29]. LOXs are dioxygenases that catalyze the reaction of incorporating an oxygen molecule into a specific position of polyunsaturated fatty acids (peroxidation reaction), mainly of arachidonic acid [30–32]. COX exhibit dual catalytic activity: dioxygenase (cyclooxygenase), responsible for the synthesis of prostaglandin G2 (PGG2) from arachidonic acid, and peroxidase, which is responsible for the reduction of PGG2 to prostaglandin H2 (PGH2) [29].

Polyunsaturated fatty acids belong to the two families of omega-3 and omega-6. The parent form of the n-3 acid family is linolenic acid (ALA; 18: 3 n-3), and the bioactive forms are the following acids: eicosapentaenoic acid (EPA; 20: 5 n-3) and docosahexaenoic acid (DHA; 22: 6 n-3). This group also includes stearidic acid (STA; 18: 4 n-3) [33]. The parent acid of the n-6 family is linoleic acid (CLA; C18: 2 n-6). Other important acids in this family are: γ-linolenic (GLA) and dihomo-γ-linolenic (DGLA) and arachidonic (AA) acids [18, 29, 34, 35]. The main component of the cell membranes of cortical neurons in the peripheral nervous system is docosahexaenoic acid (DHA) [35]. DHA is also a substrate of neuroprotection and maresin. These compounds are involved in the final stage of the inflammatory process [36]. The main source of DHA is fat from fish and marine animals [Newton, 1996]. Stearidic acid (STA) is found, for example, in borage oil, evening primrose, echinacea and some tropical plants [37]. It is also located in the fruits of black currant [38], and its content depends on the genotype of the plant and is at the level of 2–4%. The highest content of γ-linolenic acid is found in rapeseed and soybean oils. A high content of this acid is also found in the green leaves of cruciferous vegetables [39].

Oxylipin biosynthesis is initiated by dioxygenases or monooxygenases, as well as non-enzymatic autoxidative processes, and as a result contributes to the formation of plant oxylipins (PO) (phytoprostanes, isoprostanes) [40, 41]. Dioxygenases include LOK [6, 30], heme-dependent fatty acid oxygenase (plants, fungi) [2, 42] and cyclooxygenase (COK) (animals) [29]. The enzyme responsible for the oxidation of fatty acids and esters in both plant and animal organisms is the LOX enzyme [43]. As a result, hydroxides and their decomposition products are formed. There is a divalent iron ion (Fe^{2+}) in the LOX molecule, which tends to be oxidized to a trivalent ion (Fe^{3+}) by fatty acid hydroperoxides or hydrogen peroxide. In this respect, work has been carried out on soybean [44, 45], potato [18, 46, 47], pea [48], lupine [49, 50] and other plant species [51, 52]. The formation of fatty acid hydroperoxides is the first step leading to the formation of a structurally diverse group of oxidized fatty acid metabolites (oxylipins) [53]. Plants receive information from the environment based on a network of signaling pathways that are intelligently connected [54] and guarantee an appropriate response to various stresses, such as herbivore foraging or abiotic stress [55]. Lipids constituting the main component of cell membranes are the first sites to experience environmental hazards [47].

Oxylipins also occur as signaling molecules in plant defense mechanisms [56–58]. JA and jasmonates are the best-known metabolites derived from LOX as they rapidly accumulate in damaged (injured) plants [59] and play an important role in wound signaling. Methyl-JA can be released as a volatile organic compound to predict the mutual threat between plants [60]. The JA level depends on the species, physiological and chronological age of the plant, and its highest content occurs in young plant tissues and flowers. They are bioactive compounds that participate in many physiological processes in plant and animal organisms. Their results suggest that the expression of the barley cysteine proteinase inhibitor Hv-CPI2 in tomato plants activates endogenous, direct and indirect defense mechanisms [59]. The high biodiversity of oxylipins, both in terms of structure and function, reflects the complex control of their biosynthetic activity, which derives from the precise connections between different signaling pathways [56].

Although oxylipins can be synthesized from free fatty acids, they are also components of the plastid-localized lipids of the polar complex, e.g., in *A. thaliana*. Also included are oxophytiodienoic acid (OPDA), dinor-OPDA (dnOPDA), 18-carbon ketonic acids and 16-carbon ketonic acids [61].

Weber et al. [62] showed a differentiated content of oxylipins in injured and undamaged leaves of *A. thaliana* and Solanum tuberosum. The level of OPDA was significantly higher than that of JA in healthy Arabidopsis leaves, while in potato leaves the levels of these two compounds were similar. In injured leaves of *A. thaliana*, the level of JA was significantly higher than that of OPDA, while in damaged leaves of S. tuberosum, the level of OPDA was higher than that of JA. Jasmonates mediate resistance responses to insect attack, especially to certain necrotrophic fungal pathogens and non-pathogenic fungi, and to the action of *Erwinia carotovora* [63–65]. Tomato plants poor in jasmonic acid (JA) are very susceptible to the action of spider mites [60].

15.4 PLANT VOLATILES AS MULTIFUNCTIONAL WEAPON AGAINST HERBIVORES AND PATHOGENS

Plants in the AgroSystem cannot avoid the attacks of moth-forming microorganisms and pests. As a consequence, plants "arm themselves" with molecular weapons against their attackers. All plant defense responses are based on a complex signaling network in which the hormones jasmonic acid (JA), salicylic acid (SA), and ethylene (ET) are suspected of interactions between the host and the pest. It is the leaf volatile compounds (GLV), C_6 carbon particles that are very quickly produced and emitted by green plants after infection with an herbivore or pathogen. They play a very important role in plant protection. GLVs are semiochemicals used by insects to search for food. They are crucial in indirect defense and directly affect pests, but not only. These volatile substances are also able to directly trigger plant defense responses. GLV, thanks to the crosstalk with phytohormones (mainly JA), can influence the defense reaction of plants against pathogens. GLVs consist of C_6 compounds, including alcohols, aldehydes and esters, and their name derives from their smell, reminiscent of the smell of fresh, cut grass [2, 67].

GLVs are produced by herbaceous plants and their increased release may be caused by abiotic factors, pathogens or herbivores [6–10]. GLVs are also involved in inducing plant defense and inducing so-called "Priming," i.e., a state that prepares the plant for an extended response to an attack by herbivores or a pathogen [19, 66].

Due to the fact that GLVs are involved in many aspects of the adaptation of plants to their environment, they are defined as multi-faceted molecules, resulting from disturbances in the plant system, and which help them survive in a hostile environment. Their special physiological importance should be emphasized, and this proves that they play a key role in plant defense responses. GLVs are also emitted by plants under the influence of biotic stress caused mainly by pathogens. For example, after infection with the pathogenic bacterium *Pseudomonas syringae* var. *phasolicola*, lima bean leaves release E-2-hexenal and Z-3-hexenol [67]. In turn, *Nicotiana tabaccum* infected with *Pseudomonas syringae* pv. *syringae* emits E -2-hexenal [68]. In both cases, GLV secretion begins between 18 and 20 hours post infection, while bacteria grow exponentially, which takes three days [66]. *Pseudomonas syringae* v. *multiplies i*n the apoplast and is a hemibiotrophic pathogen [67]. GLVs are characterized by antimicrobial activity against bacteria [67, 68]. This applies to C6 aldehydes, of which E-2-hexenal has the highest antimicrobial activity due to the reactive, electrophilic α, β-unsaturated carbonyl group. It would be very beneficial for the plant to produce GLV shortly after being injured in order to limit infection and significantly inhibit bacterial growth [68, 69].

Herbivorous caterpillars contain effectors in their oral secretions that alter green leaf volatile substances (GLV) produced by the plants that the caterpillars feed on. These are isomerase, fatty acid dehydratase (FHD), and the heat-stable hexenal retaining molecule (HALT). GLVs function as signaling compounds in plant-insect interactions and communication between plants. Jones et al. [69] investigated the distribution and activity of the isomerase effectors, FHD and HALT in 10 species from 7 butterfly families. Six out of 10 species had all three effectors in their oral secretions. The activity of the HALT and FHD effectors was observed in all investigated caterpillars, and the activity of the isomerase effector was varied. It has been shown that GLV-altering effectors, acting on the GLV biosynthetic pathway and present in the investigated caterpillars, emphasize the importance of these effectors in changing the emission of these compounds during caterpillars herbivorousness.

Data on the antimicrobial activity of GLV are based on in vitro studies. For example, Lima bean leaves, immediately after being infected with *Pseudomonas*, release E-2-hexenal and Z-3-hexenol in concentrations that inhibit bacterial growth in vitro [66]. However, in vitro tests do not consider that bacteria are found in a living organism and are not only in contact with volatile substances, but interact with the host in other ways, or vice versa. So far, the role of HPL, a key enzyme in GLV biosynthesis, on disease development in plant-bacterial interactions has been investigated. HPL has been shown to have a beneficial effect on the growth of *P. syringae* DC3000 by inducing higher JA levels in infected *Arabidopsis* compared to HPL plants [63]. Initial treatment with E -2-hexenal increases the bacterial population, and the end result is dependent in part on coronatin and on a transcription factor that integrates both JA and ET signaling pathways [68, 69]. *Pseudomonas* exploits the antagonistic effects of JA on the SA-dependent defense mechanisms of Arabidopsis through the synthesis of coronatine that mimics JA-Ile. *Pseudomonas* benefits from inducing HPL by taking advantage of the effect on the JA pathway. However, this must be confirmed by further research [69, 70]. According to Stolterfoht et al. [70] plant extracts are used as sources of LOX and HPL. However, these processes are limited by the low enzyme concentration, stability, and specificity. Alternatively, however, recombinant enzymes can be used as biocatalysts for the synthesis of GLV.

15.4.1 Internal "Communication" of the Oxylipin Kingdom

POs are involved in plant-plant, plant-pathogen, and plant-insect interactions, and recently research is being done on lipid-mediated communication between hosts and pathogens [47]. It has been shown that organisms commonly use the oxylipin pathways as a means of communication to obtain biological responses. Fungal oxylipins (FO) modify the reactions of both plant and mammal hosts [71]. The research of Fernandez-Conradi [72] proved that fungi may be important, so far overlooked factors of interactions between plants and herbivores. They suggest a direct as well as an indirect influence of fungi on the behavior and development of insects. Many microbes, including fungi, produce eicosanoids. These substances can mediate host penetration with the pathogen by weakening the host's local defense responses and increasing their virulence [2, 71]. Plants and fungi have been suggested to communicate using the oxylipine "tongue," mainly through quorum sensing-like mechanisms [73]. Thus, a clear response to the exogenous use of PUFA derivatives purified from interacting partners should be observed. C18: 2 products (e.g., 9 (S)—and 13 (S) -HPOD) or green leaf volatile compounds (GLV) regulate fungal growth, spore development, and mycotoxin production in Aspergillus sp. And grown on various plant species [74, 75], confirming the hypothesis that FO and OP may be involved in quorum detection. Because prematurely developed sex inducer factors (psi) are similar to PO and can influence the physiological processes of fungi mimicking the action of FO [71, 74], thus facilitating cross-perception of these molecules [72]. Analyses of several genomes revealed the presence of fungal GPCR (G protein-coupled receptor). Affeldt [74] proved that GPCRs were responsible for the perception of HPO. Hence, they should be recognized as oxylipin receptors [75, 76]. This supports the hypothesis that FO, along with all stimulus forms, can be perceived by fungi through a GPCR-mediated cascade.

Future research should focus on the structural foundations of GPCR-effector interactions and the signaling conformations that will provide the missing link in order to gain a better understanding of the mechanistic underpinnings of GPCR activation and signaling.

15.4.2 Research on the Use of OP

The role of PO in plant defense signaling pathways is described in the literature, but direct interaction of PO with pathogens is also possible. Research on the

TABLE 15.1
List of Effective Non-Antimicrobial POs in "in vitro" Tests

	Strain Bacteria			Fungi								Oomycetes	
PO	Pc	Ps	Xc	Ab	Bc	Ch	Fo	Lm	Rsp	Ss	IV	Pi	Pp
ω-5(Z)-Etherolenic acid	–	++++	–	+++	– +	–	++	–	–	–	+	–	+
(±)-cis-12,13-Epoxy-9(Z)-octadecenoic acid	–	–	–	++	–	+++	–	–	+	++	–	–	+++
(±)-cis-9,10-Epoxy-12(Z)-octadecenoic acid	–	++	–	–	–	+++	–	++	+	–	–	–	++
(±)-threo-12,13-Dihydroxy-9(Z)-octadecenoic acid	–	–	–	++	–	+++	–	+++	–	+	–	–	–
(±)-threo-9,10-Dihydroxy-12(Z)-octadecenoic acid	–	– +	+	++	–	–	–	–	–	+	–	–	–
10(S),11(S)-Epoxy-9(S)hydroxy12(Z),15(Z)-octadecadienoate	–	–	–	x	–	–	–	x	–	x	x	–	–
11(S),12(S)-Epoxy-13(S)hydroxy9(Z),15(Z)-octadecadienoate	–	++	–	x	+	–	–	x	–	x	x	+	–
13(S)-Hydroperoxy9(Z),11(E),15(Z)-octadecatrienoic acid (13-HPOT)	–	–	–	++	++++	++++	+ ++	–	–	–	–	+++	+
13(S)-Hydroperoxy-9(Z),11(E)-octadecadienoic acid (13-HPOD)	–	+	–	–	–	++++	–	–	–	–	–	–	++++
13(S)(Z),11(E),15(Z)octadecatrienoic acid (13-HOT)	–	–	–	+	++++	++++	–	+++	–	–	–	–	++++
13(S)-Hydroxy-9(Z),11(E)-octadecadienoic acid (13-HOD)	–	+	–	–	+	++++	+	–	–	–	–	+	++++

[a] Oxylipins were tested at concentrations up to 100 μM and measurements were made after a 24-hour incubation.

[b] Test bacteria: *Pectobacterium carotovorum* (Pc), *Pseudomonas syringae* (Ps) and *Xanthomonas campestris* (Xc). Tested fungi: *Alternaria brassicae* (Ab), *Botrytis cinerea* (Bc), *Cladosporium herbarum* (Ch), *Fusarium oxysporum* (Fo), *Leptosphaeria maculans* (Lm), *Rhizopus* sp. (Rsp), *Sclerotinia sclerotiorum* (Ss) and *Verticillium longisporum* (VI). Test oomycetes: *Phytophthora infestans* (Pi) and *Phytophthora parasitica* (Pp). ++++, very high efficiency; +++, highly effective; ++, moderately effective; +, effective; – ineffective; x, not tested.

Source: own based on Granér, et al. [78] and Prost et al., [80], modified by D. Skiba potential antimicrobial effects of PO focuses on the in vitro effects of PO against biotrophic, necrotrophic or hemibiotrophic pathogens. Oxylipins derived from the 9-LOX and α-DOX pathways show a very strong anti-bacterial activity [67]. The in vitro activity and stability of 50 PO against 13 agriculturally important pathogens (bacteria, fungi and oomycetes) were tested [77]. All pathogens were inhibited by one or more oxylipins. They turned out to be even more effective in inhibiting the germination of fungal spores, with a very high effectiveness of such acids as: (ω-5-Z) -etherolenic acid, colnenic acid and colnelenic acid [77, 78]. It is generally accepted that divinyl-, keto- and hydroxy-FAs and HPO have very strong direct antimicrobial activity, while other JAs and some volatile aldehydes are only suggested for signaling.

As shown in table 15.1, the growth of all pathogens was inhibited by one or more oxylipins. OPs were even more effective in inhibiting fungal spore germination, especially with a very high effectiveness of (ω-5-Z) -etherolenic, colneic and colnelenic acids [77, 78]. It is assumed that divinyl-, keto- and hydroxy-FAs and HPO show a strong direct antimicrobial effect, while others, JA and some volatile aldehydes, are only suggested as signaling. Since the previously described studies were performed in vitro, it is unclear whether oxylipins can induce these defense mechanisms also under field conditions. In nature, plants do not experience isolated stress, and the reactions are controlled by various OP pathways that can interact and inhibit each other [77]. Arabidopsis plants grown in an air-conditioned chamber were pretreated with 9-LOX-derived oxylipins and then challenged with *P. syringae* DC3000. The effect of this experiment was observed in local tissues, and a significant reduction in bacterial growth was observed in distal leaves, mainly from 9-KOT, as predicted by in vitro tests. Further genetic studies also confirmed that 9-LOX influences *Pseudomonas* responsive genes that are associated with oxidative stress and hormonal responses [67]. Hence, 9-LOX as well as other active PO compounds can support the innate resistance of plants as elicitors and / or direct biocides. However, only 50 POs have been tested in vitro, so the ability of the others as direct biocides or elicitors is questionable. At the same time, the molecular mechanisms of this biocidal activity should be elucidated. Multidisciplinary approaches (e.g., metabolomics, proteomics, transcriptomics) can help to better understand how oxylipins work in plant stress responses. Moreover, the subcellular localization of OP during pathogen attack should be elucidated as it is a key element in the development of new biological control agents. An integrated biological approach should be taken where scientists mimic the actual field stresses (culture medium, strain selection, application pattern, duration and duration of stress, growth conditions, etc.).

15.5 CONCLUSIONS AND FUTURE PERSPECTIVES

The European Green Deal focuses on sustainable agriculture and a significant increase in the acreage of organic farming. Therefore, biological methods of plant protection should be introduced on a larger scale than before. This is related to building higher awareness of agricultural producers and the use of plant protection products that are safe for consumers. The implementation of the principles of biological protection into practice requires full commitment and focus on professional cultivation, commitment, and the high level of knowledge of the farmer. When using biological products in plant protection, strictly follow the recommendations for their use, which often require changes in technology. In the case of "biology," the basis is prevention and consistency in action.

Recent research using molecular genetics and biotechnological methods in both pathogens and their hosts has increased the overall level of knowledge in the field. It has been suggested that some HPO may exert antimicrobial activity through interaction with pathogen membranes, in particular 13 (S) -HPOD, which increases the concentration-dependent fluidity of yeast membrane at the level of membrane lipids. This gave rise to the notion that oxylipins can sometimes be incorporated into the two layers of the membrane, increasing its disturbance, modifying their functions, and thus influencing the contact between microorganisms and plants. The recent discovery of an RNAi and small RNA exchange between *A. thaliana* and *B. cinerea* suggests that there is a bidirectional oxylipin exchange between kingdoms. Recent discoveries therefore lead to a better understanding of how plants and innate immunity and defenses work.

The search for alternatives to intensive farming is a difficult research area. Increasing the knowledge of how plants respond to stresses at the molecular, physiological and metabolic levels will be crucial for the development of new plant varieties and even more for the development of new biopesticides.

The physiological role of different classes of oxylipins in the defense mechanisms of plants was elucidated. These findings add importance to a deeper understanding of how plants and their innate immunity and defenses work, but there are still gaps to be filled, such as:

- perception of signals related to wounds or pathogen initiators and mechanisms at the cellular level by which they induce a rapid response of damaged tissues,
- contribution of transduction signals (air, chemical, physical signals) to the systemic defense response of healthy tissues,
- discovery of the molecular mechanisms involved in the inactivation of the stress signal,
- explaining the role of unstable stress signals,
- emitting OP by damaged plants and their impact on their condition and agricultural productivity.

ABBREVIATIONS

AA	arachidonic acid
ABA	abscisic acid
ALA	linolenic acid (8:3 n-3)
Avr	avirulence factor
A. thaliana	*Arabidopsis thaliana*
C. fulvum	*Cladosporium fulvum*
CLA	linoleic acid (C18:2 n-6)
COX	cyclooxygenase
DGLA	dihomo-γ-linolenowy (DGLA)
E	effector

EPA	eicosapentaenoic acid (20:5 n-3) DHA—docosahexaenoic acid (22:6 n-3)
ET	ethylene
ETI	effector-induced resistance
ETS	effector-triggered sensitivity
FHD	fatty acid dehydratase
FO	fungal oxylipins
G. fujikuroi	*Gibberella fujikuroi*
GLA	γ-linolenic acid
GLV	green leaf volatiles
GPCR	G protein-coupled receptor
HALT	thermostable hexenal retaining molecule
H. parasitica	*Hyaloperonospora parasitica*
HPL	a key enzyme in GLV biosynthesis
HR	hypersensitivity reaction
ISR	induced systemic resistance
JA	jasmonic acid
LOX	lipoxygenase
MAMP	molecular patterns associated with microorganisms
MeJA	jasmonic acid methyl ester
MeSA	salicylic acid methyl
P450	cytochrome peroxygenase
PAMP	patterns molecular pathogen-related
PGG_2	prostaglandins G2
PGPR	plant growth-promoting bacteria
Ph. Infestans	*Phytopthora infestans*
PO	plants oxylipin
PR	pathogenesis-related proteins
PRR	molecular pattern recognition receptors
PTI	resistance induced by molecular patterns
R	resistance gene/protein
SA	salicylic acid
SAR	systemic acquired resistance
STA	stearic acid (18:4 n-3)
TD	threonine deaminase

REFERENCES

1. Blue E. Impact of phyto-oxylipins in plant defense. Trends Plant Sci. 2002, 7(7): 315–22. doi: 10.1016/s1360–1385(02)02290–2. https://pubmed.ncbi.nlm.nih.gov/12118169 (accessed 02.05.2022).
2. Brodhun F., Feussner I. 2011. Oxylipins in fungi. FEBS Journal, 2011, 278(7): 1047–1063.
3. Caligiuri S P.B., Parikh M., Stamenkovic A., Pierce G.N., Aukema H.M. Dietary modulation of oxylipins in cardiovascular disease and aging. Am. J. Physiol. Hear. Circ. Physiol., 2017, 313: 903–918.

4. Chechetkin I.R., Blufard A.S., Yarin A.Y., Fedina E.O., Khairutdinov B.I., Grechkin, A.N. Detection and identification of complex oxylipins in meadow buttercup (Ranunculus acris) leaves. Phytochemistry,2019, 157: 92–102.
5. Christensen LP. Bioactive C17 and C18 Acetylenic Oxylipins from Terrestrial Plants as Potential Lead Compounds for Anticancer Drug Development, Molecules, 2020, 25(11): 2568, doi: 10.3390/molecules25112568.
6. Porta H, Rocha-Sosa M. Plant lipoxygenases. Physiological and molecular features. Plant Physiol. 2002 Sep,130(1):15–21. doi: 10.1104/pp.010787.
7. Mastrogiovanni, M., Trostchansky, A., Naya, H., Dominguez, R., Marco, C., Povedano, M., López-Vales, R., Rubbo, H. HPLC-MS/MS Oxylipin Analysis of Plasma from Amyotrophic Lateral Sclerosis Patients. Biomedicines 2022, 10, 674. https://doi.org/10.3390/biomedicines10030674.
8. Howe GA, Schilmiller AL. Oxylipin metabolism in response to stress. Curr Opin Plant Biol. 2002, 5(3):230–6. doi: 10.1016/s1369–5266(02)00250–9
9. Dąbkowska M. Znaczenie wielonienasyconych kwasów tłuszczowych WNKT omega 3 i omega 6 w żywieniu człowieka. Acta Salutem Scientiae, 2021, 2: 19–31.
10. Göbel C, Feussner I, Hamberg M, Rosahl S. Oxylipin profiling in pathogen-infected potato leaves. Biochim Biophys Acta. 2002,1584(1): 55–64. doi: 10.1016/s1388–1981(02)00268–8
11. Hossain R, Quispe C, Saikat ASM, Jain D, Habib A, Janmeda D, Islam MT, Radha J, Daştan SD, Kumar M, Butnariu M, Cho WC, Sharifi-Rad J, Kipchakbayeva A, Calina D. Biosynthesis of secondary metabolites based on cooperation with microRNA. BioMed Research International 2022(2), DOI:10,1155/2022/9349897.
12. Christie, William W, and John L Harwood. Oxidation of polyunsaturated fatty acids to produce lipid mediators. Essays in Biochemistry 2020, 64(3): 401–421. doi:10.1042/EBC20190082
13. Sawicka B. Loss of agricultural products after harvest. [In:] Leal Filho W., Azul A., Brandli L., Özuyar P., Wall T. (ed.) *Zero Hunger. Encyclopedia of the UN's Sustainable Development Goals*. Springer, 2020, Cham DOI: https://doi.org/10.1007/978-3-319-69626-3. (accessed 24.05.2022).
14. WHO 2020, World health statistics 2020: monitoring health for the SDGs, sustainable development goals? ISBN 978–92–4-000511–2 (print version).
15. Sawicka, B., Barbaś, P., Pszczółkowski, P., Skiba, D., Yeganehpoor, F., Krochmal-Marczak, B. Climate Changes in South-Eastern Poland and Food Security. Climate, 2022, 10, 57. https://doi.org/10.3390/cli10040057
16. Scopus, 2022. A professionally selected database of abstracts and citations. www.elsevier.com/pl-pl/solutions/scopus (accessed 05.03.2022).
17. Software, V, VOSviewer 2021, www.vosviewer.com/VOSviewer (accessed 07.03.2022).
18. Starck Z. Plant physiology: what was yesterday, what is today, and what will tomorrow bring? Cosmos, Problems of Biological Sciences, 2014, 63 (4): 569–589.
19. Banasiak J. System odpornościowy roślin—model zygzakowy. Postępy Biochemii. Advances in Biochemistry, 2022, DOI: https://doi.org/10.18388/pb.2021_427 (in Polish).
20. Dangl JL, Jones JD. Plant pathogens and integrated defense responses to infection. Nature. 2001, 14,411(6839):826–33. doi: 10.1038/35081161.
21. Jones JD, Dangl JL, The Plant immune system. Nature, 2006, 444 (7117): 323–9. DOI: 10.1038/nature05286
22. Wojtasik W, Kuma A. Plant response to biotic stress factors. Postępy Biologii Komórki 2016, 43(3), 453–476. (in Polish)

23. Yu, Y., Guy, Y., Li, Z., Jiang, C., Guo, J., Niu, D. Induced Systemic Resistance for Improving Plant Immunity by Beneficial Microbes. Plants 2022, 11, 386. https://doi.org/ 10.3390/plants11030386
24. Bisgaard, J., Colombes, J., Hirt, H. Signaling Mechanisms in Pattern-Triggered Immunity (PTI). Mol. Plant 2015, 8, 521–539
25. Bisgaard, J., Colcombet, J., Hirt, H. Signaling Mechanisms in Pattern-Triggered Immunity (PTI). Mol. Plant 2015, 8, 521–539.
26. Ghanta S, Chattopadhyay S. Glutathione as a signaling molecule: another challenge to pathogens. Plant Signal Behav. 2011, 6(6): 783–788. doi:10.4161/psb.6.6.15147
27. Singh, P., Arif, Y., Miszczuk, E., Bajguz, A., Hayat, S. Specific Roles of Lipoxygenases in Development and Responses to Stress in Plants. Plants 2022, 11, 979. https://doi.org/ 10.3390/plants11070979
28. Hayward, S., Cilliers, T., Swart, P. Lipoxygenases: From isolation to application. Compr. Rev. Food Sci. Food Saf. 2016, 16, 199–211.
29. Viswanath, K.K., Varakumar, P., Pamuru, R.R., Basha, S.J., Mehta, S., Rao, A.D. Plant lipoxygenases and their role in plant physiology. J. Plant Biol. 2020, 63, 83–95.
30. Gabbs M., Leng S., Devassy J.G., Monirujjaman Md, Aukema H.M. Advances in our understanding of oxylipins derived from dietary PUFAs. American Society for Nutrition. Adv Nutr., 2015, 6: 513–540.
31. Liavonchanka A., Feussner I. Lipoxygenases: occurrence, functions and catalysis. Journal of Plant Physiology, 2006, 163(3): 348–357.
32. Offenbacher, A.R., Holman, T.R. Fatty acid allosteric regulation of C-H activation in plant and animal lipoxygenases. Molecules 2020, 25, 3374.
33. Thakur, M., Udayashankar, A.C. Lipoxygenases and their function in plant innate mechanism. In *Bioactive Molecules in Plant Defense: Signaling in Growth and Stress*, Jogaiah, S., Abdelrahman, M., Eds., Springer International Publishing: Cham, Switzerland, 2019, pp. 133–143.
34. Bałasińska B., Jank M., Kulasek G. Właściwości i rola wielonienasyconych kwasów tłuszczowych w utrzymaniu zdrowia ludzi i zwierząt. Życie Weterynaryjne, 2010, 85(9): 749–756. (in Polish).
35. Stark A.H., Crawford M.A., Reifen R. Update on alpha-linolenic acid. Nutrition Reviews, 2008, 66(6): 326–332.
36. Burdge G.C. Metabolism of α-linolenic acid in humans. Prostaglandins, leukotrienes and Essential Fatty Acids, 2006, 75(3): 161–168.
37. Łacheta D., Olejarz W., Włodarczyk M., Nowicka G. Wpływ kwasu dokozaheksaenowego (DHA) i eikozapentaenowego (EPA) na regulację funkcji komórek śródbłonka naczyniowego. Postepy Hig Med Dosw., 2019,73: 458–466. (in Polish).
38. Asadi-Samani M., Bahmani M., Rafieian-Kopaei M. The chemical composition, botanical characteristic and biological activities of *Borago officinalis*: a review. Asian Pacific Journal of Tropical Medicine, 2014, 7: 22–28.
39. Krzepiłko A., Prazak R., Skwarylo-Bednarz B., Świeciło A. Pąki, liście i nasiona porzeczki czarnej-źródło substancji bioaktywnych o prozdrowotnych właściwościach. Żywność Nauka Technologia Jakość, 2018, 25(2): 24–33. (in Polish).
40. Moyad M. 2005. An introduction to dietary/supplemental omega-3 fatty acids for general health and prevention: part I. Urologic Oncol Semin Origin Investig, 23: 28–35.
41. Schwartz S. H., Qin X., Zeevaart J.D. Characterization of a novel carotenoid cleavage dioxygenase from plants. Journal of Biological Chemistry, 2001, 276(27): 25208–25211.

42. Durand T., Bultel-Poncé V., Guy A., Berger S., Mueller M.J., Galano J.M. New bioactive oxylipins formed by non-enzymatic free-radical-catalyzed pathways: the phytoprostanes. Lipids, 2009, 44: 875–888.
43. Vicente J, et al., Role of 9-lipoxygenase and α-dioxygenase oxylipin pathways as modulators of local and systemic defense, Mol. Plant, 2012, 5, 914–928.
44. Zielińska M., Rutkowska J., Antoniewska A. Produkty utleniania lipidów-konsekwencje żywieniowe i zdrowotne. Problemy Higieny i Epidemiologii, 2017, 98(3): 203–211.
45. Kumar V., Rani A., Tindwani C., Jain M. Lipoxygenase isozymes and trypsin inhibitor activities in soybean as influenced by growing location. Food Chem, 2003, 83 : 79–83.
46. Kumar V., Rani A., Pandey V., Chauhan G.S. Changes in lipoxygenase isozymes and trypsin inhibitor activity in soybean during germination at different temperatures. Food Chemistry, 2006, 99(3): 563–568.
47. Geerts A., Feltkamp D., Rosahl, S. Expression of lipoxygenase in wounded tubers of *Solanum tuberosum* L. Plant Physiology, 1994, 105(1): 269–277.
48. Christensen S.A., Kolomiets M.V. The lipid language of plant–fungal interactions. Fungal Genetics and Biology, 2011, 8(1): 4–14.
49. Leone A., Melillo M. T., Bleve-Zacheo T. Lipoxygenase in pea roots subjected to biotic stress. Plant Science, 2001, 161(4): 703–717.
50. Szymanowska U., Jakubczyk A., Baraniak B., Kur A. Characterization of lipoxygenase from pea seeds (Pisum sativum var. Telephone L.). Food Chemistry, 2009, 116(4): 906–910.
51. Stephany M., Bader-Mittermaier S., Schweiggert-Weisz U., Carle R. 2015. Lipoxygenase activity in different species of sweet lupin (*Lupinus* L.) seeds and flakes. Food Chemistry, 174: 400–406.
52. Anese M., Sovrano S. Kinetics of thermal inactivation of tomato lipoxygenase. Food Chemistry, 2006, 95(1): 131–137.
53. Meyer D., Herrfurth C., Brodhun F., Feussner I. Degradation of lipoxygenase-derived oxylipins by glyoxysomes from sunflower and cucumber cotyledons. BMC Plant Biology, 2013, 13(1): 1–11.
54. Mosblech A., Feussner I., Heilmann, I. Oxylipins: structurally diverse metabolites from fatty acid oxidation. Plant Physiology and Biochemistry, 2009, 47(6): 511–517.
55. Scala, Alessandra et al. Green leaf volatiles: a plant's multifunctional weapon against herbivores and pathogens. International Journal of Molecular Sciences, 2013, 14(9):17781–811, doi:10.3390/ijms140917781
56. Arimura G. I., Kost C., Boland W. Herbivore-induced, indirect plant defenses. Biochemical et Biophysics Acta (BBA)-Molecular and Cell Biology of Lipids, 12005, 734(2): 91–111.
57. Santino A., Taurino M., De Domenico S., Bonsegna S., Poltronieri P., Pastor V., Flors, V. Jasmonate signaling in plant development and defense response to multiple (a) biotic stresses. Plant Cell Reports, 2013, 32(7): 1085–1098.
58. Santino A, Bonsegna S, De Domenico S, Poltronieri P. Plant oxylipins and their contribution to plant defense. Currents topic In Plant Biology. Review, 2016, 10 pp. www.researchgate.net/publication/286676547 (accessed: 25.05.2022).
59. Han G.Z. Evolution of jasmonate biosynthesis and signaling mechanisms. J. Exp. Bot., 2012, 68: 1323–1331.
60. Wasternack C., Strnad M. Jasmonates: news on occurrence, biosynthesis, metabolism and action of an ancient group of signaling compounds. International Journal of Molecular Sciences, 2018, 19(9), 2539. doi:10.3390/ijms19092539

61. Hamza, R., Pérez-Hedo, M., Urbaneja, A. et al. Expression of two barley proteinase inhibitors in tomato promotes endogenous defensive response and enhances resistance to *Tuta absoluta*. BMC Plant Biol 2018, 18, 24. https://doi.org/10.1186/s12870-018-1240-6.
62. Buseman C.M., Tamura P., Sparks A.A., Baughman E.J., Maatta S., Zhao J., Roth M.R., Esch S. W., Shah J., Williams T.D., Welti R. Wounding stimulates the accumulation of glycerolipids containing oxophytodienoic acid and dinor-oxophytodienoic acid in *Arabidopsis* leaves. Plant Physiology, 2006, 142(1): 28–39.
63. Weber H., Chételat A., Caldelari D., Farmer E.E. Divinyl ether fatty acid synthesis in late blight–diseased potato leaves. The Plant Cell, 1999, 11(3): 485–493.
64. Norman-Setterblad C., Vidal S., Palva E.T. Interacting signal pathways control defense gene expression in Arabidopsis in response to cell wall degrading enzymes from *Erwinia carotovora*. Mol Plant Microbe Int., 2000, 4: 430–438.
65. O'Donnell P.J., Schmelz E., Block A., Miersch O., Wasternack C., Jones J.B., Klee H.J. Multiple hormones act sequentially to mediate a susceptible tomato pathogen defense response. Plant Physiology, 2003, 133(3): 1181–1189.
66. Halim V. A., Vess A., Scheel D., Rosahl S. The role of salicylic acid and jasmonic acid in pathogen defense. Plant Biology, 2006, 8(03): 307–313.
67. Scala A, Allmann S, Mirabella R, Haring MA, Schuurink RC. Green leaf volatiles: a plant's multifunctional weapon against herbivores and pathogens. Int J Mol Sci. 2013, 14(9):17781–17811. doi:10.3390/ijms140917781
68. Croft K., Juttner F., Slusarenko A. Volatile products of the lipoxygenase pathway evolved from *Phaseolus vulgaris* (L.) leaves inoculated with P*seudomonas syringae* pv. *phaseolicola*. Plant Physiol. 1993,101:13–24.
69. Heiden A.C., Kobel K., Langebartels C. Emissions of oxygenated volatile organic compounds from plants Part I: Emissions from lipoxygenase activity. J. Atmos. Chem. 2003,45:143–172.
70. Jones A, Cofer TM, Engelberth J, Tumlinson J, Herbivorous Caterpillars and the Green Leaf Volatile (GLV) Quandary Journal of Chemical Ecology, 2022, 48(4). DOI: 10.1007/s10886–021–01330–6
71. Stolterfoht H, Rinnofner C, Winkler M, Harald W, Pichler H. Recombinant lipoxygenases (LOX) and hydroperoxide lyases (HPL) for the synthesis of green leaf volatiles. Journal of Agricultural and Food Chemistry, 2019, 67, 49, 13367–13392, DOI: 10.1021/acs.jafc.9b02690
72. Fischer G.J., Keller N.P. Production of cross-kingdom oxylipins by pathogenic fungi: an update on their role in development and pathogenicity, J. Microbiol. 54, 2016, 254–264.
73. Fernandez-Conradi P, Jactel H, Robin C, Tack AJM, Castagneyrol B. Fungi reduce preference and performance of insect herbivores on challenged plants, Ecology, 2018, 99(2): 300–311, https://doi.org/10.1002/ecy.2044
74. Affeldt K.J., et al., Global survey of canonical *Aspergillus flavus* GPCRs, MBio 5, 2014, e01501–e01514.
75. Brodhagen M, et al., Reciprocal oxylipin-mediated cross-talk in the *Aspergillus*–seed pathosystem, Mol. Microbiol. 67, 2008, 378–391.
76. Ghosh, E., Kumari, P., Jaiman, D. et al. Methodological advances: the unsung heroes of the GPCR structural revolution. Nat Rev Mol Cell Biol, 2016, 16, 69–81. https://doi.org/10.1038/nrm3933
77. Affeldt KJ, et al. *Aspergillus* oxylipin signaling and quorum sensing pathways depend on G protein-coupled receptors, Toxins (Basel) 4, 2012, 695–717.

78. Granér G., Hamberg M., Meijer J., Screening of oxylipins for control of oilseed rape (*Brassica napus*) fungal pathogens, Phytochemistry 2003, 63, 89–95.
79. Nakamura S, Hatanaka A, Green-leaf-derived C6-aroma compounds with potent antibacterial action that act on both Gram-negative and Gram-positive bacteria, J. Agric. Food Chem. 50, 2002, 7639–7644.
80. Prost I, Dhondt S, Rothe G, Vicente J, Rodriguez MJ, Kift N, Carbonne F, Griffiths G, Esquerré-Tugayé MT, Rosahl S, Castresana C, Hamberg M, Fournier J. Evaluation of the antimicrobial activities of plant oxylipins supports their involvement in defense against pathogens. Plant Physiol. 2005;139(4):1902–13. doi: 10.1104/pp.105.066274.

16 Techniques in Plant Oxylipins Profiling

Qadrul Nisa[*1], *Nawreen Mir*[1], *Gazala Gulzar*[1], *Khair Ul Nisa*[2, 3], *and Najeebul Tarfeen*[3]
[1] Division of Plant Pathology, SKUAST-K, Shalimar, India
[2]Department of Environmental Science, University of Kashmir, Srinagar, India
[3]Centre of Research for Development, University of Kashmir, Srinagar, India
Email: qadrul.nisa126@gmail.com
*All the authors have equal contribution

CONTENTS

16.1 INTRODUCTION

Oxylipins constitute a family of oxygenated natural products which are typically produced from polyunsaturated fatty acids (PUFA's) through a number of different processes. To make it simpler, they can be defined as compounds with comparable structures, chemistries, and physical properties that are created by adding various oxygen species to a small number of fatty acids [1]. Oxylipins are produced by the diverse group of organisms like plants, animals, and fungi. Hydroperoxy-, hydroxy-, oxo-, and epoxy-fatty acids, divinyl ethers, volatile aldehydes, and the plant hormone jasmonic acid are among the oxylipins produced by plants [2]. Dioxygenases or monooxygenases start the biosynthesis of oxylipins, however, non-enzymatic autoxidative mechanisms can also produce oxylipins. Non-enzymatic oxidation usually

DOI: 10.1201/9781003316558-16

involves the formation of reactive oxygen species (ROS), which have a preliminary role in plant defense against various biotic and abiotic stresses. In plants, these oxylipins are generally found in estrified form called glacto and phospho lipids. Their pioneer study dates back to *Arabidopsis thaliana* to the more recent study in family *Brasicacea* where a wide range of fatty acids have been classified [3]. Oxylipins affect a large number of biological processes like hormonal regulation, growth, and development, oxidative stress, and various physiological problems. They are also closely related to various biotic and abiotic stress inflicted upon the plants. A good amount of work has been done in that aspect of oxylipin profiling. Our understanding of numerous physiological or pathological processes can be greatly improved by studying variations in the number of oxylipins like drug target discovery and toxicity [4]. It can also serve as a tool for disease diagnosis and consequently various metabolic pathways affected by the disease. Though a diversified group of oxylipins have been characterized their actual biological function is still unknown. In order to investigate the functional role of plant oxylipins their accurate identification and profiling is a preliminary step. The conventional methods of plant oxylipin profiling include mass chromatography (MC) and gas chromatography (GC). This method could be conveniently used for quantification of various oxylipins [5]. The oxylipins which are sensitive to high temperatures cannot be quantified through conventional techniques, hence liquid chromatography (LC) is the better suited technique. Also, some oxylipins are present in very small concentrations and can be structurally very similar, therefore another sensitive and sophisticated technique is applied for the quantification of those analytes named high-profile liquid chromatograply (HPLC) [6]. Currently, there are several techniques available for determining the concentrations of oxylipins in various plant tissues and samples. But none of them comes clean of any drawbacks. This is largely owing to the fact that oxylipins have little stability, are found in extremely minute quantities in biological samples, and are prone to deterioration and self-oxidation. Additionally, several oxylipins, particularly those having same initial fatty acid backbone and much similar structures demand quick, very sensitive and precise analytical techniques for oxylipin analysis [7, 8] (Figure 16.1). The present chapter will briefly summarize the various techniques adopted for plant oxylipin profiling which will finally lead to our knowledge in their functional characterization.

16.2 HIGH PERFORMANCE LIQUID CHROMATOGRAPHY (HPLC)

High performance liquid chromatography (HPLC) has emerged as one of the best chromatography techniques used for oxylipin profiling, largely replacing TLC method. HPLC is a flexible technique that involves the use of different stationary phases for several oxylipin separation techniques, including reversed-phase (RP)-HPLC, normal-phase (NP)-HPLC, chiral HPLC, and hydrophilic interaction chromatography (HILIC). The primary technique for separating the analytes possessing the hydrophobic characteristics remains RP-HPLC.

For sample preparation, the approach combines protein precipitation and solid-phase extraction (SPE), which is then followed by UPLC-MS/MS [9]. From the perspective of lowering analysis time and enhancing the chromatographic resolution, using a core-shell column in place of a conventional C18 column appears fruitful

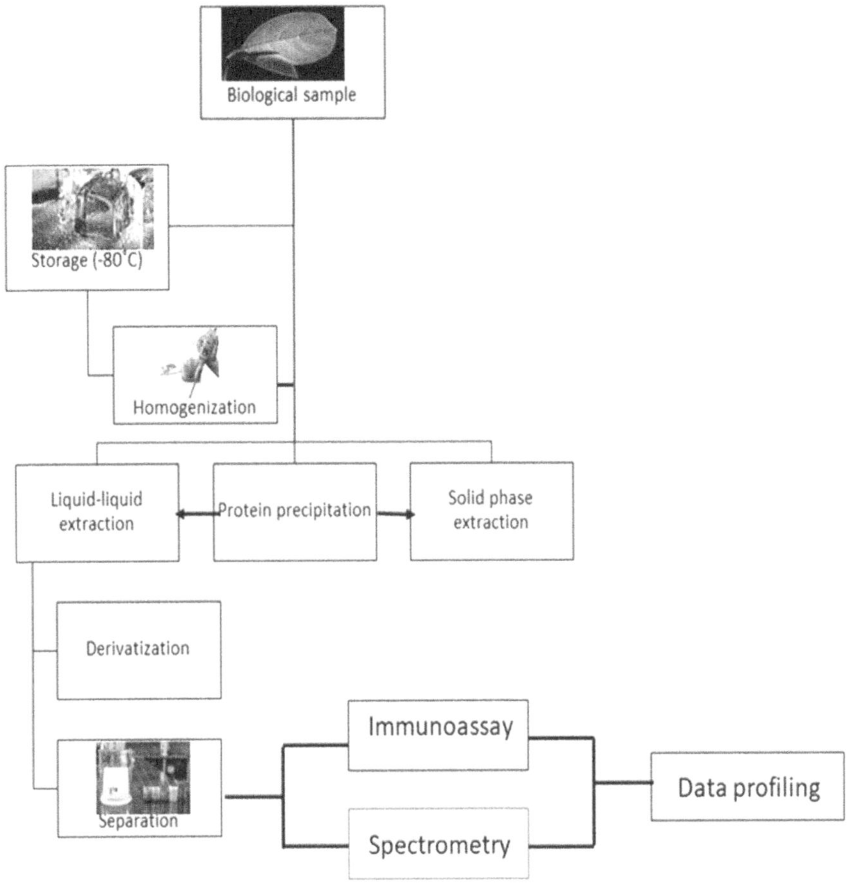

FIGURE 16.1 Steps involved in complete oxylipin profiling from a given plant/biological sample (Modified Liakh et al., 2019).

[10]. Additionally, by adjusting the mobile phase composition, gradient parameters, stationary phases, and run duration, chromatographic separation may be optimized.

The compounds' volatility at high temperatures, which would be necessary for GC separation, makes techniques based on HPLC helpful for the characterization and quantification of practically all oxylipin classes in plants. Moreover, HPLC offers resolution based on functional group positions (straight phase) or the acyl chain length or the number of unsaturated bonds (reverse phase). The technique of HPLC is very affordable, too, in comparison to other profiling techniques available.

However, despite of all the advantages HPLC has to offer, the conjugated dienes and keto groups' low UV range (235–280 nm) absorption, typical analysis employing HPLC with UV detection is a challenging operation. The lack of appropriate color imparting components, i.e., chromophores, makes most oxylipins less perceptive for their investigation in intricate cell or tissue extracts.

16.3 CHIRAL CHROMATOGRAPHY

The existence of key separation pairs (molecules with same molecular anatomy, identical fragmentation and near retention duration), and a significant number of isomers that can be produced during oxidation, are issues in the investigation of oxylipins. Chiral chromatography, which enables the use of unique chiral columns (protein-based columns/ immobilized polysaccharide columns), is employed to address this [11, 12]. From a pharmacological and toxicological perspective, determining the enantiomeric composition of alkaloid-containing plants is extremely important and has its own niche in chiral chromatography. The impact of chirality on the analysis of alkaloids in plants has been beautifully reviewed recently by Nguyen et al., in 2021 [13]. Monoterpenoids is the essential class of essential oils accumulated in various plant familes like Umbelliferae and Rutaceae. Due to their commercial applications, chemical makeup, and biological activity, their enantiomeric separation through chiral chromatography is of particular interest [14]. Thus, chiral chromatography successfully distinguishes between the isomers of oxylipins, however, due to several drawbacks like the requirement for lengthy equilibration, the usage of an isocratic gradient and consequently a prolonged time for analysis and the utilization of inaccessible inner standards it is more frequently utilized for the targeted examination of particular oxylipin species [15] (Table 16.1).

16.4 IMS (ION MOBILITY SPECTROMETRY)

A separation method that is utilized to enhance the recognition and characterization of oxylipin species in living materials, particularly for the isomers, is ion mobility (IMS). The incorporation of collision-cross-section (CCS) value and IMS administration between the chromatographic and MS steps adds additional level of separation, improving the accuracy of oxylipin identification. For the separation of 42 isomer pairs or groups in a positive or negative mode, Kyle et al. successfully adopted this technique [16]. IMS applications in agriculture have a lot of potential thanks to traits including high sensitivity, selectivity, analytical flexibility, field portability, and real-time monitoring capabilities. This method has been employed in the assessment of soil pollution, the detection of harmful substances, the monitoring of plant stress, the evaluation of food and beverage quality, etc. Diisopropyl methylphosphonate (DIMP), diazinon, aldicarb, dimethoate, malathion, dichlorovos, nitrite and nitrate are some of the toxic soil and plant chemicals screened through this technique [17].

16.5 IMMUNOAFFINITY CHROMATOGRAPHY (IAC)

In order to separate a specific molecule from living samples for analysis by GC-MS or LC-MS, immunoaffinity chromatography (IAC), a kind of LC wherein the stationary phase includes an antibody or an artificial protein-binding reagent, is an effective approach [18]. For the recognition and measurement of isoprostanes (IsoP), prostanes, and their metabolites, which frequently arise at incredibly lessser quantities in living tissues, IAC is greatly meticulous and discrete [18]. This technique was used as a means of purifying peroxidase from different vegetables like turnip, broccoli and Brussels sprouts [19]. Also, through this technique it was possible to employ antibodies to successfully purify plant proteins like legumin. Before being analyzed by HPLC, plant and plant cell culture extracts were purified using the immunoaffinity column. Taxoids could be concentrated specifically thanks to immunoaffinity chromatography, which also improved sample cleaning [20]. The broad use of IAC is, however, constrained by the scarcity of ready-made antibodies and the technical difficulty of producing them [18].

16.6 THIN LAYER CHROMATOGRAPHY (TLC)

Thin layer chromatography (TLC) is a further sample preparation method that can be employed before MS analysis. It is generally used to separate non-volatile compounds of various biological mixtures [21] The technique uses a stationary phase and a mobile phase, based on the affinity of different compounds to the mobile and stationary phase the compounds in the mixture are separated. Further the analysis is done through the well-defined separated spots on the TLC plate [22]. The technique has been widely and extensively used in various vegetable and medicinal crops. The common compounds separated through the technique are chlorophylls, carotenoids and xanthophylls [23]. The method has gained a lot of importance in pharmaceutical drug industries to study the medicinal properties in various medicinal plants like *Moringa olifera* containing antioxidants like phenolics and flavonoids. A modified method of TLC was used by Matysik et al. which they named MGD-2D TLC "Two-dimensional gradient thin layer chromatography." This modified technique can be used to separate multicomponent mixtures of various plant extracts like *Juniperus* and *Thymus*. This method in addition to isolation and identifying the compounds also maintains their purity [24].

16.7 GAS CHROMATOGRAPHY—EI/MASS SPECTROPHOTOMETRY

More sensitive analytical procedures are required for the identification of oxylipins with low abundance and phytohormones without intramolecular chromophores. These techniques are GC/MS based on either electron ionization (EI) or detection of CI. EI is crucial to the everyday investigation of small molecules. The sample that has been eluted from the column is subject to an electron beam bombardment in a vacuum, which causes electron ejection and the production of the positively charged molecular ion [M]+ and a certain amount of fragmentation that, if too great, could reduce the molecular ion's intensity but creates a "molecular fingerprint." EI is substantially less helpful for molecules with molecular masses greater than 400 Da. This is a common technique for detecting oxylipins and other low-molecular-mass compounds in biological samples [25]. F2-IsoPs from various biological sources are often quantified using GC-MS [26].

The 1980s saw the most advancement in oxylipin level research using GC-MS. Since oxylipins are not volatile and thermally stable enough for GC analysis, derivatization of carboxyl and hydroxyl groups is necessary to boost the analysis's sensitivity [27]. For the silylation of hydroxyl groups, reagents like N, O-bis(trimethylsilyl)-trifluoroacetamide (BSTFA) are utilized, followed by detection in electron impact (EI) mode [25]. GC is nearly typically combined with MS detection to boost the sensitivity of the analysis. This considerably lowers the cost of routine detection by enabling the identification of numerous analytes in a single sample.

GC/MS technique offers an advantage over LC/MS as the known LC-MS/MS methods' lower limits of quantitation (LLOQ) values are many times greater than those of the described GC-MS/MS methods [28]. Although GC-MS has long been a popular analytical method for the quantitative and structural interpretation of eicosanoids, fewer laboratories now employ it because of the high cost of equipment and the difficulty in sample preparation [27]. Additionally, to eliminate contaminants created during the derivatization process, GC-MS needs purification procedures following derivatization, which can make the analysis labor-intensive too [29].

16.8 MALDI- TOF/MS (MATRIX-ASSISTED LASER DESORPTION AND IONIZATION—TIME OF FLIGHT/MASS SPECTROMETRY)

Researchers from Germany and Japan independently created matrix-assisted laser desorption and ionization mass spectrometry around the end of the twentieth century. It is now mostly employed in protein and peptide studies; however, it is also used to analyse DNA and carbohydrates. The foundation of MALDI-TOF MS is the use of a matrix that is (typically) ultraviolet-absorbing. Nearly all commercially available MALDI machines have UV lasers, while there are additional IR lasers in use today that need entirely different matrix molecules (like glycerol, for example). This technique involves generation of quasimolecular ions, generated as a result of addition of a cation to the analyte, when the laser beam strikes the sample. High mass ions take longer to reach the detector than do low mass ions [30]. The TOF detector is highly well-liked since it has a practically infinite mass range. However, MALDI is frequently employed for the detection of big molecules. The pulsed ion production of MALDI, is best suited for the TOF detector.

MALDI analysis offers a range of advantages over the other available analysis techniques. The ease and swiftness of MALDI technique is quite unmatched whereby one sample can be analyzed in under one minute. MALDI technique does not require sample purification as it is able to bear higher amount of adulteration than other available MS methods [31, 32]. However, the sample preparation also has certain drawbacks: As opposed to all other MS procedures, MALDI-TOF MS uses a solid sample. The matrix and analyte co-crystals are almost never entirely homogenous, they do have abnormalities. Consequently, the attainable signal intensities depend on where the laser is located and fluctuates from shot to shot when it strikes the sample/matrix crystal.

16.9 ESI-MS/MS (ELECTROSPRAY IONIZATION—TANDEM MASS SPECTROMETRY)

Mass spectrometry based lipidomic studies are generally carried out using two fundamental pathways viz. CLASS (comprehensive lipidomic analysis by separation simplification) and shotgun lipidomics. Prior to mass analysis, different lipid categories are separated using various extraction and chromatographic procedures, which forms the foundation of CLASS [33]. Shotgun lipidomics, in which the sample is introduced into the mass spectrometer without separation and fragmented components are scanned in MS/MS modes, is based on ESI's capacity to analyse multiple sample components at once, enabling the profiling of numerous lipid classes in biological tissue concurrently [34]. Recently, by using ESI-MS in positive ion mode, Milic et al., 2013 reported a novel derivatization approach for the simultaneous detection of the oxidation products of DHA, ARA, LA, and oleic acid [35].

16.10 LIQUID CHROMATOGRAPHY-MASS SPECTROMETRY (LC-MS)

A potent analytical technique called liquid chromatography-mass spectrometry (LC-MS) is used to separate, identify, and quantify both known and unidentified substances as well as to clarify the structure and chemical characteristics of various molecules [36]. It is the fast and the most robust method for quantification of lipids in plant world. The method was used to study the lipidome of *Arabidopsis*, tomato, maize and other photosynthetic organisms like green alga [37–40].

The steps involve:

- Source being studied
- Source of ionization
- Detectors that use the m/z ratio to identify ions
- Data analysis [41]

Different labs have created LC-MS-based lipidomic platforms for plant study, covering a variety of lipid classes, for example, glycerolipids, sterols, sphingolipids etc. In a single sample, thousands of analytes can be found [42, 43]. This technique produces strong, comprehensive data that can be incorporated further using the outcomes of various techniques, including transcriptomics and proteomics (Table 16.1). It can help us comprehend, for instance, plant reactions to biotic and abiotic stresses [44–47].

16.11 CONCLUSION

Oxylipins from plants are an expanding family of signaling molecules composed of oxygenated fatty acids and their byproducts. Understanding of oxylipin manufacture, metabolism, and function has greatly advanced during the past ten years. The presence of oxylipins in complex lipids as esters or as free fatty acid derivatives broadens their structural diversity even more and require further sophisticated techniques for their analysis. In order to retain the purity of the compound and quantify the compounds fairly, these approaches need to be reviewed and revisited while keeping in mind the benefits and drawbacks of various methodologies.

TABLE 16.1
Merits and Deficiencies of Different Methods Employed for Oxylipin Analysis

Serial No.	Method	Merits	Deficiencies
1.	Immunoassay	EIA and RIA are easy to handle, cost effective and sensitive [48]	Analyses a single molecule at one time, only few molecules are targeted, run time is long for RIA and uncertainty due to cross reactivity [18]
2.	HPLC	Gives high reactivity and selectivity, is accurate and efficient [49]	Selectivity is low, long time required for analysis, derivatization required for HPLCs with fluorescence detectors [50]
3.	Chiral chromatography	Provides analysis of enantiomeric oxylipins [15]	Sensitivity is very less and run time is very long [15]
4.	Thin layer chromatography	Has key role in distinguishing compounds primarily [26]	More volumes of plasma are needed and waste of products during TLC [51]
5.	GC-MS	Analyses many compounds at one time, GC-MS is highly specific and sensitive [52]	Derivatization is needed, some compounds lack derivatization technique and compounds used should be thermally stable [39, 53]
6.	MALDI-TOF	Fast, simple, records mass spectra of cells and plant extracts [54]	The reproducibility of MALDI-TOF mass spectra depends significantly on homogeneity of the co-crystals between matrix and analyte, The sensitivity also varies
7.	ESI-MS	Exhibits greater signal to noise ratio, high reproducibility	Limited solvents and soloutions can be utilized, less accuracy, demands constant flow of sample
8.	LC-MS	Enhanced selection, greater accuracy and precision, and general applicability [55]	Expensive, works with volatile buffers, high maintenance cost and requires more space [56]

REFERENCES

1. Genva, M., et al., *New insights into the biosynthesis of esterified oxylipins and their involvement in plant defense and developmental mechanisms*. Phytochemistry Reviews, 2019. **18**(1): p. 343–358.
2. Dave, A. and I.A. Graham, *Oxylipin signaling: a distinct role for the jasmonic acid precursor cis-(+)-12-oxo-phytodienoic acid (cis-OPDA)*. Frontiers in Plant Science, 2012. **3**: p. 42.
3. Feussner, I. and C. Wasternack, *The lipoxygenase pathway*. Annual Review of Plant Biology, 2002. **53**: p. 275.
4. Martin, R., et al. *Rapid profiling of oxylipins for drug discovery and development nutritional and clinical research*. in *61st Conference on Mass Spectrometry and Allied Topics*. 2013.
5. Göbel, C. and I. Feussner, *Methods for the analysis of oxylipins in plants*. Phytochemistry, 2009. **70**(13–14): p. 1485–1503.
6. Boligon, A. and M. Athayde, *Importance of HPLC in analysis of plants extracts*. Austin Chromatogr, 2014. **1**(3): p. 2.
7. Hewawasam, E., et al., *A stable method for routine analysis of oxylipins from dried blood spots using ultra-high performance liquid chromatography–tandem mass spectrometry*. Prostaglandins, Leukotrienes and Essential Fatty Acids, 2018. **137**: p. 12–18.
8. Liakh, I., et al., *Modern methods of sample preparation for the analysis of oxylipins in biological samples*. Molecules, 2019. **24**(8): p. 1639.
9. Yuan, Z.-X., et al., *Lipidomic profiling of targeted oxylipins with ultra-performance liquid chromatography-tandem mass spectrometry*. Analytical and Bioanalytical Chemistry, 2018. **410**(23): p. 6009–6029.
10. Kortz, L., C. Helmschrodt, and U. Ceglarek, *Fast liquid chromatography combined with mass spectrometry for the analysis of metabolites and proteins in human body fluids*. Analytical and Bioanalytical Chemistry, 2011. **399**(8): p. 2635–2644.
11. Schneider, C., et al., *Enantiomeric separation of hydroxy and hydroperoxy eicosanoids by chiral column chromatography*. Methods in Enzymology, 2007. **433**: p. 145–157.
12. Gouveia-Figueira, S., et al., *Profiling the oxylipin and endocannabinoid metabolome by UPLC-ESI-MS/MS in human plasma to monitor postprandial inflammation*. PloS one, 2015. **10**(7): p. e0132042.
13. Nguyen, K.-N.H., et al., *The impact of chirality on the analysis of alkaloids in plant*. Pharmacia, 2021. **68**: p. 643.
14. Asztemborska, M. and J.R. Ochocka, *Chiral monoterpenoids in plants—Enantioselective chromatographic analysis, and their bioactivity*. Studies in Natural Products Chemistry, 2002. **27**: p. 361–391.
15. Bayer, M., A. Mosandl, and D. Thaçi, *Improved enantioselective analysis of polyunsaturated hydroxy fatty acids in psoriatic skin scales using high-performance liquid chromatography*. Journal of Chromatography B, 2005. **819**(2): p. 323–328.
16. Hinz, C., et al., *A comprehensive UHPLC ion mobility quadrupole time-of-flight method for profiling and quantification of eicosanoids, other oxylipins, and fatty acids*. Analytical Chemistry, 2019. **91**(13): p. 8025–8035.
17. Kafle, G.K., et al., *State of ion mobility spectrometry and applications in agriculture: A review*. Engineering in agriculture, environment and food, 2016. **9**(4): p. 346–357.
18. Tsikas, D., et al., *Divergence in urinary 8-iso-PGF2α (iPF2α-III, 15-F2t-IsoP) levels from gas chromatography–tandem mass spectrometry quantification after thin-layer chromatography and immunoaffinity column chromatography reveals heterogeneity of*

8-iso-PGF2α: possible methodological, mechanistic and clinical implications. Journal of Chromatography B, 2003. **794**(2): p. 237–255.

19. García-Padilla, S., et al., *Immunoaffinity chromatography scheme for plant peroxidase purification*. EJEAFChe, Electron. J. EnViron. Agric. Food Chem, 2007.
20. Hernández-Mesa, M., et al., *Ion mobility spectrometry in food analysis: Principles, current applications and future trends*. Molecules, 2019. **24**(15): p. 2706.
21. Geiss, F., *Fundamentals of thin layer chromatography*. 1987.
22. Sherma, J. and B. Fried, *Handbook of thin-layer chromatography*. 2003: CRC press.
23. Maróti, I. and E. Gabnai, *Separation of chlorophylls and carotenoids by thin-layer chromatography*. Acta Biol. Szeged, 1971. **17**: p. 67–77.
24. Matysik, E., et al., *The new TLC method for separation and determination of multicomponent mixtures of plant extracts*. Journal of Analytical Methods in Chemistry, 2016. **2016**.
25. Mueller, M.J., et al., *Oxylipin analysis methods*. The Plant Journal, 2006. **45**(4): p. 472–489.
26. Parker, C.E., et al., *An improved GC/MS-based procedure for the quantitation of the isoprostane 15-F2t-IsoP in rat plasma*. Molecular Biotechnology, 2001. **18**(2): p. 105–118.
27. O'Donnell, V.B., B. Maskrey, and G.W. Taylor, *Eicosanoids: generation and detection in mammalian cells*. Lipid Signaling Protocols, 2009: p. 1–19.
28. Vigor, C., et al., *Non-enzymatic lipid oxidation products in biological systems: assessment of the metabolites from polyunsaturated fatty acids*. Journal of Chromatography B, 2014. **964**: p. 65–78.
29. Rund, K.M., et al., *Development of an LC-ESI (-)-MS/MS method for the simultaneous quantification of 35 isoprostanes and isofurans derived from the major n3-and n6-PUFAs*. Analytica Chimica Acta, 2018. **1037**: p. 63–74.
30. Fuchs, B., et al., *A direct and simple method of coupling matrix-assisted laser desorption and ionization time-of-flight mass spectrometry (MALDI-TOF MS) to thin-layer chromatography (TLC) for the analysis of phospholipids from egg yolk*. Analytical and Bioanalytical Chemistry, 2007. **389**(3): p. 827–834.
31. Liébana-Martos, C., *Indications, interpretation of results, advantages, disadvantages, and limitations of MALDI-TOF*, in *The Use of Mass Spectrometry Technology (MALDI-TOF) in Clinical Microbiology*. 2018, Elsevier. p. 75–86.
32. Fukuzawa, S., et al., *On-probe sample preparation without washes for matrix-assisted laser desorption/ionization mass spectrometry using an anion exchange medium*. Analytical Chemistry, 2005. **77**(17): p. 5750–5754.
33. Harkewicz, R. and E.A. Dennis, *Applications of mass spectrometry to lipids and membranes*. Annual Review of Biochemistry, 2011. **80**: p. 301.
34. Spickett, C.M. and A.R. Pitt, *Oxidative lipidomics coming of age: advances in analysis of oxidized phospholipids in physiology and pathology*. Antioxidants & Redox Signaling, 2015. **22**(18): p. 1646–1666.
35. Milic, I., R. Hoffmann, and M. Fedorova, *Simultaneous detection of low and high molecular weight carbonylated compounds derived from lipid peroxidation by electrospray ionization-tandem mass spectrometry*. Analytical Chemistry, 2013. **85**(1): p. 156–162.
36. Lapidot-Cohen, T., L. Rosental, and Y. Brotman, *Liquid Chromatography–Mass Spectrometry (LC-MS)-Based Analysis for Lipophilic Compound Profiling in Plants*. Current Protocols in Plant Biology, 2020. **5**(2): p. e20109.
37. Tenenboim, H., et al., *VMP1-deficient Chlamydomonas exhibits severely aberrant cell morphology and disrupted cytokinesis*. BMC Plant Biology, 2014. **14**(1): p. 1–13.

38. Ichino, T., et al., *GFS 9/TT 9 contributes to intracellular membrane trafficking and flavonoid accumulation in A rabidopsis thaliana*. The Plant Journal, 2014. **80**(3): p. 410–423.
39. Halket, J.M., et al., *Chemical derivatization and mass spectral libraries in metabolic profiling by GC/MS and LC/MS/MS*. Journal of Experimental Botany, 2005. **56**(410): p. 219–243.
40. Garbowicz, K., et al., *Quantitative trait loci analysis identifies a prominent gene involved in the production of fatty acid-derived flavor volatiles in tomato*. Molecular Plant, 2018. **11**(9): p. 1147–1165.
41. Cubbon, S., et al., *Metabolomic applications of hilic–lc–ms*. Mass Spectrometry Reviews, 2010. **29**(5): p. 671–684.
42. Hummel, J., et al., *Ultra performance liquid chromatography and high resolution mass spectrometry for the analysis of plant lipids*. Frontiers in Plant Science, 2011. **2**: p. 54.
43. Bromke, M.A., et al., *Liquid chromatography high-resolution mass spectrometry for fatty acid profiling*. The Plant Journal, 2015. **81**(3): p. 529–536.
44. Markham, J.E. and J.G. Jaworski, *Rapid measurement of sphingolipids from Arabidopsis thaliana by reversed-phase high-performance liquid chromatography coupled to electrospray ionization tandem mass spectrometry*. Rapid Communications in Mass Spectrometry: An International Journal Devoted to the Rapid Dissemination of Up-to-the-Minute Research in Mass Spectrometry, 2007. **21**(7): p. 1304–1314.
45. Burgos, A., et al., *Analysis of short-term changes in the Arabidopsis thaliana glycerolipidome in response to temperature and light*. The Plant Journal, 2011. **66**(4): p. 656–668.
46. Sanchez-Arcos, C., et al., *Untargeted metabolomics approach reveals differences in host plant chemistry before and after infestation with different pea aphid host races*. Frontiers in Plant Science, 2019. **10**: p. 188.
47. Xie, L.-J., et al., *Unsaturation of very-long-chain ceramides protects plant from hypoxia-induced damages by modulating ethylene signaling in Arabidopsis*. PLoS genetics, 2015. **11**(3): p. e1005143.
48. Basu, S., *Radioimmunosassay of 8-iso-prostaglandin F2α: an index for oxidative injury via free radical catalysed lipid peroxidation*. Prostaglandins, Leukotrienes and Essential Fatty Acids, 1998. **58**(4): p. 319–325.
49. Nithipatikom, K., P.F. Pratt, and W.B. Campbell, *Determination of EETs using microbore liquid chromatography with fluorescence detection*. American Journal of Physiology-Heart and Circulatory Physiology, 2000. **279**(2): p. H857–H862.
50. Yue, H., et al., *Determination of bioactive eicosanoids in brain tissue by a sensitive reversed-phase liquid chromatographic method with fluorescence detection*. Journal of Chromatography B, 2004. **803**(2): p. 267–277.
51. Nourooz-Zadeh, J., et al., *Analysis of F2-isoprostanes as indicators of non-enzymatic lipid peroxidation in vivo by gas chromatography-mass spectrometry: development of a solid-phase extraction procedure*. Journal of Chromatography B: Biomedical Sciences and Applications, 1995. **667**(2): p. 199–208.
52. Puppolo, M., D. Varma, and S.A. Jansen, *A review of analytical methods for eicosanoids in brain tissue*. Journal of Chromatography B, 2014. **964**: p. 50–64.
53. Black, R.M., et al., *Application of gas chromatography-mass spectrometry and gas chromatography-tandem mass spectrometry to the analysis of chemical warfare samples, found to contain residues of the nerve agent sarin, sulphur mustard and their degradation products*. Journal of Chromatography A, 1994. **662**(2): p. 301–321.

54. Schiller, J., et al., *Maldi-Tof Ms in Lipidomics*. Frontiers in Bioscience-Landmark, 2007. **12**(7): p. 2568–2579.
55. De Hoffmann, E. and V. Stroobant, *Mass spectrometry: principles and applications*. 2007: John Wiley & Sons.
56. Zhang, A., et al., *Recent developments and emerging trends of mass spectrometry for herbal ingredients analysis*. TrAC Trends in Analytical Chemistry, 2017. **94**: p. 70–76.

17 The Computational Approach to Plant Oxylipins Profiling

Databases and Tools

Ambreen Hamadani[1*], *Nazir A. Ganai*[1], *and Sheikh Mansoor*[2]
[1]Sher-e-Kashmir University of Agricultural Sciences and Technology of Kashmir, Srinagar, J&K, India
[2]Division of Biochemistry, FBSc, SK- University of Agricultural Sciences & Technology of Jammu, India
*Correspondence: escritor005@gmail.com

CONTENTS

17.1 INTRODUCTION

Oxylipins are a family of oxygenated natural products formed from the automatic oxidation of polyunsaturated fatty acids through pathways that involve at least the dioxygen-dependent oxidation step [1]. They are derived from polyunsaturated fatty acids also known as PUFAs by cyclooxygenases, lipoxygenases, or cytochrome P450 epoxygenase [2]. Oxylipins are also called lipid mediators. They play a significant regulatory role in organisms.

Oxylipins are present in all aerobic organisms including plants, animals, and fungi. Oxylipins are of physiological significance [3, 4]. They are, however, not stored in tissues but are formed as and when required through the liberation of the precursor fatty acids from their esterified forms. In animals, oxylipins are called eicosanoids, and are seen to have potent effects. They affect the vasculature and

DOI: 10.1201/9781003316558-17

myometrium of smooth muscle and also blood platelets. Eicosanoids have diverse functions, e.g., some are proinflammatory (leukotrienes B4 and C4) while others are anti-inflammatory (resolvins, protectins) and are therefore involved in the process of wound healing. Plant oxylipins, on the other hand, are involved in the control of ontogenesis and various reproductive processes, and also help in providing resistance to various microbial pathogens and pests.

The analysis of oxylipins is critical for us to study changes in the number of oxylipins in living organisms. This provides valuable information on metabolites derived from various precursors. It also contributes to an understanding of various physiological and/or pathological processes taking place in organisms, both plants, and animals. Oxylipin profiling is also critical for drug target discovery so that novel drugs could be developed specifically for various metabolic pathways. Profiling is also essential for the screening of biomarkers which is critical for disease diagnosis, classification, and prognosis. Pharmacodynamics and drug toxicity assessment is yet another important aspect of the analysis. Environmental exposure studies through oxylipin analysis are also done.

Oxylipins, in nature unstable and, are present in very low concentrations, generally. This makes their analysis and profiling a challenge. Therefore, there is a need for new and advanced tools that could facilitate the same. In this regard, the latest developments in the area of oxylipin extraction and analysis are major game-changers for this area of science. This is especially true for the latest developments in the area of computational sciences viz., increased computational power, development of mega databases, etc.

17.2 ANALYTICAL TECHNIQUES

There are many methods of analysis of oxylipins, some of which have been developed and perfected over the last few years. Some of the techniques for the analysis of the oxylipins include:

1 **Immunoassay Methods**: These are easy to use and sensitive and do not require any extensive instrumentation either. Radioimmune assay when combined with the high-performance liquid chromatography (HPLC) technique is highly sensitive [5]. This technique however targets only a few compounds and is limited to a single metabolite at one time. They also require a long run time and generate wastes that could be hazardous.
2 **Chiral Chromatography** is yet another technique that allows the separation of oxylipins enantiomerically [6]. This method also has a long run time, and sensitivity is also limited. This method, however, is very sensitive to changes in mobile-phase composition.
3 **The Capillary Electrophoresis** allows the resolution of Epoxyeicosatrienoic acids (EET) and dihydroxyeicosatrienoic acids (DHET) Regio isomers [7] but can analyze only a limited number of analytes and has a long run time. Some product loss is also seen while using this technique.
4 **Thin-Layer Chromatography** is used for the preliminary separation of analytes [8] but also causes loss of products, required a large plasma volume, and can be used only on the metabolites that absorb UV light.

5 **HPLC-UV or Fluorescence Detection** is yet another technique that has good sensitivity and selectivity [9] and it is useful in getting structural information. But it is important to understand that high-performance liquid chromatography (HPLC) with fluorescence detection would also require derivatization. The analysis time is also very long.
6 **MALDI-TOF/MS** or matrix-assisted laser desorption/ionization (MALDI), and the mass analyzer is time-of-flight (TOF) is a soft ionization technique that allows for the analysis of non-volatile compounds and allows the direct quantification of prostaglandins [10]. The disadvantage includes the need for co-crystallization of the matrix with the sample. This may affect the quantification of the analyte. It also needs derivatization.
7 **GC-EI/MS Technique** or gas chromatography-mass spectrometry when coupled with the MS detection technique, gas chromatography-mass spectrometry is both highly sensitive and selective [11] but it also requires derivatization of the analytes. This technique offers the advantage that it can analyze multiple analytes in one sample. It is also highly sensitive. But this technique requires the analytes to be thermally stable and also their requirement of volatility is absolute.
8 **ESI-MS/MS** or electrospray ionization mass spectrometry is a simple, fast, technique with no sample carry-over [12] (shotgun analysis). The selectivity and sensitivity are also high. It is however difficult to separate isomers using this technique and ion suppression may also be seen.

17.3 LIPIDOMIC PROFILING

Mass spectrometry (MS) has gained importance in the last few years for protein analysis and this technique when combined with other proteomics methods generate a large amount of proteome data. it is important to archive and analyze this data using specialized bioinformatics tools. Global lipidomics analysis of mega data sets requires dedicated software tools that support the identification of lipids and their quantification along with efficient data management and lipidome visualization. The analytic workflow of the lipidomic profiling techniques is given in figure 17.1.

Lipidomic profiling is the process of systematic analysis as well as the identification of lipids in organisms, tissues, cells, and the molecules with which they interact. Some important processes covered under this approach include the following:

- Lipid function as well as metabolic regulation analysis
- Lipid metabolism pathway as well as network analysis

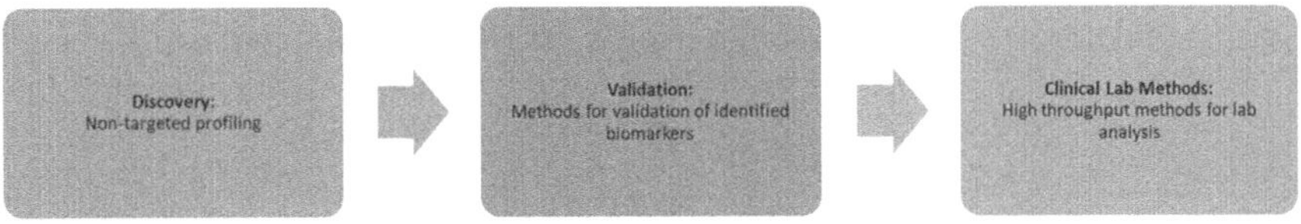

FIGURE 17.1 Analytical workflow of lipidomic studies.

- Untargeted lipidomics
- Targeted lipidomics
- Exosome lipidomics
- Maldi imaging lipidomics service

This approach is also used to understand the structure and function of lipids. This is important for the understanding of the relationship between lipid metabolism, and physiological and pathological processes inside organisms. Automation and computer-aided innovations help in simplifying the processes of analysis and profiling of various biological molecules including oxylipins. These also facilitate searching for data in known and specialized databases. For this purpose, special software is often used. These tools facilitate the automatic identification of lipids from open databases or in-house libraries. They also allow the quantification of lipids. Many such tools export the raw data received from devices for further analysis.

There are also several filtering mechanisms to minimize errors and filter out outliers and or unwanted matches. Some of the tools also allow the use of rule-based identification.

17.4 PROGRAMS AND TOOLS FOR PROFILING OF OXYLIPINS

Below, are the most popular commercial and free available programs and tools for profiling of oxylipins popularly used. Some of these tools are in open source which makes their use easy and free for all.

1. **Creative Proteomics** uses LC-MS/MS but broadens the oxylipin range to enhance the sensitivity of the technique. It is a platform that helps to better understand and monitor the physiological levels of a broad range of oxylipins [13].
2. **Lipid View** [14]: A tool for automated identification as well as the quantification of glycerophospholipid molecular species using multiple precursor ion scanning.
3. **LipidSearch** [15]: This tool is for the relative quantitation and identification of lipids from biological samples. It automatically identifies lipids and integrates the entire data set into a comprehensive report that reports the statistical differences between sample groups.
4. **SimLipid** [16]: is a high throughput lipid identification software that also quantifies lipids. This software processes raw data from thousands of LC-MS and/or MS/MS experimental runs for the detection of LC-peak, molecular feature finding, peak-picking, and retention time alignment.
5. **LipidXplorer** [17]: LipidXplorer is a software tool supporting many untargeted shotgun lipidomics experiments. It uses user-defined molecular fragmentation query language rules for the identification and quantification of lipids. This tool supports bottom-up as well as top-down shotgun experimentations on every type of tandem MS platform.

6 **LipiDex** [18]: This is a new open-source software suite for LC-MS/MS lipidomics data analysis. This tool uses multiple in silico libraries for a diversity of lipid types. It is also highly accurate for the quantitation of lipids that are co-isolated and co-eluting isobaric. It is also capable of data filtration that is streamlined downstream for lipid identifications.
7 **LIMSA** [19]: LIMSA (Lipid Mass Spectrum Analysis) is an open-source program used for the quantitative analysis of mass spectra of lipid samples. It can perform peak finding, integration, isotope correction, assigning, as well as quantitation with internal standards. LIMSA can single search lipids or batch analyze them. Either way, it can efficiently summarize results.
8 **Lipidyzer** [20]: The lipidyzer platform is an integrated and highly efficient system that quantifies over a thousand lipids across 13 different lipid classes.
9 **Lipid Data Analyzer** [21]: The algorithm is integrated into the Lipid Data Analyzer (LDA) application which also provides a statistics module for results analysis, standardization, a batch mode for analysis of several runs as well as a 3D viewer for the manual verification of the results. The statistics module additionally offers tests between sample groups, sample grouping, and export functionalities. The results can also be analyzed and visualized using heat maps and bar charts.
10 **LipidQA** [22]: this tool uses an algorithm for processing raw mass spectrometric data. it can identify and subsequently quantitate complex lipid molecules in mixtures. This is done by data-dependent scanning and searching based on fragment ion database.
11 **CEU Mass Mediator** [23]: This tool searches metabolites in various protein databases It is specially designed for performing searches through masses derived from the mass spectrometry techniques. It unifies compounds from various sources and quickly finds compounds in the databases one by one. It also allows for manual unification without the risk of getting the unification wrong.
12 **LipidLama** [24]: Makes use of Greazy which is yet another open-source tool for automated identification of phospholipids from MS/MS spectra. Greazy builds a phospholipid search space using user-defined parameters and associated theoretical MS/MS spectra. Experimental spectra can also be scored against search space lipids created with similar precursor masses. The LipidLama component of the algorithm filters the results via the methods of mixture modeling and density estimation.
13 **LipidMatch** [25]: This is a tool written in the R programming language for lipid identification for workflows from liquid chromatography-tandem mass spectrometry. LipidMatch has over 250,000 lipid species that span 56 lipid types which are contained in silico fragmentation libraries. It has unique fragmentation libraries which include oxidized lipids, sphingosines, bile acids, and previously uncharacterized adducts, including ammoniated cardiolipins.

14 **LipidMiner** [26]: A software tool for automated identification as well as the quantification of lipids from multiple liquid chromatography or mass spectrometry data files.
15 **dGOT-MS** [27]: database-assisted globally optimized targeted (dGOT)-MS, which utilizes the HMDB and METLIN databases to considerably improve both identifications as well as the metabolite coverage.
16 **ALEX** [28]: This is a new software platform that streamlines data processing, manages if, and visualizes shotgun lipidomics data that has been acquired using high-resolution Orbitrap mass spectrometry. The ALEX framework is useful for automated identification and export of lipid species intensity directly from mass spectral proprietary data files. It also has database exploration tools for sample information integration, computation of lipid abundance, and visualization of lipidomes.
17 **The Lipid Annotation Service** (LAS) [29]: the LAS programming interface service uses a representational state transfer application. It is designed for lipid annotation. It assigns levels of certainty eg. very unlikely; unlikely; likely; and very likely to putative annotations that are received as input. It also explains the rationale for providing such assignments.
18 **LOBSTAHS** [30]: LOBSTAHS is a multifunctional package for screening, annotation, and putative identification of mass spectral features in huge data sets. In silico data for a variety of oxidized lipids, lipids, and oxylipins can also be generated from user-supplied structural criteria with an additional database generation function. LOBSTAHS generates putative compound identities and assigns them to features in high-mass accuracy data sets. These can later be processed further. Evaluation is also done using this tool and confidence scores are assigned as well. This helps in the identification of potential isomers and isobars.

17.5 IMPORTANT DATABASES

A protein database is a collection of data that has been constructed from physical, chemical, and biological information on sequence, domain structure, function, three-dimensional structure, and protein-protein interactions. Collectively, protein databases may form a protein sequence database. A protein structure database is modeled around various protein structures that are experimentally determined. The aim of most protein structure databases is to organize and annotate protein structures to provide the biological community access to experimental data so that it is useful to them [31].

1 **KEGG PATHWAY**: KEGG PATHWAY is a collection of manually drawn pathway maps that represent the scientific knowledge of the molecular interaction, genetic information processing, reaction and relation networks for metabolism, cellular processes, environmental information processing, human diseases, organismal systems, and drug development [32].

2 **HMDB**: The Human Metabolome Database (HMDB) [33] is an online freely accessible, high-quality, database of small molecules. It was created by Genome Canada under the Human Metabolome Project.
3 **LipidMaps**: Lipid Metabolites and Pathways Strategy is an online portal for lipidomics resources [34]. It provides standardized methodologies for mass spectrometry analysis of lipids. The key LIPID MAPS resources include LIPID MAPS Structure Database (LMSD), LIPID MAPS In Silico Structure Database (LMISSD), and LIPID MAPS Gene/Proteome Database (LMPD).
4 **Metlin**: the METLIN Metabolite and Chemical Entity Database [35] is the largest repository of experimental tandem mass spectrometry data that has been acquired from standards. It contains data on over 860,000 molecular standards. It is useful for the identification of known molecules and is also useful for identifying unknowns.
5 **NP Atlas**: the natural products atlas open-access database of fungal and bacterial natural products. Natural Products Atlas is useful for the identification of known molecules, and exploration of structural series diversity [36].
6 **MINEs**: is an open-access database of computationally calculated enzyme promiscuity products that may fit into untargeted metabolomics [37].

17.6 CONCLUSION

Computational tools are revolutionizing the way oxylipin profiling is done and these are leading the way to new insights into the nature and function of the molecules. The globalization of data in mega databases is this crucial for the analysis of the oxylipins and other molecules using these tools.

REFERENCES

1. Mueller MJ, Mène-Saffrané L, Grun C, Karg K, Farmer E. Oxylipin analysis methods. The Plant Journal. 2006; 45(4): 472–489.
2. Strassburg K, Huijbrechts AM, Kortekaas KA, Lindeman JH, Pedersen TL, Dane A, Berger R, Brenkman A, Hankemeier T, van Duynhoven J, Kalkhoven E, Newman JW, Vreeken RJ. Quantitative profiling of oxylipins through comprehensive LC-MS/MS analysis: application in cardiac surgery. Anal Bioanal Chem. 2012 Sep; 404(5):1413–26. doi: 10.1007/s00216–012–6226-x.
3. Zhao J, Davis LC, Verpoorte R. Elicitor signal transduction leading to the production of plant secondary metabolites". Biotechnol. Adv. 2005; 23 (4): 283–333. doi:10.1016/j.biotechadv.2005.01.003.
4. Bolwell GP, Bindschedler LV, Blee KA, Butt VS, Davies DR, Gardner SL, Gerrish C, Minibayeva F. The apoplastic oxidative burst in response to biotic stress in plants: a three-component system. J. Exp. Bot. 2002; 53 (372): 1367–1376. doi:10.1093/jexbot/53.372.1367.
5. Liakh I, Pakiet A, Sledzinski T, Mika A. Methods of the Analysis of Oxylipins in Biological Samples. Molecules (Basel, Switzerland). 2020; 25(2): 349. https://doi.org/10.3390/molecules25020349

6. Bayer M, Mosandl A, Thaçi D. Improved enantioselective analysis of polyunsaturated hydroxy fatty acids in psoriatic skin scales using high-performance liquid chromatography. J. Chromatogr. B Anal. Technol. Biomed. Life Sci. 2005; 819:323–328. doi: 10.1016/j.jchromb.2005.02.008.
7. Hewawasam E, Liu G, Jeffery DW, Muhlhausler BS, Gibson RA. A stable method for routine analysis of oxylipins from dried blood spots using ultra-high performance liquid chromatography–tandem mass spectrometry. Prostaglandins Leukot. Essent. Fat. Acids. 2018; 137:12–18. doi: 10.1016/j.plefa.2018.08.001.
8. Schweer H, Watzer B, Seyberth W, Nu RM. Improved Quantiücation of 8-epi-Prostaglandin F and F -isoprostanes by Gas Quadrupole Mass Spectrometry: Partial Cyclooxygenase-dependent Formation of 8-epi-Prostaglandin F in Humans 2a. J. Mass Spectrom. 1997; 32: 1362–1370.
9. Nithipatikom K, Pratt PF, Campbell WB. Determination of EETs using microbore liquid chromatography with fluorescence detection. Am. J. Physiol. Circ. Physiol. 2000; 279: H857–H862. doi: 10.1152/ajpheart.2000.279.2.H857
10. Manna JD, Reyzer ML, Latham JC, Weaver CD, Marnett LJ, Caprioli RM. High-Throughput Quantification of Bioactive Lipids by MALDI Mass Spectrometry: Application to Prostaglandins. Anal. Chem. 2011; 83: 6683–6688. doi: 10.1021/ac201224n.
11. Puppolo M, Varma D, Jansen SA. A review of analytical methods for eicosanoids in brain tissue. J. Chromatogr. B Anal. Technol. Biomed. Life Sci. 2014; 964: 50–64. doi: 10.1016/j.jchromb.2014.03.007
12. Ståhlman M, Ejsing CS, Tarasov K, Perman J, Borén J, Ekroos K. High-throughput shotgun lipidomics by quadrupole time-of-flight mass spectrometry. J. Chromatogr. B. 2009; 877:2664–2672. doi: 10.1016/j.jchromb.2009.02.037.
13. Anonymous. 2022. Creative Proteomics. www.creative-proteomics.com/about-us.htm
14. Ejsing CS, Duchoslav E, Sampaio J, Simons K, Bonner R, Thiele C, Ekroos K, Shevchenko A. Automated Identification and Quantification of Glycerophospholipid Molecular Species by Multiple Precursor Ion Scanning. Anal. Chem. 2006; 78: 6202–6214. doi: 10.1021/ac060545x.
15. Taguchi R, Nishijima M, Shimizu T. Basic analytical systems for lipidomics by mass spectrometry in Japan. Methods Enzymol. 2007; 432: 185–211.
16. Rajanayake KK, Taylor WR, Isailovic D. The comparison of glycosphingolipids isolated from an epithelial ovarian cancer cell line and a nontumorigenic epithelial ovarian cell line using MALDI-MS and MALDI-MS/MS. Carbohydr. Res. 2016; 431: 6–14. doi: 10.1016/j.carres.2016.05.006.
17. Soares V, Taujale R, Garrett R, da Silva AJR, Borges RM. Extending compound identification for molecular network using the LipidXplorer database independent method: A proof of concept using glycoalkaloids from Solanum pseudoquina A. St.-Hil. Phytochem. Anal. 2019; 30:132–138. doi: 10.1002/pca.2798.
18. Hutchins PD, Russell JD, Coon JJ. LipiDex: An Integrated Software Package for High-Confidence Lipid Identification. Cell Syst. 2018; 6: 621–625. doi: 10.1016/j.cels.2018.03.011.
19. Haimi P, Chaithanya K, Kainu V, Hermansson M, Somerharju P. Instrument-independent software tools for the analysis of MS-MS and LC-MS lipidomics data. Methods Mol. Biol. 2009; 580:285–294.
20. Cao Z, Schmitt TC, Varma V, Sloper D, Beger RD, Sun J. Evaluation of the Performance of Lipidyzer Platform and Its Application in the Lipidomics Analysis in Mouse Heart and Liver. J. Proteome Res. 2019 doi: 10.1021/acs.jproteome.9b00289.

21. Hartler J, Trötzmüller M, Chitraju C, Spener F, Köfeler HC, Thallinger GG. Lipid Data Analyzer: Unattended identification and quantitation of lipids in LC-MS data. Bioinformatics. 2011; 27: 572–577. doi: 10.1093/bioinformatics/btq699.
22. Song H, Hsu F.-F, Ladenson J, Turk J. Algorithm for processing raw mass spectrometric data to identify and quantitate complex lipid molecular species in mixtures by data-dependent scanning and fragment ion database searching. J. Am. Soc. Mass Spectrom. 2007; 18:1848–1858. doi: 10.1016/j.jasms.2007.07.023.
23. Gil-de-la-Fuente A, Godzien J, Saugar S, Garcia-Carmona R, Badran H, Wishart DS, Barbas C, Otero A. CEU Mass Mediator 3.0: A Metabolite Annotation Tool. J. Proteome Res. 2019; 18:797–802. doi: 10.1021/acs.jproteome.8b00720.
24. Kochen MA, Chambers MC, Holman JD, Nesvizhskii AI, Weintraub ST, Belisle JT, Islam MN, Griss J, Tabb DL. Greazy: Open-Source Software for Automated Phospholipid Tandem Mass Spectrometry Identification. Anal. Chem. 2016; 88: 5733–5741. doi: 10.1021/acs.analchem.6b00021.
25. Koelmel JP, Kroeger NM, Ulmer CZ, Bowden JA, Patterson RE, Cochran JA, Beecher CWW, Garrett TJ, Yost RA. LipidMatch: An automated workflow for rule-based lipid identification using untargeted high-resolution tandem mass spectrometry data. BMC Bioinform. 2017; 18: 331. doi: 10.1186/s12859–017–1744–3.
26. Meng D, Zhang Q, Gao X, Wu S, Lin G. LipidMiner: A software for automated identification and quantification of lipids from multiple liquid chromatography/mass spectrometry data files. Rapid Commun. Mass Spectrom. 2014; 28:981–985. doi: 10.1002/rcm.6865.
27. Shi X, Wang S, Jasbi P, Turner C, Hrovat J, Wei Y, Liu J, Gu H. Database Assisted Globally Optimized Targeted Mass Spectrometry (dGOT-MS): Broad and Reliable Metabolomics Analysis with Enhanced Identification. Anal. Chem. 2019; 91:13737–13745. doi: 10.1021/acs.analchem.9b03107.
28. Husen P, Tarasov K, Katafiasz M, Sokol E, Vogt J, Baumgart J, Nitsch R, Ekroos K, Ejsing CS. Analysis of lipid experiments (ALEX): A software framework for analysis of high-resolution shotgun lipidomics data. PLoS ONE. 2013; 8:e79736. doi: 10.1371/journal.pone.0079736.
29. Fernández-López M, Gil-de-la-Fuente A, Godzien J, Rupérez FJ, Barbas C, Otero A. LAS: A Lipid Annotation Service Capable of Explaining the Annotations It Generates. Comput. Struct. Biotechnol. J. 2019; 17:1113–1122. doi: 10.1016/j.csbj.2019.07.016.
30. Collins JR, Edwards BR, Fredricks HF, Van Mooy BAS. LOBSTAHS: An Adduct-Based Lipidomics Strategy for Discovery and Identification of Oxidative Stress Biomarkers. Anal. Chem. 2016; 88:7154–7162. doi: 10.1021/acs.analchem.6b01260.
31. Laskowski RA. Protein structure databases. Mol Biotechnol. 2011; 48 (2): 183–98. doi:10.1007/s12033–010–9372–4.
32. Kanehisa M, Goto S. KEGG: Kyoto Encyclopedia of Genes and Genomes. Nucleic Acids Res. 2000; 28 (1): 27–30. doi:10.1093/nar/28.1.27
33. Wishart D S, Tzur D, Knox C, Eisner R, Guo AC; Young N et al. "HMDB: the Human Metabolobe Database. Nucleic Acids Research. 2007 January 1; 35 (D1): D521–D526. doi:10.1093/nar/gkl923.
34. Fahy E, Subramaniam S, Murphy RC, Nishijima M, Raetz CR, Shimizu T, Spener F, van Meer G, Wakelam MJ, Dennis EA. Update of the LIPID MAPS comprehensive classification system for lipids. Journal of Lipid Research. 2009 April; 50 Suppl (S1): S9–14. doi:10.1194/jlr.R800095-JLR200

35. Xue J, Guijas C, Benton H, Paul, War B, Siuzdak G. METLIN MS 2 molecular standards database: a broad chemical and biological resource. Nature Methods. 2020 October; 17 (10): 953–954. doi:10.1038/s41592–020–0942–5
36. Laskowski RA. Protein structure databases. Mol Biotechnol. 2011; 48 (2): 183–98. doi:10.1007/s12033–010–9372–4
37. Jeffryes JG, Colastani RL, Elbadawi-Sidhu M. et al. MINEs: open access databases of computationally predicted enzyme promiscuity products for untargeted metabolomics. J Cheminform. 2015; 7: 44 (2015). https://doi.org/10.1186/s13321-015-0087-1

18 Phyto-Oxylipin Bioprospecting and Biotechnology Interventions

Barbara Sawicka[1], Piotr Barbaś[2], Farhood Yeganehpoor[3], Dominika Skiba[1], and Barbara Krochmal-Marczak[4]*

[1]Department of Plant Production Technology and Commodities Science, University of Life Sciences in Lublin, 20–950 Lublin, Poland; barbara.sawicka@up.lublin.pl; dominika.skiba@up.lublin.pl

[2]Department of Potato Agronomy, Institute of Plant Breeding and Acclimatization—National Research Institute, Jadwisin, 05-140 Serock, Poland; p.barbas@ihar.edu.pl

[3]Department of Plant Eco-Physiology, University of Tabriz, 51368 Tabriz, Iraq; farhoodyeganeh@yahoo.com

[4]Department of Food Production and Safety, Krosno State College, 38-400 Krosno, Poland; barbara.marczak@kpu.krosno.pl

*Correspondence: barbara.sawick@up.lublin.pl

CONTENTS

DOI: 10.1201/9781003316558-18

18.1 INTRODUCTION

During the oxygenation of polyunsaturated fatty acids (PUFAs), various phytochemicals known as oxylipins are formed, with a developmental and defense role. This family of chemicals includes fatty acid hydroperoxides, hydroxy, keto- or oxo-fatty acids, volatile aldehydes, divinyl ethers, and the plant hormone jasmon. Many of them are bioactive compounds that participate in many physiological processes, in the defense mechanisms of plants and animals, and are responsible for adaptation and communication with other organisms. The vast variety of oxylipins, both in structure and function, reflects the complex control in their biosynthetic structure that derives from the relationship between different signaling pathways [1–5]. Oxylipins are found in all organisms in free form, esterified to phospholipids, galactolipids or they are combined with other compounds (e.g., isoleucine, methyl groups). Oxylipins participate in the development of plants and the defense against infection, pathogens, insects, and injury. The initial oxidation of substrate fatty acids is catalyzed by lipoxygenases (LOX) and α-dioxygenases, but non-enzymatic oxidation by auto-oxidation or other singlet oxygen dependent reactions may also occur. The resulting hydroperoxides are still metabolized by secondary enzymes to produce a wide variety of compounds, including the hormone jasmonic acid (JA) and green leaf short chain volatile compounds. In flowering plants, which usually lack arachidonic acid, oxilipins are formed by the oxidation of C18 polyunsaturated fatty acids, linolenic and linoleic acids [1, 6–8]. These lipids are abundant in both mammals and flowering plants, mosses, algae, bacteria and fungi [1]. They serve as signaling molecules to regulate developmental processes such as pollen formation, and mediate environmental responses such as wound healing and defense responses, or have direct antimicrobial properties [2, 9–10]. The term "oxylipin" first appeared 30 years ago. Since then, the number of publications and numerous studies on this subject has increased significantly, but still many issues, especially related to their mechanism of operation, remain unclear. Hence, the aim of this chapter is to present this issue and present the phyto-oxylipin bioperspective and the possibilities of biotechnological interventions.

18.2 THE OXYLIPIN BIOSYNTHETIC PATHWAY IN PLANTS

Oxylipin biosynthesis begins with the release of fatty acids from membrane lipids through the action of lipase. Then there is the initial oxidation reaction by different enzymes at different sites in the fatty acid skeleton (figure 18.1) [9, 11]. The oxylipin pathway can be characterized as follows: the biosynthesis of plant oxylipins begins with the conversion of polyunsaturated fatty acids such as linolenic acid (C18: 3) into hydroperoxides such as 13 (S)-hydroperoxyoctadecatrienoic acid (13-HPOT). The hydroperoxides that are produced by LOX can also be used

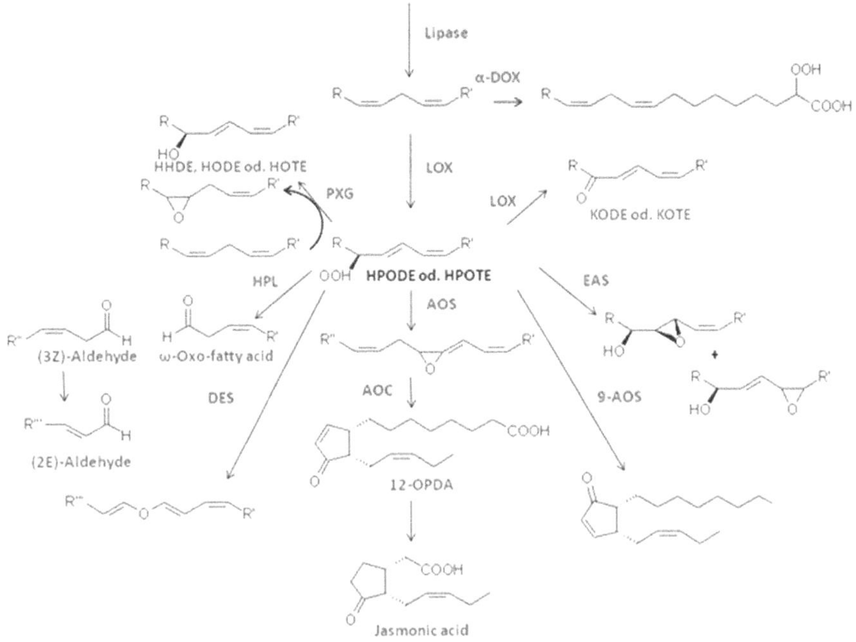

FIGURE 18.1 The oxylipin biosynthetic pathway in plants.

as substrates by other enzymes in the oxylipin pathway of these, AOS, HPL and DES formed the cytochrome P450 subfamily which has specialized in the metabolism of PUFA hydroperoxides. AOS produces 12,13- (S) -epoxy-octadecanoic acid (12,13-EOT) as the first intermediate in JA biosynthesis [11-12]. HPL then cleaves the hydroperoxides into volatile aldehydes (3-exenal) and oxo acids (12-oxo-dodecenoic acid) and finally DES catalyzes the biosynthesis of divinyl ethers as etherolenic acid. This reaction can be catalyzed by LOX or else α-dioxygenase (α-DOX). A-DOX products decompose non-enzymatically to CO_2 and aldehyde derivatives, or they are reduced chemically, i.e., with glutathione, or enzymatically – by the action of peroxygenase (PXG) [13, 14]. Hydroperoxide products produced by LOX are stable and can be further metabolized by other enzymes, i.e., members of the P450 enzyme group, the Cyp74 family, which includes: allene oxide synthase (AOS), hydroperoxide lyase (HPL) and divinylether synthase (DES), PXG or epoxy alcohol synthase (EAS) [1, 5].

18.3 SCREENING TEST

Screening tests are done to detect disease at an early stage and start treatment quickly. Prophylactic screening can only be used when there is a known method of detecting the first symptoms of a given disease or factors that may lead to its development; if we have effective, simple and fairly cheap methods of disease detection that can be applied to the entire population exposed to a given disease entity; when the method is safe, and the risk of complications is much lower than the benefits that can be obtained thanks to it.

The screening result, however, is not the final diagnosis. On the basis of analyses of medical specialists, supported by statisticians, a given group of people or a group of data that is statistically most at risk of developing the disease is usually selected to be included in the study. For this purpose, it is necessary to use epidemiological data and pay attention to the behavior and lifestyle of patients that increase the risk of developing the disease (for example, they may result from exposure to carcinogens at work). Determining how long it takes to develop the disease and how long its individual stages of development last in order to capture the changes preceding its dangerous disease process [15, 16]. These tests should be highly sensitive and have the ability to correctly detect the presence of the disease in the subjects. Screening tests are used in many of the routine tests performed during checkups [16].

18.3.1 Examples of Screening Tests

Oxylipins, as they are essential, are bioactive lipid mediators produced during inflammation or infection. They are generated by cyclooxygenases (COX), lipoxygenases (LOX) or cytochrome P450 (CYP), which are expressed in various cells and tissues. They signal through the activation of G protein-coupled receptors (GPCR). Oxylipin signaling requires deactivation. Systemic pathways for individual oxylipins, including prostacyclin and hydroxy eicosatetraenoic acids. There, the infusion of exogenous labeled lipids made it possible to determine the half-life and metabolites, some of which appear immediately and slowly disappear within minutes. Urinary metabolite analysis has become the standard for whole body oxylipin analysis. Separately, the peroxisomal β-oxidation of individual oxylipins with the aid of liver microsomes is investigated in these screening tests. Partial β-oxidation revealed truncated products called donors (minus 2 carbons) and tetranors (minus 4 carbons). They were previously identified as stable intermediates in tissues, plasma and urine [17]. The screening of linolipins, i.e., galactolipids containing esterified divinyl ether oxylipins, in leaves of several species of meadow glaucoma was conducted by Chechetkin et al. [15]. They showed that there was a rapid accumulation of linolipins in wounded, damaged leaves, while intact leaves did not contain this element. This is also confirmed by screening tests carried out on medicinal plants by Naik et al. [17]. Masoko and Eloff [18] screened 24 South African Combretum species and six Terminalia species (f. *Combretaceae*) for antioxidant and protective activity. They proved that all tested Terminalia species, extracted with acetone and methanol, showed antioxidant activity. The *T. gazensis* and *T. mollis* methanol extracts contained 11 and 14 active compounds in one of the solvent systems. Graner et al. [19] assessed the potential of various naturally occurring oxylipins found in plants for their activity as fungicides against a range of fungal pathogens interfering with Brassica cultivation. The following fungal species were tested: *Alternaria brassicae*, *Leptosphaeria maculans*, *Sclerotinia sclerotiorum*, and *Verticillium longisporum* using an in vitro plant growth inhibition test, where the relative fungal growth rate was determined in the presence of various oxylipin concentrations. Although no universal fungicidal activity has been proven for the tested compounds, examples of oxylipins with inhibitory activity have been indicated. In other cases, however, the inhibitory effects have been wiped out over time. However, several of the tested oxylipins turned out to be stable in the absence of the fungus. This effect can be explained by the induction of the degradative capacity of the fungus or its increased tolerance. Several oxylipins were also found to inhibit *L. maculans* spore sprouting, but the relative potency was different compared to the action on hyphae. The studies of these authors suggest that some selected oxylipins can be used to control Brassica plant diseases.

Hewawasam et al. [20] investigated and described the development and validation of a new system for the quantification of 21 dried spot oxylipins (DBS) using ultra-high performance tandem mass spectrometry (UHPLC-MS/MS) and stable isotope dilution analysis. The linearity and precision of the method were determined, and the stability of the 12 most abundant oxylipins was tested during two months of storage at room temperature, when added to blood and prepared as DBS on PUFAcoat™ paper. High variability of oxylipin content during the day and between days was ≤16% for all tested oxylipins. Their recovery from DBS ranged from 80 to 115%. Twelve enriched oxilipins were found to be stable for two months when stored as DBS at room temperature. This method is repeatable and precise and enables precise quantification of oxylipins in a small sample volume [20].

18.4 OXILIPIN EXPLORATION

Exploration means exploring unknown domains or areas of knowledge. Oxylipins are a series of bioactive lipid metabolites derived from polyunsaturated fatty acids, involved in, inter alia, brain homeostasis and the development of intracerebral hemorrhage (ICH). This disease is also known as cerebral bleeding, interstitial bleeding, or hemorrhagic stroke, which is sudden bleeding into the tissues of the brain, both of its chambers. Although this disease entity has been known for a long time, quantitative assessments of the oxylipin profile in ICH are still unknown.

Yuan et al. [21] performed tandem mass spectrometry with liquid chromatography to quantify the change of oxylipins in ICH. These authors detected as many as 58 oxylipins, seventeen of which increased significantly, but none of them decreased significantly in the first three days after ICH. It has been proved that the oxylipin profile changes with a decrease in ICH. These studies provided basic data on the profile of oxylipins and their enzymes in ICH. It was found that the profile of oxylipins changed with the progress of ICH and the metabolism of arachidonic and eicosapentaenoic acids in ICH, which may help to further assess the function of oxylipins and study the development of this disease, as oxilipins are found in all tissues and support homeostasis by regulating physiological processes, such as inflammation, blood clotting or blood vessel functions [21].

Oxylipins are strong biological mediators that require close control as it is still not known how they are massively removed during infection and inflammation. Misheva et al. [22] proved that lipopolysaccharide (LPS) significantly increases the removal of oxylipin through mitochondrial β-oxidation. Genetic or pharmacological targeting of palmitoyl transferase and carnitine (CPT1), the mitochondrial fatty acid importer, shows that many oxylipins are cleared by this protein during inflammation, both in vitro and in vivo. Oxylipins, or oxidized polyunsaturated fatty acids (PUFAs), are soluble mediators generated during inflammation and infection that link lipid metabolism with immunity. Monitoring and dynamic control of their removal is essential to suppress inflammation in the body. Misheva et al. [22] proved that blocking the mitochondrial enzyme CPT1 effectively doubles secreted endogenously generated oxylipins in vivo during inflammation provocation. They proposed a paradigm to exploit exogenous 12-HETE where macrophage clearance of oxylipins and their metabolites would involve the cycles of secretion and re-internalization of already partially oxidized tetranor intermediates, followed by further mitochondrial metabolism.

18.5 EXTRACTION OF OXYLIPINS

Oxylipins are strong lipid mediators derived from polyunsaturated fatty acids that play a very important role in various biological processes in the body. These compounds are an interesting subject of research, but their low or even very low stability and very low concentration of oxylipins in the samples pose a serious challenge for researchers. Hence, there is a need for continuous improvement of both the extraction techniques and the analysis techniques. Research on oxylipins is related to the development of new technological platforms based on mass spectrometry (LC-MS/MS and gas chromatography-mass spectrometry (GC-MS) / MS), as well as the improvement of the method of extracting oxylipins from biological samples [23]. However, the similar structure of oxylipins, their limited stability, and extremely low concentrations of oxylipins in the tissues place large limitations on these methods. Therefore, recently gas chromatography-mass spectrometry (GC-MS) and liquid chromatography-mass spectrometry (LC-MS) has been used recently to determine the concentration of oxylipin in biological samples [20–22]. The list of the most frequently used analytical methods in the analysis of oxylipins and their advantages and disadvantages are presented in table 18.1.

18.6 PHYTO-OXYLIPINS IN THE SERVICE OF BIOTECHNOLOGY

Lipoxygenase (LOX) is an oxidoreductase enzyme that is very widespread in the plant and animal world. Oxidation by LOX, for example, produces an aroma by regulating the biosynthesis of volatile substances. It may also function as a natural flavoring agent for food production, including as a flour bleaching agent [5, 12, 17].

18.6.1 Signaling Via Oxylipins

Oxylipins form a heterogeneous group of compounds that play various roles in the plant defense strategy. Only some of them have broad antimicrobial activity [4, 24]. Others are signaling molecules that are capable of eliciting a defense response both locally and

TABLE 18.1
Advantages and Disadvantages of Analytical Methods in the Analysis of Oxylipins

Analytical Technique	Application	Advantages	Limitations
Immunoassay methods	Eicosanoids, isops, lts, txbs, pgs	Enzyme immunoassay (EIA) and diamino assay (RIA) are easy to use, sensitive and do not require expensive instrumentation [2, 24]. RIA combined with HPLC can greatly enhance sensitivity [22].	Limited to a single metabolite at a time [21].
		RIA combined with HPLC can greatly enhance sensitivity [23].	Limited to a single metabolite at a time [22].
		ELISA is comparable to RIA and HPLC in sensitivity and selectivity [21].	Target only a few compounds [20]. Metabolite overestimation due to cross-reactivity [11, 22]. RIA requires long analysis run times and generates hazardous waste [23].
Chiral chromatography	Hetes, pgs., eets, trichomes, maresins, protections, lipoxins	Allows the enantiomeric separation of oxylipins [24].	Long equilibration and run time, and limited sensitivity [24] Reduced sensitivity (with increasing peak width and elution time, the signal/noise decreases) [25]. Not a high throughput (used for targeted analysis) [18]. Sensitive to changes in mobile-phase composition [23].
Capillary electrophoresis eats,	Diets allow the resolution of EET and DHET Regio isomers [17]	Allows the resolution of EET and DHET Regio isomers [17].	Invitation to changes in mobile-phase composition [17]. Capillary electrophoresis eats, diets allow the resolution of EET and DHET regio isomers [20]. Limited number of analytes [15]. Long run time [16].
Thin layer chromatography	Isops, pgs., keto-pgs.,	Taxes used for the preliminary separation of analytes [12, 23].	Long run time [17]. Thin layer chromatography isops, pgs., keto-pgs., tax's used for the preliminary separation of analytes [20–22]. Loss of products at the TLC stages [21].

(continued)

TABLE 18.1 (Continued)
Advantages and Disadvantages of Analytical Methods in the Analysis of Oxylipins

Analytical Technique	Application	Advantages	Limitations
HPLC-UV or fluorescence detection	Pgs., eats, hates, LT	Provides structural information [23]. Sufficient sensitivity and selectivity [15].	Limited number of UV-light absorbing analytes [22]. Sensitivity is low [1]. Requires two distinct separation methods to quantify the prostaglandin products and the HETE and leukotriene products [18]. Long analysis time required [20]. HPLC with fluorescence detection also requires derivatization [23].
Maltitol/ms	Pgs	Allows the direct quantification of prostaglandins at levels similar to ms/ms analysis [11]. Soft ionization technique allows for the analysis of non-volatile compounds [12].	Needs the co-crystallization of a matrix with the sample, which affects the quantification of the analytes [22]. Needs derivatization steps [21].
Gc-ei/ms	All classes	When coupled with ms detection, gc is both sensitive and selective [21, 22] needs derivatization of the analytes [19] multiple analytes can be detected in one sample [22]. Higher sensitivity compared to ms/ms [21].	Needs derivatization of the analytes [52]. Requires the thermal stability of the analytes [22] higher sensitivity compared to lc–ms/ms [21] there is no derivatization strategy for some compounds [23]. Absolute requirement of volatility [17].
Esi-ms/ms	All classes	Simple, fast, no sample carry-over [24] (shotgun analysis). High selectivity and good sensitivity [23].	Creates a common product ion spectrum, inability to separate the isomers [6] (shotgun analysis). Ion suppression [13] during switching of the ionization mode (negative/positive) a loss of sensitivity occurs [11].

Source: Liakh & Mika [23] modified for D. Skiba.

systemically. Some of the oxylipins may function as antimicrobial agents, influencing the growth and spread of pathogens, and as a signaling agent for compounds [25].

18.7 OXYLIPINS PRODUCED BY AOS

Jasmonates induce responses both directly (e.g., defense proteins, small molecules as alkaloids) and indirectly (through volatile compounds or non-floral nectar). Among the defense proteins, there are protease inhibitors that inhibit insect proteases, leucine aminopeptidases and threonine deaminases (TD) [15–17]. TD stands for compounds involved in the first stage of isoleucine biosynthesis, which can function as an anti-nutritional protein, interfere with the digestive process of herbivores, but also contribute to the synthesis of isoleucine and thus the production of Jasmonic acid-isoleucine (JA-Ile) [26–27]. In terms of plant defense mechanism against insects and pathogens, JA was considered the most important, key component, even though ODPA is also required for the full activation of the response. Therefore, JA and OPDA can have a positive and coordinating influence [27, 28]. In the case of A. thaliana, the rapid increase in JA-Ile biosynthesis in distal leaves co-operates with the rapid decrease in OPDA content, which suggests that this precursor may be an important control object in the biosynthesis of JA / JA-Ile [14, 27]. Recently, JA-Ile has been identified as the most important bioactive hormone involved in plant resistance to insects and pathogens [13, 17, 24, 27, 29]. Highly specific interaction of JA-Ile and other related JA conjugates (e.g., JA-Val, JA-Leu, JA-Ala, in descending order) with the COI1 unit of the E3 ubiquitin ligase complex, named as SCFcoi1 (where SCF indicates Skp / Cullin / F-box). This reaction leads to the binding of COI1 to the jasmonate ZIM (JAZ) domain protein family, to ubiquitination and their rapid degradation [2, 22, 30]. JAZ proteins are a key interface in the jasmonate signaling cascade. JAZ proteins have been shown to interact with transcription factors, each of which controls specific downstream processes. The mechanism of gene repression through JAZ has also been revealed, and the presence of JAZ proteins has been proven to be regulated by alternative splicing and interaction with proteins from other hormonal signaling pathways. These recent discoveries underline the value of studying protein-protein interactions in order to gain insight into molecular signaling pathways [30]. These proteins are repressors of JA-induced genes. Therefore, their degradation causes the activation of genes responding to JA [22, 30]. The level of JA in plant tissues varies depending on their stage of development and environmental conditions [17]. Mechanical damage causes a rapid and significant increase (25-fold) of JA and JA-Ile accumulation in places of damage to plant tissues [2, 5]. Hence, all enzymes required for their production should be in undamaged cells. There are effective mechanisms for signal suppression / deactivation. Among them are JA / JA-Ile in relation to inactive or less active compounds [16, 17, 21, 31]. For example, in wounded *A. thaliana* leaves, JA-Ile levels are approximately ten times higher and persist much longer (at least 6 hours) than in systemic tissues. Damaged leaves can be desensitized to JA-Ile by negative feedback control [30, 32]. Typically, a systemic increase in JA-Ile precedes activation of the early JA response genes. Recent reports in the case of *A. thaliana* and *N. attenuate* have shown that the synthesis of JA-Ile in distal leaves is derived from de novo synthesis [14]. Radiolabeling experiments have shown that JA / MeJA are mobile signals that can be transported through the vascular system [31, 32].

MeJA may also be considered as a volatile signal to chemical communication between damaged and undamaged plant tissues [33]. Physical signals, i.e., electrical potentials and / or hydraulic forces, have also been proposed for the rapid spread of stress signals from injured tissues to systemic tissues [5, 26, 33].

18.7.1 Volatile Oxylipins

Plant GLV levels are extremely low in undamaged plants, but they rise sharply when injured, damaged, or after feeding by herbivorous pests. Hence, GLVs are important components of the mixtures of volatile organic compounds (VOCs) released by plants in response to insect feeding. GLVs are shipped in the first phases of interaction, and other VOC components, such as terpenes, methyl salicylate and indole, are usually released later [20]. In the case of *A. thaliana*, the amount of (3Z) -hexenal increases 30-fold within five minutes after mechanical damage to the leaves [21]. GLV plays an influential role, both in the plant protection strategy, both directly and indirectly. HPL in transgenic potato plants increases the yield of aphids. *A. thaliana* plants with overexpression of HPL as well as with elevated GLV levels were more attractive to the wasp *Cotesia glomerata*, leading to higher mortality of these herbivores than those of the Brassica butterfly (*Pieris rapae*) larvae. The same plants also show higher resistance to gray mold (*Bortrytis cinerea*). Conversely, antisense HPL suppression causes lower GLV levels and greater susceptibility to the pathogen [34, 35]. Takano et al. [36] discovered that plants use (3Z) -hexenol to attract opius discitis. This compound helps wasps locate their prey, e.g., leaf miner (*Liriomyza huidobrensis*). GLVs may also stimulate the insect defense mechanism of maize by inducing the production of JA, and VOC. GLV also induces the release of VOC in tomatoes [37]. Also, the plant defense response induced by GLV can be considered moderate compared to the complete chemical protection applied after an insect or pathogen attack. Plants vaccinated with GLV are able to respond more quickly or more effectively to a subsequent attack [38], wide-ranging plant protection programs and products that can affect both plant physiology and agricultural productivity. In addition, GLV-mediated signaling is much faster than the vascular system and reaches other parts of the plant lacking or close to vascular connections to the damaged tissue but on other branches. GLVs are able to induce the expression of defense genes [21, 31, 32]. GLV and JA are also capable of inducing the secretion of extra-flora nectar as a source of carbohydrates and amino acids for ants, parasitic wasps and other herbivorous predators [39]. The induction of plant defense genes and the attraction of insect parasites negatively affect the development of herbivores [23, 39, 40]. This allows for the reduction of chemical treatments on plantations and the protection of the natural environment.

18.8 HOW CAN BIOTECHNOLOGICAL INTERVENTIONS/ TECHNIQUES BE USEFUL IN PRACTICE?

The synthesized oxylipins promote the synthesis of enzymes and proteins, and plant antibiotics may be involved in the detoxification of plants attacked by pathogens. JA is an important member of the oxylipin family. It is related to the regulation of seed formation, the germination of seeds and tubers, the development of pollen, the synthesis of methylene, as well as the genesis of tuber formation (tuberization as well as the aging of plants) [41] and the transmission of signals informing about the effects of biotic and abiotic stress [42].

Pathogenic infections and mechanical damage to plants are responsible for increasing the content of some oxylipins, which makes it easier to recognize infected tissues. It has been proven that the infection of *A. thaliana* by *Verticillium longisporum* causes e.g., a high content of several compounds, including the OPDA donor, 9,12,13-trihydroxy-10-octadecanoic acid and 9,12,13-trihydroxy-10,15-octadecadiene, which increase plant resistance to this pathogen [44].

Physiologically active oxylipin (2E) -dodecene-1,12-dicarboxylic acid (or traumatic acid) and 12-oxo-trans-10-dodecenoic acid (traumatic) may also induce cell multiplication and callus formation in damaged sites [29]. Such disorganization of plant tissues causes the release of volatile C6 and C9 aromatic compounds (smell of freshly cut grass). Both C6 compounds (hexenals and hexenol) are important antifungal and antibacterial agents that provide basic protection against pests and attackers [44]. *Nicotiana tabacum* L. infected with *Golovinomyces cichoracearum* reacts with an increased level of 2 (E) -hexenal [129]. Infection with *Botrytis cinerea* increased the level of (2Z) and (3Z) -hexenals, (3Z) -hexenilacetate and (3Z) -hexenol, which inhibited the growth of fungal infection in tomato tissues [45]. (2E) and (3Z)-nonenale (volatile compounds C9) with the smell of fresh cucumber were released as a result of mechanical damage and limited the activity of pathogens [46].

Moreover, the expression of LOX genes is regulated by pathogens and phytohormones, i.e., the AtLOX1 gene induced by JA and ABA, and the OsLOX3 gene was induced by JA [5]. The mutation in AtLOX3 and AtLOX4 led to various developmental dysfunctions in Nicotiana tabacum plants. Expression of AtLOX2, AtLOX6 and TomLoxD has been shown to be associated with wound-induced JA biosynthesis [5, 46]. Overexpression of the OsLOX2 genes shortened the germination time of seeds [47]. AdLOX from Actinidia deliciosa (kiwi) participate in the formation of the fruit aroma [48]. On the other hand, the silencing of CaLOX2 led to a reduction in JA levels and resistance to thrips. Exogenous JA application negatively influenced feeding and thrips preferences [49].

18.8.1 Biotechnological Techniques Useful for Pharmaceutical Companies

Thanks to biotechnology, the greatest revolution is currently taking place in medicine and pharmacy. It concerns all elements of medical and pharmaceutical activity, from the design and synthesis of new drugs, through the revolution in diagnostics, prevention, to the introduction of new methods of treating various diseases. Using both conventional and sophisticated methods of sophisticated molecular biology methods, genes encoding proteins with desired characteristics are now identified, and then these genes are transferred to other organisms. You can also combine gene fragments and create new hybrids with the desired features, even more marked than in the original genes [50].

Molecular biology techniques have also made significant progress in laboratory diagnostics. This mainly concerns the identification of the molecular causes of monogene and multigene diseases, as well as practical diagnostics. Kits for the determination of nucleic acids of pathogenic microorganisms (Amplicor MTB, Amplicor HPV, Roche; TBC-PCR, HPV-PCR, Oligene etc.), based on the polymerase chain reaction (PCR) technique, have already been introduced into routine use. Many diseases look for mutations or polymorphisms (genetic variations) in specific genes. Both kits produced by pharmaceutical companies and methods developed by specific laboratories serve this purpose. For example, in 2004, AmpliChip CYP450 was released for the rapid evaluation of two genes involved in the degradation of many drugs [50].

Today, approximately 17% of drug revenues are biopharmaceuticals. In the future, a further increase in the importance of biopharmaceuticals in the treatment of both humans and animals can be expected. The share of substances in preclinical studies based on biotechnology is more than 27% of all substances in preclinical studies. The most important are raw materials and products for the treatment of cancer, various metabolic disorders, and infectious diseases. Today, traditional approaches to therapy, such as RNA interference, already play a minor role in commercial drug research and development (approximately 2.0% of all preclinical biological substances). Investing in high technology such as biotechnology is crucial for highly developed countries due to a lack of raw materials. It is biotechnology that helps the pharmaceutical industry to develop new products, new processes, new methods and new services, and to improve the existing ones [51, 52]. Most of the therapeutic drugs on the market are mainly biopreparations such as antibodies, nucleic acid products, and vaccines. Bioformulations are developed in several steps, starting with understanding the basic principles of health and disease; through molecular mechanisms, functions of related biomolecules; synthesis and purification of molecules, further determining the stability, toxicity and immunogenicity of the drug; drug coordination; patenting and the final stage are clinical trials [52].

18.9 CONCLUSIONS AND A FUTURE PERSPECTIVE

Oxylipin biosynthesis can take place in plants at the level of esterified or free, polyunsaturated fatty acids. LOX, as a redox dioxygenase enzyme, catalyzes PUFAs and esters with hydroperoxide derivatives. Cis- and trans-pentadiene structures with double bonds are synthesized by adding intramolecular oxygen. Linoleic and linolenic acids, found in plants, function as LOX substrates, and these in turn mediate JA biosynthesis and function as stress biomarkers against fungal, bacterial, and pest stresses, as well as against abiotic stresses such as drought, heat, cold, or radiation. Plants use hormones and hormone-like compounds as alarm signals of stress from pathogen or insect-infested tissues to organs within the same plant or to other neighboring plants. Some of these signaling molecules, such as JA and MeJA, can be systemically translocated, others, such as GLV and MeJA, serve as airborne signals. The application of different, controlled signals and differentiated diffusion systems allow for the rapid transmission of stress signals to all tissues and the reduction of inappropriate expression and avoiding costly systemic protection. Research into molecular mechanisms in stress relief has shed new light on the physiological and biochemical changes in plants. In the near future, scientists should focus on the advances in the biosynthesis of oxylipins and their contribution to the local and systemic development of plant defense mechanisms.

ABBREVIATIONS

A. solani	*Alternaria solani*
A. thaliana	*Arabidopsis thaliana*
AM	arbuscular mycorrhiza
AOC	allene oxide cyclosis
AOS	allene oxide synthase
C. lagenarium	*Colletotrichum lagenarium*
C. perniciosa	*Crinipellis perniciosa*
DES	synthase divinyl ether
F. oxysporum, f. sp. *Lycopersici*	*Fusarium oxysporum*, f. sp. *lycopersici*
F. oxysporum, f. sp. *Cucumerinum*	*Fusarium oxysporum*, f. sp. *cucumerinum*
EAS	epoxy alcohol synthase
GC-MS	mass spectrometry
GLV	green volatile substances
GLVs	antibacterial activity
HPL	hydroperoxide lyase
ICH	intracerebral hemorrhage
JA	jasmonate
JA-Ile	Jasmonic acid-isoleucine
JAZ – ZIM	domain protein family
LC-MS	liquid chromatography-mass spectrometry
LOX	lipoxygenase
LPS	lipopolysaccharide
MeJA	methyl jasmonate
R. solani	*Rhizoctonia solani*
ROS	reactive oxygen species
OPDA	12-oxophytodienoic acid donor
P. avenae	*Pyrenophora avenae*
P. ultimum	*Pythium ultimum*
PO	oxylipin plants
pPLA-I	patatin lipase
PUFA	polyunsaturated fatty acids
PXG	peroxygenase
TD	threonine deaminases
UHPLC-MS/MS	ultra-high-performance liquid-tandem chromatography mass spectrometry
α-DOX	α-dioxygenase

REFERENCES

1. Lee, D.-S., Nioche, P., Hamberg, M., and Raman, CS. Structural insight into the evolutionary pathways of the enzymes in oxylipin biosynthesis. Nature, 2008, 455: 363–368. DOI: 10.1038/nature07307.
2. Hamberg, M. Biosynthesis of 12-Oxo-10,15 (Z) -phytiodic acid: identification of allene oxide cyclase. Biochem. Biophysics. Res. Communication. 1988, 156: 543–550. DOI: 10.1016 / S0006-291X (88) 80876-3.
3. Andreou, A., Brodhun, F. i Feussner, I. Oxylipin biosynthesis in non-mammals. Prog. Lipid Res. 2009, 48:148–170. DOI: 10.1016/j.plipres.2009.02.002.
4. Santino, A., Bonsegna S., De Domenico S., Poltronieri P. Plant oxylipins and their contribution to plant defence. Review. Current Topics in Plant Biology, 2010, 1–10, file:///C:/Users/Barbara/Downloads/Santinoetal.2011%20(1).pdf
5. Singh, P., Arif, Y., Miszczuk, E., Bajguz, A., Hayat, S. Specific Roles of Lipoxygenases in Development and Responses to Stress in Plants. Plants, 2022, 11, 979. https://doi.org/ 10.3390/plants11070979
6. Ponce LI, Mats H., Carmen C. Oxylipins in moss development and defence. Frontiers in Plant Science, 6, 2015, 486: 1–12, DOI: 10.3389/fpls.2015.00483.
7. Avis T. J., Bélanger R. R. 2001. Specificity and mode of action of the antifungal fatty acid cis-9-heptadecenoic acid produced by *Pseudozyma flocculosa*. Applied and Environmental Microbiology, 67: 956–960.
8. Liu S., Ruan W., Li J., Xu H., Wang J., Gao Y., Wang J. Biological control of phytopathogenic fungi by fatty acids. Micropathological, 2008, 166(2): 93–102.
9. Mosblech A., Feussner I., Heilmann I. Oxylipins: structurally diverse metabolites from fatty acid oxidation. Plant Physiology and Biochemistry, 2009, 47(6): 511–517.
10. Cowley T., Walters D. Local and systemic effects of oxylipins on powdery mildew infection in barley. Pest Management Science: Formerly Pesticide Science, 2005, 61(6): 572–576.
11. Granér G., Hamberg M., Meijer J. Screening of oxylipins for control of oilseed rape (*Brassica napus*) fungal pathogens. Phytochemistry, 2003, 63(1): 89–95.
12. Andreou A., Feussner I. 2009. Lipoxygenases – structure and reaction mechanism. Phytochemistry, 2009, 70(13–14): 1504–1510.
13. Ellinger, D., Stingl, N., Kubigsteltig, II, Bals, T., Juenger, M., Pollmann, S., Berger, S., Schuenemann, D. i Mueller, MJ. DONGLE and DEFECTIVE IN ANTHER DEHISCENCE1 are lipases not essential in wound and pathogen-induced jasmonate biosynthesis: excess lipases contribute to the formation of jasmone's. Plant Physiol., 2010, 153: 114–127. DOI: 10.1104/s. 110.15593.
14. Troufflard S., Mullen W., Larson T.R., Graham I. A., Crozier A., Amtmann A., Armengaud P. Potassium deficiency induces the biosynthesis of oxylipins and glucosinolates in *Arabidopsis thaliana*. BMC Plant Biology, 2010, 10(1): 1–13.
15. .Chechetkin IR, Blufard AS, Khairutdinov BI et al (2013) Isolation and structure elucidation of linolipins C and D, complex oxylipins from flax leaves. Phytochemistry 123 Phytochem Rev (2019) 18:343–358 355 96:110–116. https://doi.org/10.1016/j.phytochem.2013.08. 010
16. Genva M, Akong FO, Andersson MX, Deleu M., Lins L., Fauconnier ML, New insights into the biosynthesis of esterified oxylipins and their involvement in plant defense and developmental mechanisms. Phytochem Rev (2019) 18:343–358.
17. Naik GH, Priyadarsini, K.I., Satav, J.G., Banavalikar, M.M., Sohoni, D.P., Biyani, M.K., Mohan, H. Phytochemistry, 2003, 63(1): 97–104. https://doi.org/10.1016/S0031-9422(02)00754-9

18. Masoko P, Eloff JN. Screening of twenty-four South African *Combretum* and six Terminalia species (*Combretaceae*) for antioxidant activities. Afr J Tradit Complement Altern Med. 2006, 4(2):231–239. doi:10.4314/ajtcam.v4i2.31213
19. Granér G, Hamberg M, Meijer J. Screening of oxylipins for control of oilseed rape (Brassica napus) fungal pathogens. Phytochemistry. 2003; 63(1): 89–95. doi: 10.1016/s0031-9422(02)00724-0. PMID: 12657302.
20. Hewawasam E, Liu G, Jeffery DW, Muhlhausler BS, Gibson RA. A stable method for routine analysis of oxylipins from dried blood spots using ultra-high performance liquid chromatography-tandem mass spectrometry. Prostaglandins Leukot Essent Fatty Acids. 2018,137: 12–18. doi: 10.1016/j.plefa.2018.08.001.
21. Yuan JJ, Chen Q, Xiong XY, *et al*. Quantitative Profiling of Oxylipins in Acute Experimental Intracerebral Hemorrhage. Front Neurosci. 2020, 14: 777. doi:10.3389/fnins.2020.00777
22. Misheva, M., Kotzamanis, K., Davies, L.C. *et al*. Oxylipin metabolism is controlled by mitochondrial β-oxidation during bacterial inflammation. *Nat Commun* 2022, **13**, 139. https://doi.org/10.1038/s41467-021-27766-8
23. Liakh I, Mika A. Reprogramming of lipid metabolism in colorectal cancer cell. [in:] Science, Research and Scientific Reporting 2020. Part I. Natural and medical sciences. Publisher: Idea Knowledge Future, Świebodzice, ISBN: 978-83-953882-6-2, ISBN (full) 978-83-953882-4-8.
24. Prost I., Dhondt S., Rothe G., Vicente J., Rodriguez M. J., Kift N., Carbonne F., Griffiths G., Esquerré-Tugayé M. T., Rosahl S. Evaluation of the antimicrobial activities of plant oxylipins supports their involvement in defence against pathogens. Plant Physiol., 2005, 139: 1902–1913.
25. Rafiqi M., Jelonek L., Akum N.F., Zhang F., Kogel K.H. Effector candidates in the secretive of *Piriformospora indica*, a ubiquitous plant-associated fungus. Front. Plant Sci., 2013, 4:228. doi: 10.3389/fpls.2013.00228.
26. Studholme D.J., Harris B., Le Cocq K., Winsbury R., Perera V., Ryder L., Ward J.L., Beale M.H., Thornton C.R. Investigating the beneficial traits of *Trichoderma hamatum* GD12 for sustainable agriculture-insights from genomics. Front. Plant Sci. 2013, 4:258. doi: 10.3389/fpls.2013.00258
27. Davis J.L., Armengaud P., Larson T.R., Graham I.A., White P.J., Newton A.C., Amtmann A. Contrasting nutrient–disease relationships: potassium gradients in barley leaves have opposite effects on two fungal pathogens with different sensitivities to jasmonic acid. Plant, Cell & Environment, 2018, 41(10): 2357–2372.
28. Cipollini D.F., Redman A.M. Age-dependent effects of jasmonic acid treatment and wind exposure on foliar oxidase activity and insect resistance in tomato. Journal of Chemical Ecology, 1999, 25: 271–281.
29. Hammerbacher A., Coutinho T.A., Gershenzon J. Roles of plant volatiles in defence against microbial pathogens and microbial exploitation of volatiles. Plant, Cell & Environment, 2019, 42(10): 2827–2843.
30. Pauwels L, Goossens A. The JAZ proteins: a crucial interface in the jasmonate signaling cascade. Plant Cell. 2011, 23(9): 3089–3100. doi:10.1105/tpc.111.089300
31. Rodriguez-Saona C.R., Rodriguez-Saona L. E., Frost C.J. Herbivore-induced volatiles in the perennial shrub, *Vaccinium corymbosum*, and their role in inter-branch signalling. Journal of Chemical Ecology, 2009, 35(2): 163–175.
32. Martinez-Medina A., Fernandez I., Sánchez-Guzmán M.J., Jung S.C., Pascual J.A., Pozo M.J. Deciphering the hormonal signalling network behind the systemic resistance induced by *Trichoderma harzianum* in tomato. Front. Plant Sci. 2013, 4: 206. doi: 10.3389/fpls.2013.00206

33. Liu B., Kaurilind E., Zhang L., Okereke C. N., Remmel T., Niinemets Ü. Improved plant heat shock resistance is introduced differently by heat and insect infestation: the role of volatile emission traits. Oecologia, 2022, 1–16. https://doi.org/10.1007/s00442-022-05168-x
34. Howe, GA i Jander, G. Plant resistance to insectivorous plants. Ann. Rev. Plant Biol., 59, 2008, 41–66. DOI: 10.1146/annurev.arplant.59.032607.092825.
35. Walters D., Raynor L., Mitchell A., Walker R., Walker K. Antifungal activities of four fatty acids against plant pathogenic fungi. Mycopathologia, 2004, 157(1): 87–90.
36. Takano S.-I., Iwaizumi R , Nakanishi Y, Someya H. aboratory hybridization between the two clades of *Liriomyza huidobrensis* (Diptera: *Agromyzidae*), Applied Entomology and Zoology, 2008, 43(3): 397–402. Doi: 10.1303/aez.2008.397.
37. Scala A, Allmann S, Mirabella R, Haring MA, Schuurink RC. Green leaf volatiles: a plant's multifunctional weapon against herbivores and pathogens. Int J Mol Sci. 2013;14(9):17781–17811. Published 2013 Aug 30. doi:10.3390/ijms140917781
38. War AR, Paulraj MG, Ahmad T, et al. Mechanisms of plant defense against insect herbivores. Plant Signal Behav. 2012, 7(10):1306–1320. doi:10.4161/psb.21663
39. Allmann S., Baldwin I. T. 2010. Insects betray themselves in nature to predators by rapid isomerization of green leaf volatiles. Science, 2010, 329, 1075–1078.
40. Matsui K. Green leaf volatiles: hydroperoxide lyase pathway of oxylipin metabolism. Current Opinion in Plant Biology, 2006, 9(3): 274–280.
41. Delporte, A.; Lannoo, N.; Vandenborre, G.; Ongenaert, M.; Van Damme, E.J.M. Jasmonate response of the *Nicotiana tabacum* agglutinin promoter in *Arabidopsis thaliana*. Plant Physiol. Biochem. 2011, 49, 843–851.
42. Piotrowska, A, Bajguz, A. Conjugates of abscisic acid, brassinosteroids, ethylene, gibberellins, and jasmonates. Phytochemistry, 2011, 72: 2097–2112.
43. Künstler A, Gullner G, Ádám AL, Kolozsváriné Nagy J, Király L. The Versatile Roles of Sulfur-Containing Biomolecules in Plant Defense-A Road to Disease Resistance. Plants (Basel). 2020;9(12):1705. Published 2020 Dec 3. doi:10.3390/plants9121705
44. Skoczek A., Piesik D., Wenda-Piesik A., Buszewski B., Bocianowski J., Wawrzyniak M. Volatile organic compounds released by maize following herbivory or insect extract application and communication between plants. Journal of Applied Entomology, 2017, 141(8): 630–643.
45. Vidhyasekaran P. Plant Innate Immunity Signals and Signaling Systems. Bioengineering and Molecular Manipulation for Crop Disease Management. Copyright: 2020 Published: 16 April 2021, Publisher: Springer, Netherlands, 2020, DOI: 10.1007/978-94-024-1940-5. ISBN: 978-9-40-241939-9, 978-9-40-241940-5
46. Matsui K, Minami A, Hornung E, Shibata H, Kishimoto K, Ahnert V, Kindl H, Kajiwara T, Feussner I. Biosynthesis of fatty acid derived aldehydes is induced upon mechanical wounding and its products show fungicidal activities in cucumber. Phytochemistry. 2006 Apr;67(7):649–57. doi: 10.1016/j.phytochem.2006.01.006. Epub 2006 Feb 23. PMID: 16497344.
47. Huang J, Cai M, Long Q, Liu L, Lin Q, Jiang L, Chen S, Wan J. OsLOX2, a rice type I lipoxygenase, confers opposite effects on seed germination and longevity. Transgenic Res. 2014 Aug;23(4):643–55. doi: 10.1007/s11248-014-9803-2. Epub 2014 May 4. PMID: 24792034.
48. Cesoniene L, Daubaras R, Bogacioviene S, et al. Investigations of Volatile Organic Compounds in Berries of Different *Actinidia kolomikta* (Rupr. & Maxim.) Maxim. Accessions. Polish Journal of Food and Nutrition Sciences. 2020;70(3):291–300. doi:10.31883/pjfns/124029.

49. Sarde SJ, Bouwmeester K, Venegas-Molina J, David A, Boland W. *et al.* Involvement of sweet pepper CaLOX2 in jasmonate-dependent induced defence against Western flower thrips. Journal Integrative Plant Biology, 2019, 61(10): 1085–1098. https://doi.org/10.1111/jipb.12742
50. Anonimous 2022. Puls Medycyny. https://pulsmedycyny.pl/biotechnologiczna-rewolucja-w-farmacji-i-medycynie-880229 (accessed 30.05.2022).
51. Gaisser S, Nusser M. Stellenwert der Biotechnologie in der pharmazeutischen Wirkstoffentwicklung. Z Evid Fortbild Qual Gesundhwes. 2010, 104(10): 732–7. ndoi: 10.1016/j.zefq.2010.05.001. Epub 2010. PMID: 21147436.
52. Mallela K. Pharmaceutical biotechnology - concepts and applications. Hum Genomics. 2010;4(3): 218–219. doi:10.1186/1479-7364-4-3-218

19 Antimicrobial Activities of Oxylipins in Plants

Olugbemi T. Olaniyan[1*], *Peter Onyebuagu*[2] *and Charles O. Adetunji*[3]
[1*]Laboratory for Reproductive Biology and Developmental Programming, Department of Physiology, Rhema University Aba, Abia State, Nigeria
[2]Department of Physiology, Federal University of Technology, Owerri, Nigeria
[3]Applied Microbiology, Biotechnology and Nanotechnology Laboratory, Department of Microbiology, Edo State University Uzairue, Edo State, Nigeria
*All correspondence: +2348055763933; olugbemiolaniyan@binghamuni.edu.ng

CONTENTS

19.1 INTRODUCTION

Over the last few decades, several studies have highlighted the important role of plant oxylipins in prevention and inhibition of microbial development and growth. Oxylipins like jasmonates, green leaf volatiles, and divinylethers have stimulated a lot of interest due to their active role as antimicrobial agents. Muhammad et al. [1] wrote extensively on the antimicrobial activity of plant oxylipins as defense system through the production of reactive oxygen species against pathogens. Isabelle et al. [2] also revealed that plant oxylipins are involved in defense mechanisms through antimicrobial activities, stimulation of plant defense gene expression, and control of plant cell death against pathogens. The authors utilized in vitro growth inhibition assays to analyze some individual oxylipins for their antimicrobial actions. They worked on 43 oxylipins and about 13 microbes including oomycetes, fungi, and bacteria, thus reported that many of the oxylipins were able to significantly suppress the plant microbe's growth, block mycelial development with inhibition of spore germination. Oxylipins as antimicrobial agent can activate transcription factors, hormone related genes, and signaling cascade of events like oxidative stress in plant pathogen interactions [3].

DOI: 10.1201/9781003316558-19

Studies have shown that oxylipins have different physiological functions such as biological mediators, signaling molecules, and defense mechanisms. These functions include enhancing the plasticity of plasma membranes, the production of hydroxy fatty acids and mobilization of lipids that are involved in molecular communication and antibiosis effect. The antimicrobial activity of oxylipins has led to discovery of other novel polyesters, referred to as estolides, which form a novel group of lubricants and green emulsifiers [4]. Recently, several scientists have reported interest in the utilization of natural antimicrobial agents in combating many pathogenic diseases. Though, many of these natural antimicrobial agents' mechanism of action is yet to be elucidated but the popularity in public health safety have been spectacular. Therefore, this book chapter highlights the antimicrobial activity of oxylipins against several pathogenic organisms like fungi, oomycetes, and bacteria.

19.2 ANTIMICROBIAL ACTIVITIES OF OXYLIPINS IN PLANTS

Claus and Ivo, [5] reported that oxylipins plants are known to possess substantial amounts of bioactive agents such as metabolites, hydroxyl fatty acids, and oxygenated fatty acids with enormous pharmacological actions. Over the last few decades, several oxylipins plants such as jasmonates have been explored for possible mechanism of action in several physiological functions. Many of the enzymes derived from these plants are tested and evaluated for possible bio-signaling activity like cross-talk. Estelle et al. [6] revealed that plant oxylipins possess biocidal activity against pathogenic organisms owing to their structural—functional configuration in elucidating reactive oxygen species and activation of defense-related genes. The authors attributed the biocidal properties of oxylipins to the antimicrobial activity such as membrane pore formation, nucleic acid, or protein denaturation, membrane destabilization, oxidative bursts, detergent-like action, exhibit growth-inhibitory activity, and excessive production of electrophilic molecules.

Nilgün and Şeniz, [7] showed that natural antimicrobial agents derived from bioresources are beginning to generated public interest owing to their efficacy and lower side effects as compared with many synthetic drugs. The authors revealed that plant-based antimicrobial agents are known to inhibit the growth of pathogenic food microbes against food borne disease. Studies have revealed that food borne diseases have increased globally causing serious public health concern. Food spoilage is a critical factor for food insecurity and disease development resulting in poor health status, thus so many food industries utilize food preservatives to fight against saprophyte microorganisms and increase food shelf life. Reports have shown that several conventional methods or approaches such as chilling, drying, freezing, heat treatment, gamma irradiation, high pressure, modified atmosphere packaging, and additives have been used over the decades with little or no improvement and more damage to the food organoleptic properties, thus recently a search for replacement or alternative food preservatives has been seen.

Noteworthy is the detrimental effect of chemical or synthetic preservatives on human health resulting in cancer and other metabolic diseases. This has resulted in increases in utilization of plant-based antimicrobials agents such as oxylipins for food preservatives. Some of the proposed mechanisms of action of these plant-based antimicrobial agents include perturbation of the membrane with phenolic compounds, chelating metals with flavonols or flavonoids, leakage of cell contents, active transport, disruption of metabolic enzymes, loss of ATP, degradation of the cell wall, proteins, coagulation of cytoplasm, inhibition of the cytoplasmic membrane and depletion of proton motive force and interacting genetic materials. Estelle et al. [6] revealed that phyto-oxylipins are biocidal agents due to the structural and chemical configuration, with the ability to induce reactive oxygen species, stimulate defense-related gene expression, and electrophile species. The chemical ability is strong enough to break pathogenic membranes, to generate active metabolites and cause serious enzymatic reaction. Phyto-oxylipins has been shown to act as systemic acquired resistance and in vitro effects on pathogenic organisms like biotrophic, hemibiotrophic, and necrotrophic with strong antimicrobial activities.

Oxylipins have been shown to be derived from a-DOX and 9-LOX pathways like 9-Keto-10(E), 12(Z), 15(Z)-octadecatrienoic acid from linoleic acid acting as strong potential as antibacterial. Oxylipins have been shown to possess strong in vitro activity with antimicrobial potential against pathogenic organisms like fungi, bacteria, and oomycetes. Oxylipins as antimicrobial agents are able to induce membrane pore formation, protein or nucleic acid denaturation, oxidative bursts, detergent-like action, reactive electrophiles species, and membrane de-stabilization. Many types of plants oxylipins that exhibit antimicrobial activity include u-5(Z)-etherolenic acid, (G)-cis-12,13-epoxy-9(Z)-octadecenoic acid, (G)-cis-9,10-epoxy-12(Z)-octadecenoic acid, G)-threo-12,13-dihydroxy-9(Z)-octadecenoic acid, (G)-threo-9,10-dihydroxy-12(Z)-octadecenoic acid, 10(S),11(S)-epoxy-9(S)-hydroxy-12(Z), 15(Z)-octadecadienoate, 11(S),12(S)-epoxy-13(S)-hydroxy-9(Z), 15(Z)-octadecadienoate, 13(S)-hydroperoxy-9(Z),11(E),15(Z)-octadecatrienoic acid (13-HPOT, 13(S)-hydroperoxy-9(Z),11(E),15(Z)-octadecatrienoic acid (13-HPOT, 13(S)-hydroxy-9(Z),11(E),15(Z)-octadecatrienoic acid (13-HOT), 13(S)-hydroxy-9(Z),11(E)-octadecadienoic acid (13-HOD), 13-keto-9(Z),11(E)-octadecadienoic acid (13-KOD), 13-keto-9(Z),11(E),15(Z)-octadecatrienoic acid (13-KOT), 9(S)-hydroperoxy-10(E),12(Z),15(Z)-octadecatrienoic acid (9-HPOT), 9(S)-hydroperoxy-10(E),12(Z)-octadecadienoic acid (9-HPOD), 9(S)-hydroxy-10(E),12(Z),15(Z)-octadecatrienoic acid (9-HOT), 9(S)-hydroxy-10(E),12(Z)-octadecadienoic acid (9-HOD), 9-keto-10(E),12(Z)-octadecadienoic acid (9-KOD), 9-keto-10(E),12(Z),15(Z)-octadecatrienoic acid (9-KOT), colneleic acid, colnelenic acid, anacardic acid, 12-oxo-10,15(Z)-phytodienoic acid (OPDA), 2(E)-nonenal, 3(Z)-nonenal, 2(E)-hexenal, and 3(Z)-hexenal. Studies have revealed that secondary metabolites of fatty acid breakdown possess antibacterial activity responsible for peroxidation process and reactive oxygen species through short chain aldehydes and oxylipins.

Eliana et al. [8] reported that plants possess antimicrobial lipids as natural compound with great potential in pharmaceutical industry. The authors demonstrated that through lipidomics bioprospecting, isolation, and characterization of these antimicrobial lipids can be done. Many of these antimicrobial lipids are reported to be abundant in marine organisms, plants, and marine vertebrates. Eliana et al. [8] revealed that oxylipins are from oxidation of polyunsaturated fatty acids with antifungal activity that can cause damage to several mold species and yeast due to increased movement on the cell membrane. Oxylipins have been shown to have 1–3 hydroxyl groups effective against bacteria, fungi, and mold. Oxylipins according to these authors are derived from polyunsaturated fatty acids of plant secondary metabolites with antibacterial action. Oxylipins cause membrane leakage and protein synthesis inhibition on pathogenic organism bacterial, cancer, parasitic infections, through inflammation.

Eliana et al. [8] revealed that oxylipins are generated from stems, roots and leaves of Alternanthera brasiliana (Brazilian joyweed) and endophytic Bacillus strains through extraction using ethanol or ethyl-acetate. This production reveals a crosstalk interface between plant and bacteria. It is revealed that oxylipins are present in almost every organism occurring as a free molecule. They are produced from a complex reaction of network of signaling cascade of events in the tissues involving G protein-coupled receptors (GPCR), psi-producing oxygenase (Ppo) and protein kinase (Pka) proteins. Oxyliins are formed from the fatty acid hydroperoxides from non-enymatic and enzymatic reactions in racemic mixtures. The biological activity of oxylipinds against *Lycopersicon esculentum* is through signaling process involving acidic moiety. Deboever et al. [9] showed that plant oxylipins are fatty acid hydroperoxides which act as a signaling molecule against pathogenic organisms. The mechanism of defense involves biocidal action against gram negative bacteria like *Pectobacterium carotovorum*, *Xanthomonas translucens*, and *Pseudomonas syringae*. The authors conducted integrative biophysical methods using in silico and in vitro methods to investigate the antibacterial activity of oxylipins against pathogenic organisms. From their study, it was demonstrated that the amphiphilic molecules target the lipid membrane resulting into membrane damage through cardiolipin and phosphatidylethanolamine on the bacteria membrane. The authors noted that many amphipathic molecules can interact well with lipid membranes to produce a detergent-like mechanism and distribution of membrane proteins.

Isabelle et al. [2] demonstrated that oxylipins are important antibacterial agents produced from plant polyunsaturated fatty acids as metabolites. Through in vitro growth inhibition assays, the authors were able to reveal the mechanism of its antimicrobial action against bacteria (*P. syringae* pv syringae, *P. syringae* pv tomato, *P. syringae* pv maculicola, *P. syringae* pv tabaci, *X. campestris* pv campestris, and *E. carotovora* subsp. carotovora), fungi (*A. brassicicola*, *F. oxysporum*, *F. radicis-lycopersici*, *B. cinerea*, *C. herbarum*, and *Rhizopus spp.*) and oomycetes (*P. infestans* and *P. parasitica* var. nicotianae) through inhibition of mycelial growth and spore germination. Montillet et al. [10] noted that oxylipins act as antibacterial agents by stimulating innate immunity against pathogenic organisms. The authors were able to reveal this mechanism by utilizing genetic, pharmacological, and biochemical approaches. Ponce et al. [11] showed that oxylipins participate in the defense mechanisms of plant against pathogenic organisms through reactive oxygen species generation like hydroperoxides, hydroxides, keto acids, aldehydes, and oxoacids, divinyl ethers, oxidation, and enzymes production. Studies have revealed that fatty acids form the major building block of many complex lipid structures with several physiochemical properties. In eukaryotic organisms, the polyunsaturated fatty acids form oxylipins which are secondary metabolites.

Oxylipins are also produced in mammals in form of prostanoids along the inflammatory pathways. During the production of oxylipins, fatty acids are converted into fatty acid hydroperoxides through non-enzymatic or enzymatic pathways. Linoleic (18:2), hexadecatrienoic acid (16:3) and α-linolenic acid (18:3) are the major substrate for oxylipins production in plants. Sucharitha and Uma [12] reported that phyto-oxylipins have been revealed to possess antimicrobial properties due to the role of 9 and 13-lipoxygenase (LOX) products against several pathogenic organisms. The authors utilized in vitro growth inhibition assays to analyze the antimicrobial actin of LOX hydroperoxides products like 9-hydroperoxy octadecatrienoic acid (9-HPOTrE) and 9-hydroperoxy octadecadienoic acid (9-HPODE) against fungi and bacteria. In their conclusion, the authors reported that the antimicrobial activity of 9-hydroperoxy octadecatrienoic acid (9-HPOTrE) is the strongest as compared with 9-hydroperoxy octadecadienoic acid (9-HPODE). LOX metabolites such as fatty acid hydroperoxides, 9-HPOTrE, 13-HPOTrE and 9-HPODE and 13-HPODE, colnelenic acid and colneleic acid are known to act as antimicrobial agents. The antimicrobial action causes cell apoptosis, generation of reactive species, and necrosis. Other studies have highlighted the importance of oxylipins against pathogenic organism in preventing diseases.

Oxylipins are shown to induce chemotroic reaction and chemo-attractants in beneficial fungus *T harzianum*. Oxylipins induce inflammatory response and hyperresponsiveness in host respiratory air ways resulting into disruption of airway epithelial cells related calcium homeostasis, mitochondrial structural dysfunction, bronchial cell injury, severe airway remodeling, enhanced airway neutrophilia, and elevated stress-related pro-inflammatory cytokine mediators [13]. Jorge et al. [14] reported that oxylipins are derived from metabolites of lipids such as linoleic acids and linolenic through the action of lipoxygenases (13-LOX and 9-LOX) which play a significant role in defense system of plants against pathogenic organisms. The authors showed that jasmonic acid as oxylipin is an important antimicrobial agent through signals regulating gene expression, generation of antimicrobial products, and cell death. The authors utilized different types of oxylipins in their study with antibacterial activity such as a-DOX derivatives, 2(R)-hydroxy-9(Z),12(Z),15(Z)-octadecatrienoic acid, 2(R,S)-hydroxy-9(Z)-octadecenoic acid, 8(Z),11(Z),14(Z)-heptadecatrienal, 2(R)-hydroxy-azelaic acid, 9-LOX derivatives, 9(S)-hydroxy-10(E),12(Z)-octadecadienoic acid, 9(S)-hydroxy-10(E),12(Z),15(Z)-octadecatrienoic acid, 9-keto-10(E),12(Z)-octadecadienoic acid, 9-keto-10(E),12(Z),15(Z)-octadecatrienoic acid, 2(E)-nonena, 3(Z)-nonenal, 9-oxononanoic acid, 10(S),11(S)-epoxy-9(S)-hydroxy-12(Z),15(Z)-octadecadienoatea, 9(S),10(S),11(R)-trihydroxy-12(Z)-octadecenoic acid, 9(S),12(S),13(S)-trihydroxy-10(E)-octadecenoic acid, 9(S),12(S),13(S)-trihydroxy-10(E),15(Z)-octadecadienoic acid, 9-hydroxy-10-oxo-12(Z)-octadecenoic acid, azelaic acid, peroxygenase/epoxygenase derivatives, cis_9,10,epoxyoctadecanoic acid, 9(R),10(S)-epoxy-12(Z)-octadecenoic acid, (6)-threo-9,10-dihydroxy-12(Z)-octadecenoic acid, and (6)-threo-9,10-dihydroxy-12(Z),15(Z)-octadecadienoic acid.

Muhammad et al. [1] reported that plants have numerous defense mechanisms to cope with pathogenic attack and stress. The authors highlighted that some of the pathogenic chemicals are endogenously produced, such as oxylipins like jasmonates (12-oxo-phytodienoic acid, jasmonic acid and methyl jasmonate), green leaf volatiles (C6 and C9 aldehydes, esters and alcohols) and divinylethers. Many of these oxylipins have been reported to play a significant role as antimicrobial agents through inhibition of pathogen's propagation and growth like bacteria, fungi, and viruses. Muhammad et al. [1] showed that oxylipins are very active against gram negative and positive bacteria. Tatyana et al. [15] showed that oxylipins exist in both animals and plants. In their study, the authors identified analogous molecular structures of plant oxylipins in animal as eicosanoids, playing corresponding roles in stress-signaling cascades of events. The authors further demonstrated that octadecanoids are plant oxylipins, generated through oxidative pathways from linolenic acid mainly in form of jasmonate.

Tatyana et al. [15] explained further that jasmonate plays a significant biological activity in plants as antimicrobial agents. Also in animal eicosanoids, including prostaglandins, lipoxins, leukotrienes, and other related compounds have huge biological activity similar to oxylipins in plants. The authors enumerated the biological functions of eicosanoids as control of wound responses, immune responses, and inflammation mediators. They suggested that the structural analogue of eicosanoids and oxylipins with a functional similarity between these two molecules validated their similarities in terms of secretion, responses, and regulation.

Ignacio et al. [16] demonstrated that oxylipins antimicrobial activity is through facilitating cell membrane plasticity, mobilization of lipids, antibiosis effect, and generation of hydroxy fatty acids utilized as cellular communication. The authors in their study revealed that TriHOME compounds are a type of plant oxylipin that possess powerful antifungal activity. Furthermore, the authors demonstrated that oxylipins are powerful antimicrobial agents showing strong activity against phytopathogenic fungal strains like *Colletotrichum gloeosporioides*, *Drechslera teres*, and *Fusarium oxysporum* through growth inhibition, and caused *Escherichia coli*, *Micrococcus luteus*, *Staphylococcus aureus*, *Bacillus subtilis* growth inhibition. Oxylipins like 12-oxophytodienoic acid and jasmonic acid are known to modulate the expression of numerous genes and control specific aspects of plant development and growth, responses and development to stresses. Robert and Rao, [17] reported that oxylipins do not act along but stimulate and induce a crosstalk with other cascades of signaling molecules, salicylic acid and ethylene.

Marília et al. [18] reported that oxylipins were isolated from the *Alternanthera brasiliana* plant utilizing dereplication strategies. The plant oxylipins were tested for their antimicrobial activity and were confirmed by the authors to demonstrate a strong antibacterial action against endophytic bacteria. Also, oxylipins were reported to display strong anti-inflammatory, antibiotic and anti-cancer properties in a similar fashion in animal oxylipins such as leukotrienes, prostaglandins, dihomo-γ-linolenic acid, docosahexaenoic acid, epoxyeicosatrienoic acids, arachidonic acid, and eicosapentanoic acid.

Chanel et al. [19] reported that phyto-oxylipins are involved in plant defense mechanisms through the oxylipins structural characteristics, such as the number of double bonds, *cis*-double bonds and a free carboxylic acid moiety with the ability to interact with pathogens cell membrane causing detrimental effects. These result in membrane fluidity, leakage of the cytoplasmic contents, destabilization of the membrane, lysis, disruption in energy production, and oxidative phosphorylation. The pathogenic organism membrane oxidative phosphorylation occurs in two forms; it causes disturbance in the proton gradient, thus inhibiting the conversion of ADP to ATP to generate energy and through direct binding with attenuation of ATP enzyme synthase activity, thus restricting the capability to generate ATP. Oxylipins have been shown to obstruct nutrient intake linked to transport proteins and also inhibit both cytosol and membrane enzyme activity.

Chanel et al. [19] revealed that oxylipins can act as antibacterial agents owing to their structural configuration such as double bonds, a free carboxylic acid moiety, and the number of double bonds. Oxylipins interact with bacterial cell membranes; causing disruption/penetration of the membrane structure, which causes several detrimental roles on bacterial cell vitality and viability. Badrunnisa et al. [20] reported that oxylipins and eicosanoids like prostaglandins, leukotrienes, thromboxanes, and lipoxygenase are important pharmacological products derived from plants with physiological activities. The authors reported that these compounds are very detrimental to fungi, oomycetes, and bacteria survival. Some of the actions of oxylipins against *P. aeruginosa* include inhibition of flagellum-driven motility and upregulate type IV pilus-dependent twitching motility.

19.3 CONCLUSION

This book chapter has highlighted various roles of oxylipins as antimicrobial agents in the inhibition of fungi, oomycetes, and bacteria. Oxylipins and eicosanoids are known to be produced from plants, marine algae, and animals as prostaglandins, leukotrienes, thromboxanes, and lipoxygenase. The antimicrobial pathways of oxylipins actions include inhibition of nutrient intake linked to transport proteins, inhibition of cytosol and membrane enzyme activity, membrane fluidity, leakage of the cytoplasmic contents, destabilization of the membrane, lysis, disruption in energy production, and oxidative phosphorylation. The oxylipin action is based on the number of double bonds, *cis*-double bonds and a free carboxylic acid moiety with the ability to interact with pathogens cell membrane causing detrimental effects.

REFERENCES

1. Muhammad Naeemul Hassan, Zamri Zainal and Ismanizan Ismail (2015). Green leaf volatiles: biosynthesis, biological functions and their applications in biotechnology. Plant Biotechnology Journal, 13, pp. 727–739.
2. Isabelle Prost, Sandrine Dhondt, Grit Rothe, Jorge Vicente, Maria Jose´ Rodriguez, Neil Kift, Francis Carbonne, Gareth Griffiths, Marie-The´re`se Esquerre´-Tugaye, Sabine Rosah, Carmen Castresana, Mats Hamberg, and Joe¨lle Fournier (2005). Evaluation of the Antimicrobial Activities of Plant Oxylipins Supports Their Involvement in Defense against Pathogens 1(W). Plant Physiology, 139, pp. 1902–1913.
3. Tsitsigiannis DI and Keller NP (2007). Oxylipins as developmental and host–fungal communication signals. Trends Microbiol, 15, pp. 109–118.
4. Biermann, U., Bornscheuer, U., Meier, M. A. R., Metzger, J. O., Schäfer, H. J. (2011). *Angew.* Chem. Int. Ed., 50, p. 3854.
5. Claus Wasternack and Ivo Feussner (2017). The Oxylipin Pathways: Biochemistry and Function. Annual Review of Plant Biology, 12, p. 22.

6. Estelle Deboever, Magali Deleu, Se´ bastien Mongrand, Laurence Lins, and Marie-Laure Fauconnier (2019). Plant–Pathogen Interactions: Underestimated Roles of Phyto-oxylipins, Trends in Plant Science, pp. 1–13. https://doi.org/10.1016/j.tplants.2019.09.009.
7. Nilgün Öncül, and Şeniz Karabıyıklı (2016). Mechanism of antibacterial effect of plant-based Antimicrobials. Food Technologies. 5 (3), pp. 541–549.
8. Eliana Alves, Dias M, Lopes D, Almeida A, Domingues MDR, Rey F. (2020). Antimicrobial Lipids from Plants and Marine Organisms: An Overview of the Current State-of-the-Art and Future Prospects. Antibiotics (Basel), 9 (8), p. 441. doi: 10.3390/antibiotics9080441. PMID: 32722192; PMCID: PMC7459900.
9. Deboever Estelle, Lins Laurence, Ongena Marc, De Clerck Caroline, Deleu Magali, Fauconnier Marie-Laure (2020). Linolenic fatty acid hydroperoxide acts as biocide on plant pathogenic bacteria: Biophysical investigation of the mode of action. Bioorganic Chemistry, 100, p. 103877.
10. Montillet J-L, Nathalie Leonhardt, Samuel Mondy, Sylvain Tranchimand, Dominique Rumeau, Marie Boudsocq, Ana Victoria Garcia, Thierry Douki, Jean Bigeard, Christiane Lauriere, Anne Chevalier, Carmen Castresana, Heribert Hirt (2013). An Abscisic Acid-Independent Oxylipin Pathway Controls Stomatal Closure and Immune Defense in Arabidopsis, PLoS Biol, 11(3), p. e1001513. doi:10.1371/journal.pbio.1001513.
11. Ponce de León I, Hamberg M and Castresana C (2015). Oxylipins in moss development and defense. Front. Plant Sci, 6, p. 483. doi: 10.3389/fpls.2015.00483.
12. Sucharitha A. and Uma Maheswari Devi P. (2010). Antimicrobial properties of chilli lipoxygenase products. African Journal of Microbiology Research, 4(9), pp. 748–752.
13. Fischer, G. J., and Keller, N. P. (2016). Production of cross-kingdom oxylipins by pathogenic fungi: an update on their role in development and pathogenicity. J. Microbiol, 54, pp. 254–264. doi: 10.1007/s12275–016–5620-z
14. Jorge Vicentea, Tomas Cascona, Begonya Vicedob, Pilar Garcıa-Agustınb, Mats Hambergc and Carmen Castresanaa, (2012). Role of 9-Lipoxygenase and a-Dioxygenase Oxylipin Pathways as Modulators of Local and Systemic Defense. Molecular plant, 5 (4), pp. 914–928.
15. Tatyana Savchenko, Justin W. Walley, E. Wassim Chehab, Yanmei Xiao, Roy Kaspi,a Matthew F. Pye, Maged E. Mohamed, Colin M. Lazarus, Richard M. Bostock, and Katayoon Dehesh (2010). Arachidonic Acid: An Evolutionarily Conserved Signaling Molecule Modulates Plant Stress Signaling Networks. The Plant Cell, 22, pp. 3193–3205.
16. Ignacio Martin Arjol, Montserrat Busquets and Àngels Manresa (2015). Production of bacterial oxylipins by *Pseudomonas aeruginosa* 42A2. Recent Advances in Pharmaceutical Sciences V, pp. 149–165.
17. Robert A. Creelman and Rao Mulpuri (2002). The Oxylipin Pathway in *Arabidopsis*. The Arabidopsis Book. The American Society of Plant Biologists, pp. 1–24. https://doi.org/10.1199/tab.0012.
18. Marília Almeida Trapp, Marco Kai, Axel Mithöfer, Edson Rodrigues-Filho (2015). Antibiotic oxylipins from Alternanthera brasiliana and its endophytic Bacteria. Phytochemistry, 110, pp. 72–82.
19. Chanel J. Pretorius, Dylan R. Zeiss and Ian A. Dubery (2021). The presence of oxygenated lipids in plant defense in response to biotic stress: a metabolomics

appraisal, Plant Signaling & Behavior, 16 (12), p. 1989215, DOI: 10.1080/15592324.2021.1989215.
20. Badrunnisa S, Divvya Reddy, Chandrika P, Jeevitha Palatli (2013) Isolation of Oxylipins from Rice Bran as Antibacterial Principle against Pseudomonas Aeuruginosa. International Journal of Research Studies in Biosciences, 1 (1), pp. 1–7.

Index

U

V